MAYO CLINIC PREVENTIVE MEDICINE AND PUBLIC HEALTH BOARD REVIEW

Mayo Clinic Scientific Press

Mayo Clinic Atlas of Regional Anesthesia and Ultrasound-Guided Nerve Blockade
Edited by James R. Hebl, MD, and Robert L. Lennon, DO

MAYO CLINIC PREVENTIVE MEDICINE AND PUBLIC HEALTH BOARD REVIEW

Edited by

Prathibha Varkey, MBBS, MPH, MHPE

Consultant, Division of Preventive, Occupational and Aerospace Medicine
Mayo Clinic, Rochester, MN
Associate Professor of Preventive Medicine, of Medicine, and of Medical Education
College of Medicine, Mayo Clinic, Rochester, MN

MAYO CLINIC SCIENTIFIC PRESS   OXFORD UNIVERSITY PRESS

MAYO CLINIC

The triple-shield Mayo logo and the words MAYO, MAYO CLINIC, and MAYO CLINIC
SCIENTIFIC PRESS are marks of Mayo Foundation for Medical Education and Research.

OXFORD
UNIVERSITY PRESS

Oxford University Press, Inc., publishes works that further
Oxford University's objective of excellence
in research, scholarship, and education.

Oxford   New York
Auckland   Cape Town   Dar es Salaam   Hong Kong   Karachi
Kuala Lumpur   Madrid   Melbourne   Mexico City   Nairobi
New Delhi   Shanghai   Taipei   Toronto

With offices in
Argentina   Austria   Brazil   Chile   Czech Republic   France   Greece
Guatemala   Hungary   Italy   Japan   Poland   Portugal   Singapore
South Korea   Switzerland   Thailand   Turkey   Ukraine   Vietnam

Copyright © 2010 by Mayo Foundation for Medical Education and Research.

Published by Oxford University Press, Inc.
198 Madison Avenue, New York, New York 10016
www.oup.com

Oxford is a registered trademark of Oxford University Press

Library of Congress Cataloging-in-Publication Data

Mayo Clinic preventive medicine and public health board review / edited by Prathibha Varkey.
   p. ; cm.
  Includes bibliographical references and index.
  ISBN 978-0-19-974301-8
 1. Medicine, Preventive. 2. Public health. I. Varkey, Prathibha. II. Mayo Clinic.
III. Title: Preventive medicine and public health board review.
  [DNLM: 1. Preventive Medicine. 2. Public Health. WA 108 M473 2010]
  RA425.M385 2010
  362.1—dc22
                                                            2009048777
ISBN-13 978-0-19-974301-8

9 8 7 6 5 4 3 2 1

Printed in China
on acid-free paper

For my parents, Varkey M. Chacko, MD, and Leelamma Varkey, MD,
two incredibly caring and giving physician leaders.

FOREWORD

Prevention intuitively makes sense. However, intuition is not the same as evidence. Having worked in the field of preventive medicine for a number of years, I have observed the field progress and develop the evidence base to support the intuition associated with prevention. Yet some confusion still remains in many areas of prevention, and finding evidence-based knowledge and practical information can be challenging.

In this book, Dr Prathibha Varkey has assembled a group of authors who know the field of preventive medicine well. Of this I am sure because I have worked with most of them at Mayo Clinic, and many are within the Division of Preventive, Occupational and Aerospace Medicine, which includes physicians representing all 3 sections of the American Board of Preventive Medicine: Public Health and General Preventive Medicine, Occupational Medicine, and Aerospace Medicine. Within the Division of Preventive, Occupational and Aerospace Medicine, our clinicians have expertise in toxicology, safety, correctional medicine, immigration medicine, quality improvement, nutrition, public health, and other areas. I can think of no better group to write about these and other topics in preventive medicine. The Mayo Clinic Executive Health Program is one of our key clinics where we provide clinical preventive medicine to patients across the United States and the world. Our Section of Occupational Medicine/Employee Health Services delivers care to more than 30,000 Mayo Clinic employees in Rochester, Minnesota, and many others outside of the clinic. Our Section of Aviation and Aerospace Medicine provides Federal Aviation Administration examinations for complex medical situations to help keep pilots flying, as appropriate, and we have a state-of-the-art hyperbaric and altitude chamber that is part of our practice. We also provide public health consulting to the Olmsted County Public Health Services. We are very committed to training future preventists. Dr Varkey has directed our Preventive Medicine training program in the past and is very familiar with the core curriculum for Preventive Medicine and Public Health. We also recently started an Aerospace Medicine training program.

This book will be important to you and others, not only as a review text for the examination of the American Board of Preventive Medicine, but also because it contains the knowledge and credible practical information that many health care providers can and should use in their own clinical, public health, and academic settings. In this way, we hope that the intuition you possess regarding prevention will be supported by current evidence from the literature and will ultimately benefit your patients and community.

Donald D. Hensrud, MD, MPH
Chair, Division of Preventive, Occupational and
Aerospace Medicine, Mayo Clinic, Rochester, Minnesota;
Associate Professor of Preventive Medicine and Nutrition,
College of Medicine, Mayo Clinic

PREFACE

With the burgeoning number of uninsured persons in the United States (including many of the working poor), catapulting health care costs, and an aging population, the need for more preventive medicine and public health services is ever critical. Our specialty physicians have been on the front lines managing recent national emergencies, be it the H1N1 influenza pandemic, the New Orleans flood disasters, or the anthrax attacks. Preventive medicine and public health physicians have also been at the forefront managing chronic diseases and environmental disasters and aiding new ventures in aerospace.

With this first edition of *Mayo Clinic Preventive Medicine and Public Health Board Review*, we hope to provide a foundation of essential knowledge in preventive medicine, public health, occupational medicine, environmental medicine, and aerospace medicine. The need to write this book became apparent during my tenure as Program Director of the Preventive Medicine Fellowship at Mayo Clinic, as evidenced by the many fellows who were studying for the board examinations without a suitable textbook that contained all the necessary core knowledge. With that underlying intention, this book is primarily for preventive medicine physicians-in-training who are preparing for board certification, and it is also for preventive medicine and public health practitioners who are preparing for recertification. This book is also a concise review for internal medicine physicians, residents, and medical students who wish to learn more about preventive medicine and public health.

The book is organized by subspecialty sections, and bullet points are provided throughout each chapter to summarize key points. Multiple-choice questions and annotated answers are provided to enhance learning and retention of knowledge. Numerous figures are used to illustrate the text. Chapter authors are all Mayo Clinic physicians who spend most of their time providing clinical care to patients and assisting with public health operations in Olmsted County, Minnesota. They also are key educators of our medical students, residents, preventive medicine fellows, and allied health staff.

I am indebted to all the authors for their immense effort and contributions to this first edition of the book. I thank the staff of the Section of Scientific Publications, Dr Joseph G. Murphy, Dr June Oshiro, Roberta Schwartz, Susan R. Miller, and Ann Ihrke; the Section of Illustration and Design, Deb Veerkamp, Joanna King, and Ryan Ledebuhr; and the incredible faculty of the Division of Preventive, Occupational and Aerospace Medicine for their contributions to this edition. The support of the publisher, Oxford University Press, is also greatly appreciated.

We welcome comments from our readers, especially about how this textbook could be improved and about any errors that you may find.

Best wishes,
Prathibha Varkey, MBBS, MPH, MHPE

CONTENTS

CONTRIBUTORS

Muktar H. Aliyu, MBBS, DrPH
Fellow in Preventive Medicine
Mayo School of Graduate Medical Education
Assistant Professor of Preventive Medicine
College of Medicine Mayo Clinic
Rochester, MN
Presently, Assistant Professor of Preventive Medicine
Vanderbilt University School of Medicine
Nashville, TN

Kodjo M. Bossou, MD, MPH
Fellow in Preventive Medicine
Mayo School of Graduate Medical Education
College of Medicine, Mayo Clinic, Rochester, MN

Brian C. Brost, MD
Consultant, Division of Maternal and Fetal Medicine
Mayo Clinic, Rochester, MN
Associate Professor of Obstetrics and Gynecology
College of Medicine, Mayo Clinic

Darryl S. Chutka, MD
Consultant, Division of Preventive, Occupational and
  Aerospace Medicine
Mayo Clinic, Rochester, MN
Associate Professor of Medicine
College of Medicine, Mayo Clinic

Clayton T. Cowl, MD, MS
Consultant, Division of Preventive, Occupational and
  Aerospace Medicine, Mayo Clinic, Rochester, MN
Associate Professor of Medicine
College of Medicine, Mayo Clinic

Philip T. Hagen, MD
Consultant, Division of Preventive, Occupational and
  Aerospace Medicine
Mayo Clinic, Rochester, MN
Assistant Professor of Medicine
College of Medicine, Mayo Clinic

Donald D. Hensrud, MD, MPH
Chair, Division of Preventive, Occupational and
  Aerospace Medicine and Consultant, Division of
  Endocrinology, Diabetes, Metabolism, and Nutrition
Mayo Clinic, Rochester, MN
Associate Professor of Preventive Medicine
  and Nutrition
College of Medicine, Mayo Clinic

Kurtis M. Hoppe, MD
Consultant, Department of Physical Medicine and
  Rehabilitation
Mayo Clinic, Rochester, MN
Instructor in Physical Medicine and Rehabilitation
College of Medicine, Mayo Clinic

Salma Iftikhar, MD
Consultant, Division of General Internal Medicine
Mayo Clinic, Rochester, MN
Instructor in Medicine
College of Medicine, Mayo Clinic

Mary Jo Kasten, MD
Consultant, Division of General Internal Medicine
Mayo Clinic, Rochester, MN
Assistant Professor of Medicine
College of Medicine, Mayo Clinic

Cindy Kermott, MD, MPH
Consultant, Division of Preventive, Occupational and
  Aerospace Medicine
Mayo Clinic, Rochester, MN
Instructor in Medicine
College of Medicine, Mayo Clinic

Kyle J. Kircher, MD
Consultant, Department of Family Medicine
Mayo Clinic, Rochester, MN
Assistant Professor of Family Medicine
College of Medicine, Mayo Clinic

Paul J. Limburg, MD
Consultant, Division of Gastroenterology and
  Hepatology
Mayo Clinic, Rochester, MN
Associate Professor of Medicine
College of Medicine, Mayo Clinic

William J. Litchy, MD
Consultant, Department of Neurology
Mayo Clinic, Rochester, MN
Medical Director, MMSI
Mayo Clinic Health Solutions

Andrew J. Majka, MD
Consultant, Division of General Internal Medicine
Mayo Clinic, Rochester, MN
Instructor in Medicine
College of Medicine, Mayo Clinic

Mark A. Matthias, BA
Chief Financial Officer
Mayo Clinic Health Solutions
Rochester, MN

Martha P. Millman, MD, MPH
Consultant, Division of Preventive, Occupational and
  Aerospace Medicine
Mayo Clinic, Rochester, MN
Instructor in Preventive Medicine
College of Medicine, Mayo Clinic

Robin G. Molella, MD, MPH
Consultant, Division of Preventive, Occupational and
  Aerospace Medicine
Mayo Clinic, Rochester, MN
Instructor in Preventive Medicine
College of Medicine, Mayo Clinic

M. Hassan Murad, MD, MPH
Senior Associate Consultant and Director of Preventive
  Medicine Fellowship, Division of Preventive,
  Occupational and Aerospace Medicine
Mayo Clinic, Rochester, MN
Assistant Professor of Medicine
College of Medicine, Mayo Clinic

Richard D. Newcomb, MD, MPH
Consultant, Division of Preventive, Occupational and
  Aerospace Medicine
Mayo Clinic, Rochester, MN
Instructor in Preventive Medicine
College of Medicine, Mayo Clinic

Robert R. Orford, MD, MS, MPH
Consultant, Division of Preventive, Occupational and
  Aerospace Medicine
Mayo Clinic, Scottsdale, AZ
Assistant Professor of Medicine
College of Medicine, Mayo Clinic

Hamid Rehman, MD, MPH
Consultant, Division of Preventive, Occupational and
  Aerospace Medicine
Mayo Clinic, Rochester, MN
Instructor in Medicine
College of Medicine, Mayo Clinic

Heidi K. Roeber Rice, MD, MPH
Fellow in Preventive Medicine, Mayo School of Graduate
  Medical Education, College of Medicine
Mayo Clinic, Rochester, MN
Presently, Research Fellow, Project San Francisco Rwanda
Emory University, Atlanta, GA

Qian Shi, PhD
Research Associate, Department of Health
  Sciences Research
Mayo Clinic, Rochester, MN
Assistant Professor of Biostatistics
College of Medicine, Mayo Clinic

Lawrence Steinkraus, MD, MPH
Senior Associate Consultant, and Director of Aerospace
  Medicine Fellowship
Division of Preventive, Occupational
  and Aerospace Medicine
Mayo Clinic, Rochester, MN
Assistant Professor of Preventive Medicine
College of Medicine, Mayo Clinic

Jan Stepanek, MD, MPH
Consultant, Division of Preventive, Occupational and
  Aerospace Medicine
Mayo Clinic, Scottsdale, AZ
Assistant Professor of Medicine
College of Medicine, Mayo Clinic

Claudia L. Swanton, RN, MS, CNP
Nurse Practitioner, Division of Preventive, Occupational
  and Aerospace Medicine
Mayo Clinic, Rochester, MN
Instructor in Preventive Medicine
College of Medicine, Mayo Clinic

Zelalem Temesgen, MD
Consultant, Division of Infectious Diseases
Mayo Clinic, Rochester, MN
Professor of Medicine
College of Medicine, Mayo Clinic

Warren G. Thompson, MD
Consultant, Division of Preventive, Occupational and
  Aerospace Medicine
Mayo Clinic, Rochester, MN
Associate Professor of Medicine
College of Medicine, Mayo Clinic

Barbara J. Timm, RN, MS, CNP
Nurse Practitioner, Division of Preventive, Occupational
  and Aerospace Medicine
Mayo Clinic, Rochester, MN

Prathibha Varkey, MBBS, MPH, MHPE
Consultant, Division of Preventive, Occupational and
  Aerospace Medicine
Mayo Clinic, Rochester, MN
Associate Professor of Preventive Medicine, Medicine,
  and Medical Education
College of Medicine, Mayo Clinic

Richard J. Vetter, PhD
Consultant, Division of Preventive, Occupational and
  Aerospace Medicine
Mayo Clinic, Rochester, MN
Professor of Biophysics
College of Medicine, Mayo Clinic

MAYO CLINIC PREVENTIVE MEDICINE AND PUBLIC HEALTH BOARD REVIEW

BIOSTATISTICS 1: BASIC CONCEPTS

M. Hassan Murad, MD, MPH; Qian Shi, PhD

Biostatistics involves the application of statistical methods to medical and biological phenomena. In this chapter, we present the basic concepts and principles of biostatistics. Knowledge of these concepts is necessary to appraise the medical literature and understand results of biomedical research. Throughout this chapter, we have attempted to use the bare minimum of formulas, complicated calculations, and technical terms and to focus on presenting the concepts that are relevant to clinicians in relatively simple and straightforward language. Concepts introduced in this chapter include descriptive and inferential biostatistics, probability and odds, estimation and hypothesis testing, type I and type II errors, *P* value, and power and sample size calculation.

Descriptive Statistics

Descriptive statistics is the process of **summarizing or displaying sample data** in a way that concisely illustrates the general features of the data set. In a medical manuscript, descriptive statistics first are presented to familiarize readers with the sample data and to provide the rationale underlying the choice of analytic methods and study design. Descriptive statistics present only sample data and do not attempt to generalize conclusions to populations. Descriptive statistics can be presented in various formats, including tables, graphs, and numeric summary measures.

Data Type (Measurement Scales)

Data usually are described as being discrete or continuous. **Discrete data** consist of variables with a finite set of possible values; they often take the values of integers or counts. The possible values of some discrete data have no possible intermediate values (eg, the number of times a woman has given birth). In contrast, **continuous data** can assume an infinite number of values, including fractions (eg, serum cholesterol level). A special case of discrete data is dichotomous (binary) data, in which a variable has only 2 possible levels or categories.

Discrete data can be nominal or ordinal. **Nominal data** have possible values that fall into unordered categories or classes (eg, sex [male, female]). **Ordinal data** are discrete data that can be categorized in a natural or logical order. For example, frequency of depression is ordinal because it could be categorized as never, infrequent, sometimes, very often, and always.

Continuous data are subdivided into **interval-scale data** (data with no true 0) and **ratio-scale data** (data with real 0 value). For example, temperature is an interval-scale variable because 0 is an arbitrary data point (0°F does not mean "absence of temperature"). In contrast, serum mercury level is a ratio-scale variable (0 ng/mL means no mercury was measured in the sample).

To get a complete picture of data characteristics, various types of descriptive statistics need to be considered together. In descriptive statistics, data are described by their central tendency (the point about which the observations tend to cluster) and their dispersion (spread or variability).

Central Tendency

The **arithmetic mean** (also termed **mean** or **average**) is the sum of all observations divided by the number of observations. The mean can be used as a summary measure for continuous data. In general, however, it is not appropriate for nominal or ordinal data. The mean is the most commonly used measure of central tendency because it is easily calculated and most intuitive.

The **median** is the number that represents the midpoint of a distribution, with an equal number of observations on each side. The median is a good summary measure for ordinal data because only the rank matters. It also is used to describe skewed continuous data because it is not sensitive to the value of each observation. If the distribution of data is symmetric, the mean and median are identical.

The **mode** is the most frequently occurring value among observations. If data have more than 1 mode (eg, bimodal or trimodal), it might be better to report these modes, rather than the mean or median. Alternatively, data could be divided into subgroups, with means or medians of each mode reported separately. The mode is not commonly used in statistics because of its intractable mathematical properties.

The **geometric mean** often is used in skewed (asymmetric) distributions. It is calculated by transforming observations to a logarithmic scale to make the distribution of observations more symmetric. The arithmetic mean of the log values is calculated after transformation (thus, the geometric mean is the antilog of the arithmetic mean of the logs). Any base can be used to compute logarithms for the geometric mean. The geometric mean will be the same, regardless of which base is used.

Example 1. Patients with influenza presenting to a primary care clinic.

Nine patients with influenza presented to a primary care clinic in January. Their ages are shown in the Table. How can the likely or average age of patients be described?

Example 1 Table. Patient Age

	Patient								
	A	B	C	D	E	F	G	H	I
Age, y	2	2	2	3	4	5	6	6	25

If we sum the age values (2+2+2+3+4+5+6+6+25=55) and divide the sum by 9 (the number of patients), the mean is 6.1 years. The median is the fifth value in the ordered series, 4 years (4 patients were older and 4 younger than 4 years). The mode

is 2 years, the value repeated more than any other (3 times).

As this example shows, the mean is sensitive to extreme values. The 25-year-old patient shifted the mean age from the median of 4 years to the older age of 6.1 years. The odd number of observations in this example (9 children) allowed us to identify the median, the value in the middle of the ordered observations. However, if the number of observations was even, the median would be calculated by averaging the central 2 observations. The mode is rarely used in statistics because it is not always the central value (in this example, it is misleading to assume that the age most commonly afflicted by influenza is 2 years). The geometric mean is calculated as follows:
$$\sqrt[9]{2\times2\times2\times3\times4\times5\times6\times6\times25} = 4.23.$$

Skewed Distributions

An example of a skewed distribution is the distribution of survival time of patients with aggressive malignancies (Figure 1). Most patients die early, but a few have considerably longer survival. Thus, this survival distribution has a longer tail to the right of the median and is termed a **right-skewed** (or **positively skewed**) distribution, with a mean that is greater than the median.

Measures of Dispersion (Spread)

The **range** is the difference between the largest and smallest observation in a sample. In Example 1 above, the range for the age of patients who presented with influenza is 25−2=23 years.

Quantile (**percentile**) is defined such that $p\%$ of observations in a sample are less than or equal to the value of pth percentile. Interquartile range, the range between the 25th and 75th percentiles, is frequently used with the

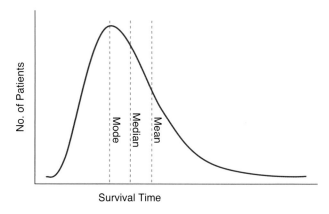

Figure 1 Survival of Patients With Malignancy. The example shows a right-skewed distribution.

median to describe data. In Example 1 above, the 75th percentile of age is calculated by multiplying 0.75 by the number of observations ($0.75 \times 9 = 6.75$) and rounding to the nearest integer (6.75 rounds to 7). Thus, the seventh value (6 years) is the 75th percentile for patients presenting with influenza (75% of observations are ≤6 years). Similarly, the 25th percentile is 2 years. Therefore, the interquartile range is $6 - 2 = 4$ years.

The **variance** of a population is calculated by summing the squared deviations of observations from their mean and dividing the sum by the number of observations (n). If the data are from a sample and not a population, the sum is divided by (n–1) instead of by n. In a sample or data set with n observations, 1 observation is fixed (not variable) because after all the other observations are known, the last observation becomes known and has no freedom to vary. Thus, degree of freedom is defined as (n–1).

The **standard deviation** (SD) is the squared root of the variance; it is more intuitive and easier to understand than the variance because it has the same units as the original observations, whereas the variance has squared units. When comparing data sets with the same units of measure, a smaller SD indicates that the observations are more homogeneous, whereas a larger SD means the observations are more dispersed. The SD is often presented with the mean to describe the characteristics of the entire distribution of the data.

The **coefficient of variation** is defined as the ratio of the SD to the mean, expressed as a percentage. It is useful when comparing the variability of several data sets with different units of measure. For example, a coefficient of variation with a value of 14% in a sample indicates that this particular sample has greater variability than a sample with a coefficient of variation of 5%.

- Discrete data consist of variables with a finite set of possible values. Nominal data can be organized in unordered categories, whereas ordinal data can be categorized in a logical order.
- Continuous data can assume an infinite number of values. Interval-scale data have no true 0, whereas ratio-scale data have real 0 value.
- Data can be described by their central tendency (eg, mean, median, mode, etc) and their dispersion (eg, range, quantile, variance, etc). Distributions may also be skewed.

Probability and Odds

Probability is frequently used to express **risk** of a particular disease or outcome. (The numeric value of a probability is between 0 and 1.) The probability of an event is the relative frequency of the event occurring over an indefinitely large number of trials conducted under virtually identical conditions. It is estimated by the sample proportion, which is calculated by counting the number of times the event has occurred and dividing it by the number of times the event could have occurred. For example, if the mumps vaccine is given to 600 children in a school of 800, the probability of a given child being vaccinated is 600/800=0.75 (ie, 75%).

When the probability of 2 events occurring is described, it is important to define the relationship between these 2 events. **Independent events** have no influence on each other (ie, the probability of the first event occurring is the same whether the second event does or does not occur). **Mutually exclusive** events cannot occur simultaneously. **Exhaustive events** encompass all possible outcomes. For example, serum cholesterol levels ≤200 mg/dL and >200 mg/dL are mutually exclusive and exhaustive outcomes.

Multiplication and Addition Laws of Probability

The multiplication law of probability states that the probability of 2 events (A and B) occurring is equal to the probability of A occurring multiplied by the probability of B occurring, given that A has already happened. If A and B are independent events, the probability of both events occurring is calculated by multiplying the individual probabilities. For example, if the mumps vaccine is given to 600 children in a school of 800, the probability that 2 children playing together would be vaccinated is 0.75×0.75=0.56, assuming that the 2 vaccination events are independent.

The addition law of probability states that the probability of either of 2 events occurring is determined by summing the probabilities of individual events occurring minus the probability of both events occurring. For example, in the previous paragraph, the probability of any child being vaccinated was 0.75. Assuming event independence, the probability that at least 1 of 2 children playing together would be vaccinated is 0.75+0.75–(0.75×0.75)=0.94. It is important to note that when 2 events are mutually exclusive, the probability of both events occurring together is 0. In this case, the probability of either event occurring equals the sum of the probabilities of the individual events.

Odds, Odds Ratio, and Relative Risk

Odds represent a ratio of the probability that the event occurs to the probability that it does not. For example, if 1 of 4 people has hypertension, the odds of having hypertension is 1:3. (In contrast, the probability or risk of having hypertension is 1/4.) The mathematical relationship between probability and odds is as follows:

$$\text{Probability} = \text{odds}/(\text{odds} + 1)$$
$$\text{Odds} = \text{probability}/(1 - \text{probability})$$

Odds ratio (OR), a common measure relating 2 proportions, is defined as the odds in favor of the event (eg, disease) among one group (eg, exposed group) divided by the odds of the same event among another group (eg, unexposed group). OR is an appropriate measure of association for different types of studies, including case-control studies, cohort studies, and cross-sectional studies.

In cohort studies, to compare the risk of disease in 2 different groups (eg, exposed and unexposed), another common measure is the relative risk (RR). RR is defined by dividing the probability of disease in the exposed group by the probability of disease in the unexposed group. When the disease is a rare event, the estimated OR is very close to the RR. Moreover, the concepts of probability and risk are more intuitive for physicians and patients compared with the concept of odds.

Probability Distributions

In scientific experiments, observational studies, and randomized clinical trials, variables are the characteristics that are measured or classified. When the possible outcomes of a variable occur with certain likelihood (probability), this means that a particular outcome will not be observed all the time (thus the variable is termed **random**). If the possible outcome values of a continuous random variable observed in a sample of data are plotted against the relative frequency of the outcome, the plot shows the frequency distribution for the random variable. Increasing the number of measurements will refine (smooth) the plot to form the probability distribution curve.

The probability distribution is a collection of the probabilities of all possible outcomes of a random variable. Certain functions (formulas) allow estimation of probabilities from probability distributions. In a **continuous probability distribution**, the y-axis represents the probability density function, and the area under the curve between 2 points is the probability itself (the area under the whole curve equals 1.0). In a **discrete probability distribution**, the y-axis value is the exact probability of the possible outcome occurring (termed **probability mass function**). The cumulative-distribution function gives the probability that the observed value of a random variable is less than or equal to a prespecified value.

A **Bernoulli trial** is a single experiment with a random variable that has only 2 mutually exclusive outcomes: "success" (with probability of p) and "failure" (with probability of $1-p$). An example of a Bernoulli trial is a coin toss. If a Bernoulli trial is repeated independently n times, then the total number of successes is said to be a **binomial random variable**. The distribution associated with this kind of random variable is called a **binomial distribution**. There are 3 assumptions behind the binomial distribution: 1) the number of Bernoulli trials, n, is fixed; 2) the outcomes of the n trials are independent; and 3) the probability p of success is constant for each trial. Another discrete distribution is the **Poisson distribution**. This model is used for rare events that take place in a unit of time (eg, probability of lung cancer development in a year).

A common continuous distribution is the **normal (Gaussian) distribution**, a symmetric, unimodal, and bell-shaped distribution in which the median equals the mean. Most biologic and natural phenomena (eg, height, weight, blood pressure, etc) that are caused by multiple independent factors (eg, genetics, environment, nutrition, etc) can be assumed to have a normal distribution. Because the normal distribution is very easy to work with, it sometimes provides an approximation to other distributions (eg, binomial and Poisson distributions) when the observations of interest are from a study with a sufficiently large sample size. In the normal distribution, roughly 68.3% of data points are within 1 SD of the mean, and 95.4% and 99.7% of the data are within 2 and 3 SDs, respectively.

The normal distribution is defined by its mean and variance. Any random variable assumed to follow a normal distribution, with any mean and variance, can be transformed to a standard normal distribution with a mean of 0 and an SD of 1. The transformed value (termed **z score**) is calculated as follows:

$$z \text{ score} = (\text{original value} - \text{mean})/(\text{SD})$$

This standardization facilitates calculation of probabilities and obviates use of statistical software; only a table of standard normal distribution (found in statistics textbooks) is needed.

Example 2. Systolic blood pressure.

In a sample of patients, the systolic blood pressure is approximately normally distributed (Figure), with a mean (SD) pressure of 120 (10) mm Hg. What is the probability of a patient having a systolic blood pressure less than 140 mm Hg?

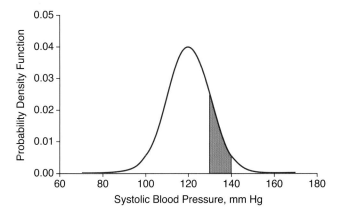

Normal Distribution of Systolic Blood Pressure. The shaded area equals the probability that an individual's blood pressure is between 130 and 140 mm Hg.

The calculation can be performed as follows:

1. The value of 140 mm Hg is transformed to the z score: $(140 - 120)/10 = 2$.

2. Using a standard normal distribution table, the corresponding probability of a z score being less than or equal to 2 is 0.98. Hence, the probability of someone in this population having a blood pressure below 140 mm Hg is 98%.

3. This can alternatively be calculated with Microsoft Excel. The function NORMSDIST(2) returns the probability of 0.98. Moreover, the function NORMDIST(140,120,10,TRUE) can also be used.

Note that the probability of someone having blood pressure greater than 140 mm Hg would be 1−0.98=0.02. To determine the probability of someone having blood pressure between 130 and 140 mm Hg (see shaded area in the figure), the above steps are repeated to calculate the probability of blood pressure below 130 mm Hg (probability, 0.84). This value is subtracted from the probability of blood pressure below 140 mm Hg:
$0.98 - 0.84 = 0.14$.

- Probability is a measure of risk for an outcome. If the probability of 2 events is described, the relationship between the events (eg, independent, mutually exclusive, or exhaustive) must be considered.
- The odds ratio (OR) and relative risk (RR) are measures used to compare the likelihood of an outcome between 2 groups (comparing odds and probabilities, respectively).
- The probability distribution is a collection of the probabilities of all possible outcomes of a random variable.
- Discrete probability distributions include the binomial distribution (used to describe outcomes of Bernoulli trials) and the Poisson distribution (used to describe rare events that take place in a unit of time).
- A common continuous distribution is the normal (Gaussian) distribution. It is a unimodal, bell-shaped distribution (used to describe most biologic and natural phenomena).
- Any random variable with a normal distribution can be transformed to a standard normal distribution with a mean of 0 and an SD of 1. Transformed values are termed z scores.

Estimation and Sampling Error

To determine, for example, the proportion of the US population with hypertension, the most accurate method is to measure the blood pressure of every person in the country and identify the number of people with hypertension. However, this process would be time consuming and costly and thus is neither practical nor feasible. Therefore, characteristics of the population usually are studied on the basis of information from a **sample** of people, and the results may be **extrapolated** to characterize the population. The process of drawing conclusions about an entire population, based on the information in a sample, is known as **statistical inference**. Statistical inference includes estimation of population parameters and hypothesis testing.

A population **parameter** is commonly estimated by a sample **statistic**. The population parameter is a particular unknown quantity, whereas the sample statistic (an estimator) is usually a real-valued function of the observations in the random sample. For example, the sample mean $\bar{x}$ is calculated by dividing the sum of all observations by the total number of observations in the random sample of data. When an experiment is repeated several times, the sample statistic will be different each time because a different group of observations from the same population will be used with every trial. This leads to some uncertainty about the sample statistic. Therefore, sample statistics are also random variables. They can be characterized by a probability distribution, in which case they are described as a sampling distribution.

If the selected samples are representative of the entire population, the sample statistics are likely to be similar to each other. In addition, any errors committed by researchers when they repeat sampling become more predictable; this error, which is due to chance, is termed **sampling error** or **random error**. Random error is bidirectional, meaning that it does not lead to systematic overestimation or underestimation of the measured values. Random error is different from **bias**, which is unidirectional.

The sampling error can be described by the **standard error**, defined as the SD of the distribution of the sample statistics. The formula for estimating standard error for a sample mean (assuming that σ is the population's SD and n is the sample size) is $\sigma/\sqrt{n}$; for a sample proportion (assuming that p is the population proportion and n is the sample size), the formula is $\sqrt{p(1-p)/n}$. A larger sample inherently will have less standard error and more precision. However, larger samples that are biased may provide false or misleading results by underestimating or overestimating the true effect. Note that increasing the sample size does not reduce nonrandom error or bias.

Estimation and Confidence Intervals

Two commonly used methods of estimation are **point estimation** and **interval estimation**. All the examples mentioned in this chapter thus far (eg, calculating mean and median) are point estimations. The point estimation itself does not reflect the uncertainty existing in the sample. The interval estimation, which accounts for the randomness of the random sample, therefore is preferred. Using the point estimate (or sample statistic), one can generate a **confidence interval** (CI) by adding and subtracting a margin of error that consists of several standard errors. The confidence coefficient is a percentile of the standard normal distribution that corresponds to how confident one wants to be. Thus, if an experiment is performed repeatedly with the same sample size and exactly identical conditions, the population parameter will be contained in the interval with a certain level of confidence. In medicine, the **arbitrary confidence limit of 95%** typically is used. This means that if 100 random samples are selected from a population and used to calculate 100 different CIs for the population parameter, approximately 95 intervals would cover the true population parameter. For a parameter with normal distribution, 95% of the values are within 2 (actually, 1.96) standard errors of the mean; hence, the confidence coefficient for a 95% CI is 1.96. The 95% CI consists of a range defined by the point estimate (eg, mean) plus or minus 1.96 standard errors.

The **central limit theorem** sometimes can be used to facilitate estimation. The central limit theorem indicates that the distribution of sample means is approximately normal when the sample size is sufficiently large, even if the variables observed in the original population are not normally distributed. Hence, when normality in the distribution of sample means is assumed, inference using the normal distribution becomes possible. In reality, the population SD (σ) is usually unknown, just like the population mean. In this situation, the CI is calculated in much the same way but is based on the Student t distribution. Like the standard normal distribution, the **Student t distribution** is unimodal and symmetric around a mean of 0 (Figure 2). Each Student distribution is defined by a degree of freedom (sample size–1). When degrees of freedom increase, the t distribution approaches the standard normal distribution.

- Statistical inference is the process of drawing conclusions about an entire population on the basis of information from a randomly selected sample from the population.
- Sampling error can be described by the SD of the distribution of the sample statistics. It does not lead to systematic overestimation or underestimation of measured values.
- In medicine, a confidence limit of 95% typically is used. The 95% confidence interval (CI) consists of a range defined by the point estimate plus or minus 1.96 standard errors.
- The central limit theorem indicates that the distribution of sample means is approximately normal when the sample size is sufficiently large, even if the variables observed in the original population are not normally distributed.

Hypothesis Testing

When investigators conduct an experiment, they begin by establishing a **null hypothesis** (H$_0$; the hypothesis they hope to reject) and an **alternative hypothesis** (H$_a$; the hypothesis they hope to prove). They also specify an acceptable threshold value for the probability of rejecting H$_0$ when in fact it is true. This threshold **significance level** (α) is traditionally set at 5%. After a random sample from the population is obtained, data can be measured and a statistical test conducted (the specific test is determined by the data distribution, eg, normal distribution). This test produces a ***P* value**, the probability of finding a value in the population that is as extreme as the sample statistic. The comparison between the *P* value and α allows investigators to reject or accept the null hypothesis. CI estimation and hypothesis testing are different ways of expressing the same information (95% CI is analogous to a significance level α of 5%). Hypothesis testing leads to a dichotomous decision (accept or reject a hypothesis), whereas estimation is used to assess the magnitude of the population parameters of interest. Although clinical studies **traditionally use a significance level of 5%**, note that this cutoff value is selected arbitrarily. The α value should be determined on the basis of what is the acceptable level of incorrectly rejecting the null hypothesis when it is actually true, and it should be established before the experiment is performed.

When conducting hypothesis testing, 4 scenarios are possible by accepting or rejecting the null and alternative hypotheses (Figure 3). These scenarios include type I and type II errors that result in false conclusions. In a **type I error**, the null hypothesis is rejected when it is actually true (eg, erroneously concluding that experimental and control treatments have different effects). A false-positive finding is a type I error. The probability of making type I error (α) usually is compared with the significance level.

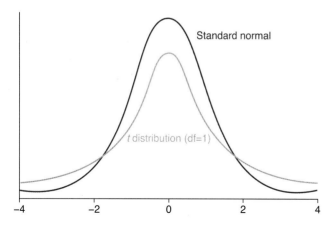

Figure 2 The Standard Normal Distribution and Student t Distribution With 1 Degree of Freedom (df).

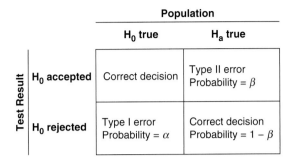

Figure 3 The 4 Scenarios of Hypothesis Testing. α denotes the probability of making a type I error; β, the probability of making a type II error; H_0, null hypothesis; H_a, alternative hypothesis.

In a **type II error**, the null hypothesis is accepted when the alternative hypothesis is true (eg, erroneously concluding that experimental and control treatments have similar effects). A false-negative finding is a type II error. The probability of making a type II error is denoted β.

Example 3. Hypothesis testing with a continuous variable.

A random sample of 9 influenza patients was identified from a primary care clinic; their mean age was 6.1 years. The mean (SD) age of all patients in the clinic was 35 (42) years. The hypothesis is that influenza infects younger patients. (H_a: The age of patients with influenza is less than the age of general patients in this primary care clinic. Specifically, the mean age of patients with influenza is <35 years.) The null hypothesis therefore is that patients with influenza are the same age or are older than that of general patients in this clinic. (H_0: Mean age of patients with influenza is ≥35 years.) The critical probability at which H_0 would be rejected was set at $\alpha=0.05$.

To calculate the standard error of the sample mean, use the formula $\sigma / \sqrt{n} = 42/3 = 14$. The sample statistic (sample mean, 6.1 years) is standardized by converting it to a z score: $z=(6.1-35)/14=-2.06$. Because the normal distribution is symmetric, the negative sign can be ignored. A standard normal distribution table or a software package is used to determine the probability of obtaining z values as extreme as the test statistic ($z \geq 2.06$): the probability is 0.02. Because the probability of finding a value as extreme as 6.1 is below 0.05, the null hypothesis is rejected and the alternative hypothesis is accepted. Influenza patients are in fact younger than the typical patients in the clinic (although there is a 5% chance that this is an erroneous conclusion).

To summarize, the probability of finding a sample with the mean age of 6.1 years in a population with a mean (SEM) age of 35 (14) is quite low (only 2%). Therefore, the random sample is unlikely to belong to the population under null hypothesis, and patients with influenza are likely younger than the general patients attending this clinic.

In the example above, 1-sided hypothesis testing is used because we would not expect influenza patients to be older than the general population; hence, we are interested only in proving that they are younger. In most cases, however, 2-sided testing is used. For example, what if it is unknown whether the mean age of influenza patients is older or younger than that of the general patients? In that case, the null hypothesis is that the mean age of patients is 35 years, and the alternative hypothesis is that the mean age of patients is not 35 years. We would then multiply the probability (0.02) by 2 and compare it against the predetermined rejection level of $\alpha=0.05$ (Figure 4).

Example 4. Hypothesis testing with a dichotomous variable.

The goal for a program immunizing patients in the community against hepatitis B is 70%. To determine whether the target has been reached, the sera of 100 randomly selected patients are tested for protective antibodies. Laboratory test results show that 75/100 patients are immunized. Was the target goal achieved? How compatible are the results from this sample (75%) and the population target of 70%?

To answer these questions, we begin by following the same steps described in Example 3. The null hypothesis is that the proportion of the community immunized (p) is 70%. The alternative hypothesis is that p does not equal 70%. Because we do not know whether the immunization rate is above or below the target rate, a 2-sided test is appropriate. We set the rejection rule as $\alpha = 0.05$.

Using the formula to calculate the standard error for a proportion ($\sqrt{p(1-p)/n}$), $\sqrt{0.70(1-0.70)/100} = 0.046$. The sample statistic is converted to a z score: $(0.75 - 0.70)/0.046 = 1.09$, assuming that the normal approximation is appropriate. A standard normal distribution table or a software package is used to determine the probability of obtaining a z score as extreme as the test statistic ($z>1.09$), which is 0.14. Because this is a 2-sided test, the probability is multiplied by 2: $P = 2 \times 0.14 = 0.28$. Because the P value exceeds .05, we cannot reject the null hypothesis. Thus, we lack statistically significant evidence supporting the alternative hypothesis (in this case, we cannot

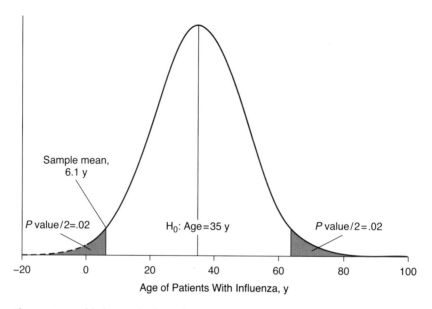

Figure 4 Two-sided Hypothesis Testing for Mean Age of Influenza Patients.

conclude that the immunization rate is greater than 70%).

- Hypothesis testing leads to a dichotomous decision (accept or reject a hypothesis), whereas estimation is used to assess the magnitude of the population parameters of interest.
- The threshold significance level (α) for the probability of falsely rejecting the null hypothesis is traditionally 5%. The *P* value is the probability of finding a value in the population that is as extreme as the sample statistic. The comparison between the *P* value and α allows investigators to reject or accept the null hypothesis.
- A type I error occurs when the null hypothesis is rejected when it is actually true (false-positive finding). A type II error occurs when the null hypothesis is accepted when the alternative hypothesis is true (false-negative finding).

Power and Sample Size Calculations

Study power is defined as the **probability of correctly rejecting the null hypothesis** (eg, showing treatment effects after an intervention but not after a placebo treatment); it is calculated as $1-\beta$, where β is the probability of making a type II error (false-negative conclusion). A study with very high power can detect trivial differences that may not have clinical significance. A study with low power may not detect an important treatment effect. Medical studies commonly use an **arbitrarily established study power of at least 80%**.

Many factors can affect study power. Power increases when sample size increases (ie, a larger sample is more likely to detect a fixed difference between 2 treatments). Power also increases when the difference between the alternative mean and the null mean increases (ie, when the difference between the effects of 2 treatments is sizable, the study is more likely to detect a difference with a fixed sample size). Power decreases when the SD of sample data increases (ie, if data have great variability, a study is less likely to detect a difference between 2 treatments). Power also decreases as the significance level (α) decreases (ie, if one is unwilling to accept a high rate of false-positive results, the likelihood of finding a true-positive answer decreases).

The formulas used to calculate a CI require the input of sample size, a point estimate (eg, mean), SD, and significance level. Hence, for a given CI of a sample with known SD, one can determine the smallest sample size (*n*) that would satisfy the CI. In medical studies, an α level of 0.05 and a β level of 0.20 (ie, significance of 0.05 and power of 0.80) typically are chosen. However, this decision should be changed depending on the type of error (false-positive or false-negative results) that has greater clinical relevance to study participants. The Table shows formulas used to estimate sample size for commonly used statistical tests.

Example 5. Sample size calculation.
In a politician approval rate poll, a 95% CI with a maximum width of 6% (ie, a margin of error of ±3%) typically is chosen. The sample size needed is $(1.96/0.03)^2 \times 0.25 = 1,067$. Hence, these types of polls usually recruit slightly more than a thousand participants to provide sufficient precision of estimating a proportion.

Table Sample Size Calculation

Sample mean	$$n = \frac{\sigma^2(z_{1-\alpha/2} + z_{1-\beta})^2}{(\mu_0 - \mu_1)^2}$$
Sample proportion	$$n = (\frac{z_{1-\alpha/2}}{m})^2 \times p(1-p)$$

Abbreviations: n, sample size; σ^2, variance; $z_{1-\alpha/2}$ and $z_{1-\beta}$, standard normal distribution quantiles for type I and type II error rates; μ_0, null hypothesis; μ_1, alternative hypothesis; m, margin of error (defined as half the width of a confidence interval); p, proportion.

Note: If the significance is established at 0.05 and a power of 0.80 is needed $(z_{1-\alpha/2} + z_{1-\beta})^2 = (1.96+0.84)^2 = 7.84$. The highest (most conservative) value of $p(1-p)$ is $0.5 \times 0.5 = 0.25$.

- Study power is defined as the probability of correctly rejecting the null hypothesis; medical studies commonly use an arbitrarily established power of at least 80%.
- Sample size can be calculated if the confidence interval, acceptable margin of error, and estimated prevalence are known.

SUGGESTED READING

DeGroot MH, Schervish MJ. Probability and statistics. 3rd ed. Boston (MA): Addison-Wesley; c2002.

Jekel JF, Katz DL, Elmore JG, Wild D. Epidemiology, biostatistics and preventive medicine. 3rd ed. Philadelphia (PA): Saunders/Elsevier; c2007.

Pagano M, Gauvreau K. Principles of biostatistics. 2nd ed. Pacific Grove (CA): Duxbury; c2000.

Rosner BA. Fundamentals of biostatistics. 6th ed. Belmont (CA): Thomson-Brooks/Cole; c2006.

Questions and Answers

Questions

1. The height of 10 people is shown in the table:

	Individual									
	1	2	3	4	5	6	7	8	9	10
Height, cm	155	160	170	170	172	175	180	181	182	185

Calculate the measures of descriptive statistics for this data set:
   a. Mean
   b. Median
   c. Mode
   d. Range
   e. Interquartile range

2. The variance of the data set in question 1 is 854. Indicate whether the following statements are true or false:
   a. The unit for this variance is centimeters.
   b. If we consider this data set a population, the SD is calculated by dividing the variance by 9 and obtaining the square root of the product.
   c. If we consider this data set a sample, the SD is calculated by dividing the variance by 10 and obtaining the square root of the product.
   d. If some of the subjects in this data set were very tall and some were very short, the variance, SD, and coefficient of variation would all be smaller numbers.
   e. If most patients were tall but a few were very short, the median would be a better measure of centrality than the mean.

3. If 120 of 150 students in a class were vaccinated against influenza, what is the probability that at least 1 of 2 students sitting next to each other would be vaccinated (assuming independence)?
   a. 99%
   b. 96%
   c. 80%
   d. 64%
   e 50%

4. Describe the data type (nominal, ordinal, interval-scale, ratio-scale) for each of the following variables:
   a. Temperature in Fahrenheit scale
   b. Temperature in Kelvin scale
   c. Pain level using a 10-point scale
   d. Color
   e. Height

5. All the following statements about the normal distribution are correct *except*:
   a. Data representing natural phenomena such as height, age, and weight are assumed to follow the normal distribution.
   b. The mean, median, and mode of the normal distribution are equal.
   c. The probability of exactly obtaining any single point value in the normal distribution is 0.
   d. In a standard normal distribution, the probability of obtaining a value ≥ 2 is equal to that of a value ≤ -2.
   e. Occasionally, the normal distribution can be bimodal or trimodal.

6. A study demonstrated that simvastatin lowered cholesterol level in a group of 10 volunteers by 35 mg/dL ($P=.03$). Indicate whether the following statements are true or false (or cannot be determined):
   a. If we repeat this study 100 times under the same conditions, on 3 occasions, this reduction will be because of random error or chance.
   b. Because most studies use a significance level of 0.05, these results are not statistically significant.
   c. This study has a 97% chance of finding the true effect of simvastatin.
   d. If we increase the sample size to 1,000 volunteers, this P value will increase.
   e. It is unlikely that this study is biased.

7. The cholesterol-lowering effect of simvastatin was shown to be 35 mg/dL, with a 95% CI of 20 to 50 mg/dL. Indicate whether the following statements are true or false:
   a. This result means that there is a 95% probability that the true cholesterol reduction caused by simvastatin is between 20 and 50 mg/dL.
   b. If we chose a larger sample size, the CI would be wider.
   c. If we change the confidence level to 99%, the CI will become narrower.
   d. These results are not statistically significant because the CI does not include the value of 0.0 mg/dL.
   e. Hypothesis testing with a significance level of 0.05 is likely to yield similar results to estimation with a 95% CI.

Answers

1. **Answers.**
   a. Mean: 173. The sum of all observations is divided by 10, the number of observations.
   b. Median: 173.5. The median is calculated by averaging the fifth and sixth observations.
   c. Mode: 170. The value 170 is repeated twice, more than any other observation.
   d. Range: 30. The range is obtained by subtracting the smallest from the largest observation (ie, 185–155).
   e. Interquartile range: 11. The interquartile range is obtained by subtracting the 25th percentile value from the 75th percentile value (ie, 181–170).

2. **Answers.**
   a. False. The unit for variance is centimeters squared.
   b. False. The denominator for the SD formula is n when data represent a population.
   c. False. The denominator for the SD formula is $(n-1)$ when data represent a sample.
   d. False. If data have considerable variability, the variance, SD, and coefficient of variation would be larger.
   e. True. In skewed distributions, the median is a better measure of central tendency than the mean.

3. **Answer b.**
   The probability of 1 student being immunized is 120/150 = 0.80. The probability of either 1 of 2 students being immunized is $0.80 + 0.80 - (0.80 \times 0.80) = 0.96$.

4. **Answers.**
   a. Interval-scale. Data have no true 0.
   b. Ratio-scale. Data have a true 0.
   c. Ordinal. Pain levels have a natural order, although they are not true continuous variables.
   d. Nominal. Colors have no numeric or ordered characteristics.
   e. Ratio-scale. Data have a true 0.

5. **Answer e.**
   The normal distribution never has more than 1 mode.
   Note that statement c is correct because probability calculations are based on intervals, not fixed points. For statement d, normal distribution is symmetric, and the sign of an observation thus can be ignored when probability is calculated.

6. **Answers.**
   a. True. We expect to obtain false-positive results on 3 occasions.
   b. False. Results are significant because $P < .05$.
   c. Cannot be determined. The question as presented has no data about power.
   d. False. Increasing sample size would decrease this P value.
   e. Cannot be determined. The question as presented has no data about bias.

7. **Answers.**
   a. False. Defining a 95% CI as an interval that has 95% probability of containing population parameter is a very common mistake. The population parameter is either contained in the interval or not; there is no probability to be estimated.
   b. False. Increasing sample size would make the CI narrower.
   c. False. Increasing confidence level would make the CI wider.
   d. False. These results are significant because the CI does not include the value 0, which would have indicated no change from baseline.
   e. True. Hypothesis testing with a significance level of 0.05 is analogous to estimation with a 95% CI.

2

BIOSTATISTICS 2: ADVANCED CONCEPTS

M. Hassan Murad, MD, MPH; and Qian Shi, PhD

In this chapter, we describe several statistical techniques that are based on the concepts presented in Chapter 1. The purpose of this chapter is to give a general overview of these statistical techniques and describe when to use them and how to interpret the results. We hope that this knowledge will enhance the readers' understanding of the medical literature and help physicians apply and interpret statistical tests in their practice of preventive medicine and public health.

Determining the Appropriate Statistical Method

In Chapter 1, hypothesis testing was described by comparing a value obtained from a sample (eg, a mean or proportion) to a value obtained from the general population or to a historical value. These tests were the **1-sample t test** (for the mean) and the **1-sample proportion test** (for the proportion). However, the more common research question is to compare the parameters of 2 groups (eg, recurrence rates between groups receiving new chemotherapy vs standard care). Many classic statistical methods can be applied to make these comparisons.

The determination of appropriate statistical method depends on 4 questions: 1) What is the type of data? 2) Are observations dependent or independent? 3) What data distribution assumptions can be made? and 4) How many variables are being investigated?

First, how are the data characterized (data type)? Observations can be continuous, categorical, or measurements with censoring (eg, time to event).

Second, did the observations come from dependent or independent samples? If each observation in the first group has a corresponding observation in the second group, samples are considered **paired** and the observations are **dependent**. Paired samples frequently are used to control for variables that can influence the comparisons of interest. Examples of paired data include tumor size in a particular patient before and after treatment (self-pairing) or age- or sex-matched patients. When the underlying populations of 2 compared groups are completely different, the samples are considered **independent** (eg, serum iron levels in healthy children vs children with cystic fibrosis).

Third, can certain assumptions be made about the data distribution? The normality assumption might be reasonable for a large sample of continuous observations.

Fourth, how many variables are being investigated? **Bivariable analysis** explores the association between 2 variables. Often, the 2 variables may have a cause-and-effect relationship (eg, the use of a cholesterol-lowering medication [**explanatory variable**] reduces the risk of myocardial infarction [**response or outcome variable**]). **Multivariable analysis** explores the association between a response variable and multiple explanatory variables. The appropriate choice of statistical test on the basis of these 4 questions (data type, dependence, distribution assumption, and number of variables) is summarized in Table 1 for bivariable analyses and Table 2 for multivariable analyses.

- What is the type of data?
- Are observations dependent or independent?

Table 1 Appropriate Statistical Significance Test for Bivariable Analysis (Analysis of 1 Independent Variable and 1 Dependent Variable)

Variables to Be Tested			
First Variable	Second Variable	Example	Appropriate Test(s) for Significance
Continuous	Continuous	Age (C) and systolic blood pressure (C)	Pearson correlation coefficient (r); linear regression
Continuous	Ordinal	Age (C) and satisfaction (O)[a]	Group the continuous variable and calculate Spearman correlation coefficient (ρ); possibly use 1-way analysis of variance (F test)
Continuous	Dichotomous unpaired	Systolic blood pressure (C) and sex (DU)	Student t test
Continuous	Dichotomous paired	Difference in systolic blood pressure (C) before vs after treatment (DP)	Paired t test
Continuous	Nominal	Hemoglobin level (C) and blood type (N)	Analysis of variance (F test)
Ordinal	Ordinal	Correlation of satisfaction with care (O)[a] and severity of illness (O)	Spearman correlation coefficient (ρ); Kendall correlation coefficient (τ)
Ordinal	Dichotomous unpaired	Satisfaction (O) and sex (DU)	Mann-Whitney U test
Ordinal	Dichotomous paired	Difference in satisfaction (O) before vs after a program (DP)	Wilcoxon matched-pair signed rank test
Ordinal	Nominal	Satisfaction (O) and ethnicity (N)	Kruskal-Wallis test
Dichotomous	Dichotomous unpaired	Success/failure (D) in treated/untreated groups (DU)	χ^2 test; Fisher exact probability test
Dichotomous	Dichotomous paired	Change in success/failure (D) before vs after treatment (DP)	McNemar χ^2 test
Dichotomous	Nominal	Success/failure (D) and blood type (N)	χ^2 test
Nominal	Nominal	Ethnicity (N) and blood type (N)	χ^2 test

Abbreviations: C, continuous; D, dichotomous; DP, dichotomous paired; DU, dichotomous unpaired; N, nominal; O, ordinal.

[a] An example of satisfaction described by an ordinal scale: *very satisfied, somewhat satisfied, neither satisfied nor dissatisfied, somewhat dissatisfied,* and *very dissatisfied.*

Adapted from Jekel et al (2007). Used with permission.

- What data distribution assumptions can be made?
- How many variables are being investigated?

Continuous Data (Comparison of Means)

Many commonly used measurements in medical research are continuous (eg, blood pressure, serum cholesterol level, height). Comparison of means is a sensible way to detect potential differences in this kind of observation. It is important to note that these observations are reasonably assumed to have a normal distribution in usual practical applications. If the sample size is large enough, the central limit theorem can be assumed. The statistical methods or test procedures discussed in this section are based on a common assumption of normality.

Independent Samples

When observations come from 2 independent groups and the data are assumed to have a normal distribution, the most commonly used statistical method is the **2-sample *t* test**. For example, study investigators give growth hormone or placebo to children to study the effect of hormone on height. The appropriate statistical test is the 2-sample *t* test because the 2 groups (hormone vs placebo) are independent, the outcome (height) is continuous, and the outcome can be assumed to be normally distributed.

Recall that 2 parameters, mean and variance, define a normal distribution. In practice, population variances of observations in 2 groups are usually unknown. This leads to using the *t* distribution as the fundamental sampling distribution for hypothesis testing. However, 2 variations of the 2-sample *t* test exist for estimating 2 population variances; one variation has equal variances, the other has unequal variances. Standard statistical software can perform both 2-sample *t* tests. An *F* test can be performed to determine the equality of the 2 variances.

When means of more than 2 groups are compared, the 1-way **analysis of variance** (ANOVA), an extension of the 2-sample *t* test, can be used. In this case, although the potential differences are tested among 3 or more groups,

Table 2 Appropriate Procedure for Multivariable Analysis (Analysis of 1 Dependent Variable and More Than 1 Independent Variable)

Characterization of Variables to Be Analyzed		
Dependent Variable	Independent Variables[a]	Appropriate Procedure(s)
Continuous	All are categorical	Analysis of variance
Continuous	Some are categorical and some are continuous	Analysis of covariance
Continuous	All are continuous	Multiple linear regression
Ordinal	. . .	There is no formal multivariable procedure for ordinal dependent variables. Either treat the variables as if they were continuous (see above procedures) or perform log-linear analysis
Dichotomous	All are categorical	Logistic regression; log-linear analysis
Dichotomous	Some are categorical and some are continuous	Logistic regression[b]
Dichotomous	All are continuous	Logistic regression or discriminant function analysis
Nominal	All are categorical	Log-linear analysis
Nominal	Some are categorical and some are continuous	Group the continuous variables and perform log-linear analysis
Nominal	All are continuous	Discriminant function analysis, or group the continuous variables and perform log-linear analysis

[a] Categorical variables include ordinal, dichotomous, and nominal variables.
[b] If the outcome is a time-related dichotomous variable (eg, live/die), proportional hazards (Cox) models are best.
Adapted from Jekel et al (2007). Used with permission.

only 1 factor or characteristic distinguishes the various groups from each other (hence the term "1-way"). In this method, the null hypothesis (ie, the means across groups are not different) is satisfied when the ratio of within-group variance to between-group variance is close to 1. **Within-group variance** is defined as the variance of the individual observations around each group mean and the **between-group variance** is defined as the variance of group means around the overall mean.

- The 2-sample t test commonly is used to analyze normally distributed observations from 2 independent groups.
- One-way analysis of variance (ANOVA) is used to compare data from more than 2 groups.

Paired Samples

In the case of subjects who are paired or matched (ie, dependent samples) a **paired t test** is used. In the paired t test, the difference in means within each pair is calculated and then analyzed using a 1-sample t test. The null hypothesis is that the difference in means equals zero. Consider an example of paired samples: blood pressure measurements observed before and after a patient receives an antihypertensive medication. The samples are not independent

because pretreatment blood pressure will likely be correlated with posttreatment blood pressure. A paired t test would be appropriate to use when studying the effects of the medication.

- The paired t test is used when subjects are matched and observations are dependent.

Analogous Nonparametric Methods of Analyzing Continuous Data

Two-sample t tests, 1-way ANOVA, and paired t tests belong to the class of parametric methods and were developed with the assumption that the data were approximately normally distributed. However, normality is not always a reasonable assumption. For example, ordinal data have a natural order, but differences between the ranks cannot be quantified. Thus, common arithmetic statistics such as mean and standard deviation are not meaningful measures, nor is the normality assumption appropriate. Other instances in which the normality assumption should not be made are when sample size is limited or when the distribution of observations is skewed.

Nonparametric methods are used when normality cannot be assumed (ie, they relax the assumption of a specific underlying distribution). One common characteristic of nonparametric methods is that tests are conducted using data ranks rather than the actual values of observations. Importantly, when the assumption of normal distribution is valid or the central limit theorem is applicable, nonparametric methods have less power than parametric tests to detect differences between groups. Another disadvantage associated with nonparametric procedures is difficulty with interpretation of results. Statistically significant differences may exist, but the magnitude of the difference is not always obvious (not easy to quantify).

- Nonparametric tests are used when normality cannot be assumed.

Independent Samples

The **Wilcoxon rank sum test** (also termed the **Mann-Whitney U test**) is analogous to the 2-sample t test for independent samples. The procedure of the Wilcoxon rank sum test can be summarized as follows: 1) combine data from both groups and order the values from lowest to highest; 2) assign ranks to ordered individual values; and 3) compare the sum of ranks in one group to the other group. The **Kruskal-Wallis test** can be used if more than 2 groups are being compared and the normality assumption is not satisfied.

- For independent samples, the Wilcoxon rank sum test is analogous to the 2-sample t test.
- The Kruskal-Wallis test can be used if more than 2 groups are being compared. This is analogous to the 1-way analysis of variance (ANOVA).

Paired Samples

If investigators want to examine patient satisfaction with a quality improvement project conducted in their clinic, they can measure the level of satisfaction by using an ordinal scale. Each patient would provide a satisfaction value before and after the intervention. These values clearly are paired or matched, and 2 statistical tests can be used to make comparisons: the Wilcoxon signed rank test or the sign test. Both tests are analogous to the paired t test.

The procedure of conducting a Wilcoxon signed rank test is as follows: 1) find the differences between each pair of ordinal measures; 2) rank the differences in the order of absolute value by ignoring the observations with 0 difference; 3) compute the sum of rank (R_1) of the positive differences; and 4) compute the test statistic by comparing the observed R_1 to the expected value under null hypothesis and scaling by the expected standard deviation. In this test, the direction and the magnitude of the difference of the scores of individual pairs are used to conduct the significance test.

If investigators are interested only in knowing whether the quality improvement project is effective (without caring about the magnitude of change), they can conduct the sign test. For each pair, a (+) sign is assigned if the intervention is effective and a (–) sign is assigned if the intervention is ineffective. The null hypothesis (ie, no difference between groups) is that the proportion of pairs with (+) signs and (–) signs is 0.5. The sign test is less sensitive than the Wilcoxon signed rank test, but it is very simple and easy to conduct.

- For paired samples, the Wilcoxon signed rank test and the sign test can be used to show effectiveness of an intervention.

Comparison of Proportions

In Chapter 1, we used the normal approximation to the binomial distribution to make inferences about a proportion and provided an example comparing a proportion obtained from a sample against a proportion obtained from the general population. More commonly, investigators compare 2 proportions (eg, derived from sample populations that received an intervention or a placebo). In the case of 2 proportions, the same normal approximation methods can be applied, although alternative methods (eg, χ^2 test) are more commonly used.

Independent Samples

One of the most common tests used to compare 2 independent proportions (2 dichotomous variables) is the χ^2 **test**. Consider a group of 175 smokers and 25 nonsmokers (Table 3). Of the smokers, 95 (54.3%) had lung cancer. Of the nonsmokers, only 5 (20%) had lung cancer. Do these data show whether smoking status is significantly associated with lung cancer? Do significantly more smokers have lung cancer than nonsmokers?

In Table 3, the data are shown in a 2 × 2 table format (a **contingency table**). To compare proportions of subjects with lung cancer between smokers and nonsmokers, the χ^2 test compares the observed counts (O) to expected counts (E) if the null hypothesis is true (ie, the proportions of subjects with lung cancer are identical among smokers and nonsmokers). If the null hypothesis is true, the classification of smoker status is ignored and all 200 subjects are treated as a single, homogeneous sample. The expected count for each cell is calculated by multiplying the row and the column marginals (totals) and dividing by the total number of subjects. For example, in upper left cell, the observed value is 95 and the expected value is $100 \times 175/200 = 87.5$.

The χ^2 statistic is the sum of $\dfrac{(O-E)^2}{E}$ that is calculated for each cell in the contingency table. If r and c are the

Table 3 Contingency Table Showing Lung Cancer and Smoking Status

Smoking	Lung Cancer		
	Yes	No	Total
Yes	95	80	175
No	5	20	25
Total	100	100	200

numbers of rows and columns in the contingency table, respectively, the probabilities associated with this statistic can be assumed to have a χ^2 distribution with degrees of freedom=$(r-1)\times(c-1)$ if the sample size is large enough. In Table 3, the degrees of freedom=$(2-1)\times(2-1)=1$, and the χ^2 statistic is 10.29. Using statistical software or a χ^2 distribution table, we can determine that the associated P value is .001, which means that if $\alpha=0.05$, we can reject the null hypothesis and declare that it is unlikely that the difference between these 2 proportions is attributable to chance.

The φ coefficient adjusts the χ^2 statistic for the sample size and represents the proportion of χ^2 that was explained by the association, helping further to quantify the strength of association. The φ coefficient is calculated using the equation $\varphi = \sqrt{\dfrac{\chi^2}{N}}$. In this example, $\varphi = \sqrt{\dfrac{10.29}{200}} = 0.23$. Hence, smoking is associated with lung cancer and explains 23% of its occurrence. It is important to recognize that even a strong association does not always confer causality. Other causality criteria need to be satisfied (eg, biological plausibility) to make such an inference.

It is also important to note that the approximation to the χ^2 distribution works best when the expected cell counts are sufficiently large. If at least 1 cell in the contingency table has an expected count less than 5, the χ^2 test is not appropriate. In such a case, another test—the **Fisher exact test**—can be used. The Fisher exact test is more conservative (gives higher P values), which is appropriate when there is uncertainty associated with small expected cell counts.

- The χ^2 test is commonly used to compare 2 independent proportions (2 dichotomous variables).
- The φ coefficient represents the proportion of χ^2 that was explained by the association.
- The Fisher exact test should be used when at least 1 cell in a contingency table has an expected count less than 5.

Paired Samples

When the 2 proportions being compared are independent, the χ^2 analysis can be conducted. However, proportions also can come from paired observations. For example, if blood pressure is measured before and after administration of an antihypertensive medication, these observations are not independent because the pretreatment blood pressure will likely influence the degree of response to the medication. The **McNemar test** for paired proportions is most appropriate when comparing dependent proportions.

- The McNemar test is most appropriate when comparing dependent proportions.

Correlation and Regression

In the preceding sections, we described statistical methods for comparing population parameters (eg, mean or proportion) between 2 groups. The groups were defined by a **categorical variable** with distinct values (eg, sex [male or female] or exposure status [not exposed, possibly exposed, definitely exposed]). However, researchers frequently encounter situations in which 2 **continuous variables** are analyzed (eg, the effect of age on annual income). The commonly used statistical techniques for evaluating 2 continuous variables in bivariable analysis are correlation and linear regression.

Pearson and Spearman Correlations

Before conducting any type of association analyses for continuous random variables, the data should be plotted on a 2-dimensional graph. Figure 1 shows the plot of a fictional data set that included the height and weight of study subjects. Each point on the plot represents the combination of height and weight that is specific to a particular subject. The plot clearly shows a positive relationship between the 2 variables (weight increases as height increases). Furthermore, this relationship can be summarized by a straight line.

When considering the relationship between 2 variables, the degree to which this relationship is linear can be quantified by determining the correlation between variables. The **Pearson correlation coefficient** (r), the estimator of the population correlation, represents the strength of the linear relationship. Pearson correlation coefficient ranges from −1 (perfect negative correlation; value of one variable decreases as another increases) to +1 (perfect positive correlation; value of one variable increases as another increases). A coefficient of 0 indicates no linear relationship between the 2 variables. An absolute value of correlation of ≥0.7 is usually considered a strong linear relationship; 0.4–0.7 is moderate; and <0.4 is weak. Nevertheless, the clinical context should supersede the arbitrary values of the coefficient.

Inferences about a population parameter can be made with correlation analysis from a sample. After following the steps of hypothesis testing, a P value is generated that

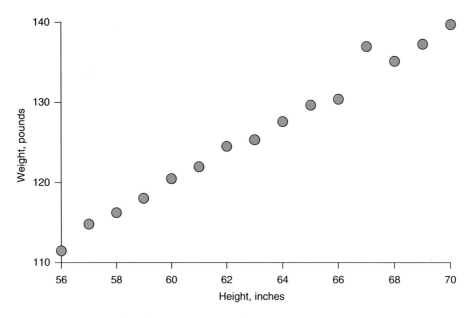

Figure 1 Scatter Plot of Weight vs Height. A straight line can represent this relationship.

can show statistical significance. The Pearson correlation does have several important limitations. First, it is only a measurement of linear relationship, but meaningful nonlinear relationships can also exist between variables. Second, the Pearson correlation coefficient is sensitive to outliers. Third, the inference from correlation analysis is not always accurate when extrapolated beyond the observed range of data. Fourth, a strong linear relationship does not imply causality.

The **Spearman correlation coefficient** is an extension of the Pearson correlation coefficient. It is used when the normality assumption is not reasonable or valid, and it depends on comparing rank order. As a nonparametric method, it does not make assumptions about the underlying distribution of data.

- The Pearson correlation coefficient is used to estimate the strength of the linear relationship between 2 variables.
- The Spearman correlation coefficient is used when data are not normally distributed.
- Variables can have meaningful nonlinear relationships, and a strong linear relationship does not imply causality.
- The Pearson correlation can be sensitive to outliers.
- Inference from correlation analysis should not be extrapolated beyond the observed range of data.

Simple Linear Regression

Correlation measurements can determine whether a linear relationship exists between 2 continuous variables;

however, sometimes this information is not sufficient. Investigators may want to quantify this relationship by knowing how much a change in one variable (explanatory variable) causes change in the other variable (response or dependent variable). The appropriate technique to quantify this relationship is **simple linear regression**. A simple linear regression line is estimated by using the formula: $y=a+bx$, where y is the response (dependent) variable, x is the explanatory (independent) variable, a is the intercept (the value of y when $x=0$), and b is the slope (determines how much y will increase for every 1-unit increase of x).

Regression is more informative than correlation for several reasons: 1) it can estimate the mean value of the response variable for a group of subjects with a given value of the explanatory variable; and 2) it can predict the value of the response variable for a future subject who has a given value of the explanatory variable. In simple linear regression, the amount of variation of the dependent variable that can be explained by the independent variable is determined by the **coefficient of determination** (R^2), which describes how well the regression line fits the observed data. It is calculated by squaring the Pearson correlation coefficient r after fitting the simple linear regression line to the data. The value of R^2 ranges from 0 through 1 (eg, R^2 of 0.45 means that 45% of the changes in y are explained by changes in x). To enable inference from regression analysis, several assumptions are made in addition to the assumption of a linear relationship. We assume **independence** (the response variables were observed independently among subjects), **normality** (normal distribution of a response variable, given a specified value for the explanatory variable, measured without error), and **homoscedasticity** (constant variance of the response, analogous to equal variances in 2-sample *t* test).

- Estimations and predictions of a response variable with respect to particular values of an explanatory variable can be conducted using regression analyses.
- The amount of variation of the response variable that can be explained by the explanatory variables can be quantified by coefficient of determination.
- To make inferences on the basis of linear regression analysis, data must be independent, normally distributed, and homoscedastic.

Logistic Regression

Linear regression is a special case of regression that is characterized by a continuous and normally distributed response variable. However, when the response variable is dichotomous, the normality assumption is violated and the **logistic regression** method should be used. In medical research, logistic regression is often used to control for variables that can affect the outcome of interest and to control for possible confounders. It estimates the **likelihood** of the occurrence of the response variable, not the actual value of this outcome (as is calculated in linear regression analysis). Logistic regression is a technique of fitting a linear model for the transformed mean of a binomially distributed response variable. The transformation here is termed **logistic function**—taking the natural logarithm of the odds in favor of the outcome of interest. In logistic regression analysis, the inference is usually based on calculating the **odds ratio** (OR) and determining the associated **confidence interval** (CI). For example, logistic regression is the appropriate method of analysis to determine whether the likelihood of surviving a heart attack (yes/no answer, dichotomous response) can be predicted by knowing 1) the time elapsed between symptom onset and presentation to the emergency department (continuous explanatory variable); 2) blood pressure at the time of symptom onset (continuous explanatory variable); or 3) whether the patient has diabetes mellitus (yes/no answer, dichotomous explanatory variable).

The OR is a measure of association—a quantification of the relationship between explanatory and response variables. For dichotomous explanatory variables, the OR is calculated as follows: OR = exp(estimated slope). The percentage of variability of the outcome variable that is explained by the model is indicated by R^2. For example, if $R^2 = 0.66$, the linear relationship expressed by the model between the logarithm of the odds of the response variable and the explanatory variables explains two-thirds of the variability of the outcome. One-third of the variability therefore is attributed to other sources not identified in the model.

- Logistic regression is used when the response variable is dichotomous. It can control for possible confounders of the outcome of interest.
- Logistic regression estimates the likelihood of the occurrence of the outcome. Inference is usually based on odds ratios (OR) and associated confidence intervals (CI).

Time-to-Event Analysis

Frequently, the effect of a medical intervention is measured in terms of the length of time between the intervention and the outcome (eg, from randomization to receive a particular treatment until death). The event of interest is usually termed failure. Although survival time is continuous, it has very different properties compared with other continuous measurements such as blood pressure or height. Distribution of survival time tends to be right-skewed (ie, most patients will die early, but a few will have unusually long survival). Furthermore, not every subject will experience the event of interest within the study period. For example, if the outcome of interest is death and a patient was alive at the end of the study, the survival time of the patient is known only to the extent that it was greater than the time observed. This partial (observed) time to event is termed **censoring time**. Ignoring censoring times will create bias when the relationships between survival time and other factors are assessed. Therefore, a special analytic technique is needed.

The distribution of survival time is characterized by the **survival function**, defined as the probability of an individual subject encountering an event of interest beyond a given time point. The **Kaplan-Meier analysis**, a nonparametric method, is the most common method of estimating the survival function. In a Kaplan-Meier graph, each segment of time is portrayed as a horizontal line that represents an event-free period; this line drops by an interval whenever 1 or more patients experience the event of interest. Figure 2 is a typical Kaplan-Meier estimate of survival function. Notice the 2 notches on the curve: these represent censoring times. At these 2 points, the curve does not drop because censoring cannot be counted as failures. The detailed steps of obtaining the Kaplan-Meier curves are not described here because the curves can be easily generated with standard statistical software packages.

In survival analysis, the censoring mechanism is usually assumed to be independent of the rate of event of interest occurring. At the end of the study, the survival rate is equal to the product of all the survival rates of the individual time segments. As implied by the nonparametric property, no assumptions are made about the functional form of the distribution of survival times when estimating the Kaplan-Meier curves.

The Kaplan-Meier curve is a descriptive method for characterizing survival data. For inferential methods, the

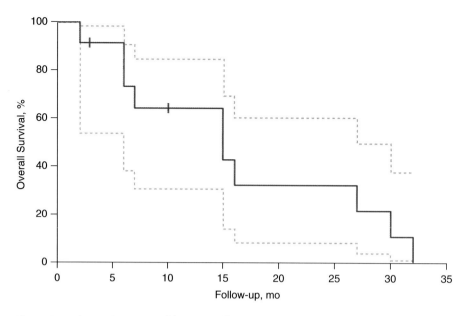

Figure 2 Kaplan-Meier Curve With 95% Confidence Interval. The survival curve is shown as the solid line; the confidence interval is between the dotted lines. The curve shows survival of 12 patients with hemophilia and AIDS in the mid to late 1980s.

nonparametric **log-rank test** can be used to compare survival functions of 2 or more groups. The **Cox proportional hazards model**, a semiparametric method, is a more flexible regression method of assessing the relationship between the time-to-event response variable and single or multiple explanatory variables. The explanatory variables can be continuous or categorical, and they can be time-dependent (ie, the values of explanatory variable change with time [eg, age]) or non–time-dependent (ie, the values of explanatory variables are fixed [eg, sex or race]).

- The survival function is the probability that an individual encounters an event of interest beyond a fixed time point.
- The nonparametric Kaplan-Meier analysis commonly is used to estimate the survival function.
- In Kaplan-Meier analysis, the censoring mechanism is assumed to be independent of the rate of the event of interest occurring.
- The survival rate is equal to the product of all the survival rates of the individual time segments.

Multivariable Analysis

Bivariable analysis explores the association between the response variable and 1 explanatory variable. In contrast, multivariable analysis explores the association between the response variable and 2 or more explanatory variables. The linear regression, logistic regression, and Cox proportional hazards model all have the capability of performing multivariable analyses (ie, simultaneous inclusion of several explanatory variables in the regression model). The basic differences among these methods are attributable to the different data types of the response variable. ANOVA is the common method used in multivariable analysis of more than 1 categorical explanatory variable (if the model has 2 categorical explanatory variables, it is called 2-way ANOVA). **Analysis of covariance** is used for multivariable analysis if some of the explanatory variables are not categorical.

When data are analyzed, several regression models are tested by including and excluding different variables; the objective is to find the best model that allows good prediction without **overfitting**. Overfitting is when the model incorporates a large number of explanatory variables and consequently matches the sample too well; overfitted models are too complex to generalize to a population. Usually, at least 10 subjects per explanatory variable are needed to prevent overfitting.

When many explanatory variables need to be analyzed, the process of model selection becomes complicated (details of the process are beyond the scope of this textbook). There is no absolutely correct way to build a model based on the observed data; an appropriate model must achieve a balance between parsimony and data-fitting adequacy. As mentioned above, overfitting will make the model too complex for interpretation and likely will reduce its generalizability. Analysis involving model selection is considered to be exploratory analysis; thus, its results should always be interpreted with caution.

- Multivariable analysis can be conducted with linear regression, logistic regression, and Cox proportional hazards model.

- Analysis of variance is commonly used for datasets with more than 1 categorical explanatory variable.
- Overfitting can occur when the model incorporates numerous explanatory variables. Because overfitted models match the sample too well, they are not easily generalized to a population.

Measures of Association

When assessing the association between a treatment or exposure and a binary (dichotomous) outcome (eg, effect of hormone replacement therapy on development of breast cancer), the strength of the association must be quantified. The **relative risk** (RR), also termed **risk ratio**, is the most intuitive association measure. It is a ratio of the risk of having the outcome with exposure versus the risk of having the outcome without the exposure (eg, the risk of breast cancer development in patients who did vs did not receive hormone replacement therapy). If the risk of breast cancer in an exposed group is 4 in 10,000 and the risk in an unexposed group is 2 in 10,000, the RR=0.0004/0.0002=2. Thus, in this example, hormone replacement therapy doubles the risk of breast cancer. RRs of 1, 1.2, or 0.5 mean that the exposure is not associated with the outcome, increases risk by 20%, or decreases risk by 50%, respectively.

Risk difference (RD) is another measure of association, calculated by subtracting one risk from the other. Unlike RR, which is a relative measure of association, the RD is an absolute measure of association. It is important to recognize that RR may exaggerate the perception of risk compared with RD. For example, if a woman is advised that hormone replacement therapy will double her risk of breast cancer, she likely would refuse treatment, whereas if she is told that her risk will increase by 2 in 10,000, she may opt to receive treatment. Both risks are in fact correct, but the first (doubled) risk is the RR and the second (2 in 10,000) risk is the RD. One of the downfalls of RD is applicability; RD is applicable to populations with similar baseline risk factors, whereas RR can be used to compare populations with varying baseline risks.

- Relative risk (RR) is the ratio of the risk of having the outcome with exposure versus the risk of having the outcome without the exposure, whereas risk difference (RD) is an absolute measure of association.
- RR may exaggerate the perception of risk compared with RD.
- RD is applied to populations with similar baseline risk factors, whereas RR is used for populations with varying baseline risks.

The OR is another relative measure of association that is analogous to RR (it is a ratio of odds instead of risks). In the example from the previous paragraph, an OR of 2 would mean that hormone replacement therapy doubled the odds (not risk) of breast cancer development. Because patients and physicians are more familiar with the concept of risk than with that of odds, OR is likely less intuitive than RR or RD. OR can be used in case-control studies, in which subjects are sampled on the basis of disease status instead of exposure status. Furthermore, the OR is equally valid for data from case-control, cohort, or cross-sectional studies. In all of these designs, the calculated ORs are estimating the same population parameter. In a case-control study, RR cannot be estimated without additional information. When analysis requires adjusting or controlling for several confounders and logistic regression is used, results usually are presented as ORs.

Like RR exaggerates the perception of risk compared with RD, OR exaggerates the perception of risk compared with RR. This exaggeration is particularly prominent when the event rate is high. However, in the special situation when the disease of interest is rare and a 2×2 contingency table shows that the values of A and C are small relative to the values of B and D, the OR is an approximation to the RR.

Formulas for computing commonly used measures of association are presented in Table 4. The standard error of the association is needed to assess the CIs and statistical significance.

- The odds ratio (OR) can be used in case-control, cohort, or cross-sectional studies. However, the relative risk (RR) is not estimable in case-control studies.
- When logistic regression is used and analysis requires controlling for confounders, results usually are presented as ORs.
- The OR exaggerates the perception of risk compared with relative risk (RR), particularly when the event rate is high. However, the OR is an approximation to the RR when the event rate is very low.

OR in Matched-Pair Study Design

Case-controlled studies occasionally match a patient with disease (case) to a patient without the disease (control) to provide direct control for possible confounding conditions. Hence, the unit of analysis is a pair of subjects, not an individual. Matching may also improve the efficiency of the investigation by providing more precise risk estimates. Table 5 shows an example study that evaluated the association between smoking and lung cancer, in which researchers matched each patient with lung cancer to a subject without lung cancer.

Pairs can be concordant in terms of their exposure (ie, both case and control smoked [cell *a*] or neither smoked [cell *d*]). However, concordant pairs do not provide data that can be used to calculate OR; obviously, when both subjects are smokers or nonsmokers, no conclusions can be drawn about smoking as a cause of lung cancer. Pairs

Table 4 Formulas to Calculate Common Measures of Association

	Status		
Exposure or Intervention	Diseased	Healthy	Total
Yes	A	B	$N_{exposed}$
No	C	D	$N_{unexposed}$

Association Measure	Formula
Risk of disease with exposure (also termed *EER*)	$A/N_{exposed}$
Risk of disease without exposure (also termed *CER*)	$C/N_{unexposed}$
Relative risk (also termed *risk ratio*)[a,b]	EER/CER
Relative risk reduction	1−relative risk; equivalent to (CER−EER)/CER
Risk difference (also termed *AAR or attributable risk*)[a,c]	EER−CER
Number needed to treat	1/ARR
Odds of outcome in the exposed group	EER/(1−EER); equivalent to A/B
Odds of outcome in the unexposed group	CER/(1−CER); equivalent to C/D
Odds ratio[a,d]	(A/B)÷(C/D); equivalent to AD/BC

Abbreviations: ARR, absolute risk reduction; CER, control event rate; EER, experimental event rate; SE_{lnOR}, standard error of ln(odds ratio); SE_{lnRR}, standard error of ln(risk ratio); SE_{RD}, standard error of risk difference.

[a] The SE_{lnRR}, SE_{lnOR}, and SE_{RD} are based on normal theory approximations.

[b] $SE_{lnRR} = \sqrt{(B/A)/N_{exposed} + (D/C)/N_{unexposed}}$

[c] $SE_{RD} = \sqrt{AB/\left(N_{exposed}\right)^3 + DC/\left(N_{unexposed}\right)^3}$

[d] $SE_{lnOR} = \sqrt{(1/A)+(1/B)+(1/C)+(1/D)}$

Table 5 Matched-Pair Design

Lung Cancer	No Lung Cancer	
	Smoker	Nonsmoker
Smoker	a	b
Nonsmoker	c	d

Relevant formulas:

$$OR = b/c$$

$$SE_{lnOR} = \sqrt{\frac{1}{b} + \frac{1}{c}}$$

Abbreviations: OR, odds ratio; SE_{lnOR}, standard error of ln(odds ratio).

can be discordant (ie, one smoked and the other did not [cells *b* and *c*]). If the number of discordant pairs in which the patients with lung cancer smoked and the controls did not (cell *b*) was higher than the number of pairs in which the patients with lung cancer did not smoke and the controls smoked (cell *c*), we can conclude that smoking causes lung cancer. The ratio of *b*/*c* is the OR for a matched case-control study. If the number of discordant pairs (*b*+*c*) is ≥20, the McNemar test can be used to test the null hypothesis, which in this case would indicate the lack of association between the 2 variables. Case-control matching sometimes induces selection bias. In such a case, the Mantel-Haenszel test can be used to account for the matching and thus remove the selection bias.

- Matched pairs can be concordant or discordant.
- Discordant pairs are needed to identify associations between variables.

Hazard Ratio

The **hazard rate** is the probability that an event will occur in a time interval, divided by the length of that interval. The time interval is made very short so that the hazard rate represents an instantaneous rate. The **hazard ratio** (HR), a measure of association, is an estimate of the ratio of the hazard rate in the treated group versus the control group. It usually is generated by proportional hazard regression models, in which the assumption is made that HR is constant over time.

HRs are used in analysis of time-to-event outcomes. HR is analogous to RR in that it is a ratio of 2 risks, but HR incorporates the element of time. An HR of 1 indicates no difference in hazard rates (similar to an RR of 1), whereas values exceeding 1 indicate increased risk and values less than 1 indicate decreased risk. Theoretically, if censoring did not occur, HR can be converted to odds by applying the same formulas used to convert RR to OR.

- The hazard rate represents an instantaneous rate (the probability that an event will occur within a very short time).
- The hazard ratio (HR) is analogous to the relative risk but incorporates the element of time.

CIs for Measures of Association

In Chapter 1, we described how CIs consist of a point estimate (best guess obtained from the sample) plus or minus a margin of error (determined by the confidence level). The margin of error is calculated by obtaining a confidence coefficient and multiplying it by the standard error. For a typical 95% CI based on normal approximation, the confidence coefficient is 1.96.

For measures of association, CIs show the uncertainty of the point estimates (eg, RR, RD, OR). The distribution of relative association measures (RR and OR) is very asymmetric because values indicating lower risk are between 0 and 1, and values indicating higher risk are between 1 and ∞. One way to calculate the CIs of RR and OR is to make the distribution more symmetric before calculating CIs, ie, RR and OR undergo transformation by conversion to a natural logarithm. To generate the upper and lower boundaries of a CI for the logarithm of the RR or OR, the standard error of the logarithm is added to and subtracted from the point estimate, respectively. Next, the upper and lower limits of the CI of the logarithm are exponentiated (the antilog function) to generate CI for RR or OR. This process makes the CI around RR and OR asymmetric, but that does not cause inferential consequences in most scenarios. RD values range from −∞ to +∞; it has a symmetric distribution and does not need logarithmic transformation. To calculate the 95% CI for an RD, the interval is 1.96 standard errors on either side of the RD.

When the CIs of an RR or OR contain the value 1, or when the CI of an RD contains the value 0, the estimation of the measure of association is not statistically significant. Either the exposure (or treatment) is not truly associated with the outcome or the study was insufficiently powered (not enough events) and thus generated wide (imprecise) CIs. Precision for association measures of categorical outcomes is driven mainly by the number of events (eg, patients with the outcome of interest); it is affected to a lesser extent by the sample size.

- The distribution of relative risks (RRs) and odds ratios (ORs) are asymmetric and may be transformed with a natural logarithm before confidence intervals (CIs) are calculated.
- Although the CI may be asymmetric about the point estimate, this usually does not cause inferential consequences.
- An estimated RR or OR is not statistically significant if the CI contains the value 1. An RD is not significant if the CI contains the value 0.

Diagnosis

Diagnostic tests (eg, laboratory or radiographic tests) are not usually 100% accurate. When a test is used to diagnose a condition, it is critical for physicians to know the accuracy of the assay when confirming or excluding a condition. Diagnostic tests are usually compared against a confirmatory test (also termed reference test, gold standard, or criterion standard) to evaluate accuracy. Table 6 shows a typical diagnosis table that compares a diagnostic (index) test with the reference standard.

The most commonly used diagnostic probabilities are **sensitivity** (SN), **specificity** (SP), **positive predictive value** (PPV), and **negative predictive value** (NPV). SN is the

Table 6 Diagnosis Table

Diagnostic (Index) Test	Reference (Criterion) Standard	
	Diseased	Healthy
Positive	TP	FP
Negative	FN	TN

Test Attribute	Formula
Sensitivity	TP/(TP+FN)
Specificity	TN/(TN+FP)
Positive predictive value	TP/(TP+FP)
Negative predictive value	TN/(TN+FN)
Prevalence	(TP+FN)/(TP+FP+TN+FN)
Diagnostic likelihood ratio for a positive test	SN/(1−SP)
Diagnostic likelihood ratio for a negative test	(1−SN)/SP
Diagnostic odds ratio	(TP/FP)/(FN/TN); equivalent to DLR+/DLR−
Diagnostic yield[a]	TP/(TP+FP+TN+FN)
Accuracy[a]	(TP+TN)/(TP+FP+TN+FN)

Abbreviations: DLR−, diagnostic likelihood ratio for a negative test; DLR+, diagnostic likelihood ratio for a positive test; FN, false-negative; FP, false-positive; SN, sensitivity; SP, specificity; TN, true-negative; TP, true-positive.
[a] These diagnostic expressions are less commonly used.

probability of having a positive test result among the subjects who truly have the disease of interest (the true-positive rate). SP is the probability of having a negative test result among the healthy (the true-negative rate). A test with high SN is better for excluding a diagnosis, whereas a test with high SP is better for including a diagnosis; the mnemonics "SNOUT" and "SPIN" are used for "sensitivity-out" and "specificity-in," respectively. PPV is the probability of having the illness, given a positive test result. Note that PPV has the same numerator as SN (the true-positive rate). NPV is the probability of being healthy and having a negative test result. Note that NPV has the same numerator as SP (the true-negative rate).

Another way to think of these probabilities is that SN and SP are helpful to consider when ordering a test because they indicate the likelihood that the test will give a correct answer. Thus, they are often used to describe test performance. In contrast, PPV and NPV are more helpful when interpreting test results (to know what results mean). Importantly, PPV and NPV are affected by **prevalence** (PREV). If a disease is rare and the diagnostic test is positive, the results might be false-positive. Similarly, if a disease is common and the test is negative, the results may be false-negative. Low PREV leads to low PPV and high PREV leads to high PPV; the opposite is true for NPV.

PPV represents the posttest probability of disease when the test is positive; it can be calculated if clinicians know the pretest PREV of a particular disease in their practice and the diagnostic characteristics (SN, SP) of a test. PPV is calculated using the following formula:

$$PPV = \frac{PREV \times SN}{(PREV \times SN) + (1-PREV)(1-SP)}$$

- The most commonly used diagnostic probabilities are sensitivity (SN), specificity (SP), positive predictive value (PPV), and negative predictive value (NPV).
- A test with high SN is better for excluding a diagnosis, whereas a test with high SP is better for including a diagnosis.
- Low prevalence (PREV) leads to low PPV and high PREV leads to high PPV. The opposite is true for NPV.

Example 1. Positive predictive value.
What is the probability of coronary artery disease in a 20-year-old woman who presents to the emergency department with chest pain and has positive findings after an isotope stress test? The test is known to have 95% sensitivity and 90% specificity. The prevalence of coronary artery disease in 20-year-old women is 1 in 1,000.
Answer:

$$PPV = \frac{0.001 \times 0.95}{(0.001 \times 0.95) + (1-0.001)(1-0.90)} = 0.01$$

Despite the excellent diagnostic characteristics of the isotope stress test (very high sensitivity and specificity), a positive result in a very low-risk population still is consistent with a very low probability of disease (1%).

Diagnostic Likelihood Ratios

The **diagnostic likelihood ratio** (DLR) for a test is the ratio of the likelihood of the observed test result in the diseased vs nondiseased populations. DLRs are true likelihood ratios in the statistical sense. The positive DLR is the ratio of the probabilities of having a positive test in the diseased vs nondiseased population, and the negative DLR has an analogous definition, except that it applies to negative tests. Both DLRs can have values that range from 0 to ∞. A useless test (ie, one that provides results with no relationship to true disease status) will have a value of 1 for both positive and negative DLRs. A positive DLR of ∞ and a negative DLR of 0 indicate a perfect, 100% accurate test. Generally, useful tests have positive DLRs greater than 1 (diseased subjects are more likely to have positive results; the higher the positive DLR, the better) and negative DLRs less than 1 (nondiseased subjects are more likely to have negative results; the lower the negative DLR, the better).

DLRs quantify changes in the risk of disease from **pretest odds** (ie, odds before test results are known) to **posttest**

odds (ie, odds after test results are known). The formula to transform pretest odds to posttest odds is as follows:

posttest odds = pretest odds × likelihood ratio

In fact, most clinicians subconsciously consider this transformation on a daily basis when performing a diagnostic evaluation.

- Useful tests have positive diagnostic likelihood ratios (DLRs) greater than 1 (diseased subjects are more likely to have positive results) and negative DLRs less than 1 (nondiseased subjects are more likely to have negative results).
- DLRs quantify the change in the risk of disease before and after test results are known.

Example 2. Likelihood ratios in clinical practice.
A nursing home resident presented with a fever. Previous experience suggests that 70% of nursing home residents who present with fever have a urinary tract infection. Urinalysis results were consistent with an infection. If urinalysis has a positive diagnostic likelihood ratio of 5, what is the probability that this patient has a urinary tract infection?

Pretest probability: 0.70
Pretest odds: 0.7/(1−0.7)=2.33
Posttest odds: 2.33×5=11.66
Posttest probability: 11.66/(1+11.66)=0.92

Therefore, the positive urinalysis result increased the probability of having a urinary tract infection from 70% to 92%.
In this example, a likelihood ratio was provided, which necessitated calculations using odds. Hence, we converted probability to odds, converted pretest odds to posttest odds, and converted posttest odds back to probability. In contrast, calculations from Example 1 were conducted using probabilities alone.

The **diagnostic odds ratio** (DOR) is the odds of positivity in disease to the odds of positivity in health (the ratio of positive DLR to negative DLR). A larger DOR indicates a more discriminatory (better) test. DLRs and DORs are not dependent on disease prevalence, which is a major advantage over PPV and NPV.

- A larger diagnostic odds ratio (DOR) indicates a more discriminatory test.
- Diagnostic likelihood ratios (DLRs) and DORs are not dependent on disease prevalence.

Estimation of Diagnostic Measures

The probabilities and diagnostic measures presented in this chapter generally are obtained from a sample of patients in a study. As with other study statistics, CIs are used to describe uncertainty about these point estimates (ie, by adding and subtracting a margin of error to the estimate). This margin of error consists of the product of the standard error multiplied by a confidence coefficient. For a 95% CI, the margin of error is the standard error multiplied by 1.96, if the normal approximation is applicable.

Receiver Operating Characteristic Curve

Results of diagnostic tests frequently are reported as continuous (not dichotomous) variables. For example, a fasting glucose test result is a number that ranges from 0 to ∞ (a dichotomous result would be yes/no). Thus, a threshold value must be used to decide whether a person has diabetes mellitus. If a high threshold (eg, 200 mg/dL) is used, the test will have poor SN because fewer cases of diabetes mellitus will be diagnosed and many who likely have the disease (eg, those with serum glucose 160 mg/dL) will not be identified. However, the test will have high SP because all identified cases invariably will have diabetes mellitus. Conversely, if a low threshold (eg, 120 mg/dL) is used, the test will have high SN by identifying most subjects with diabetes mellitus, including those with borderline glucose values, but the test will have poor SP because it also will identify a large number of people who do not have the disease. Each threshold has its own SN, SP, PPV, NPV, positive DLR, and negative DLR (ie, each threshold can be depicted with a unique 2×2 diagnostic table).

To determine the best threshold value and to characterize the overall performance of a diagnostic test, the true-positive rate (SN) is plotted on the y-axis against the false-positive rate (1−SP) on the x-axis. The resulting plot is called the **receiver operating characteristic** (ROC) curve (Figure 3). The ROC curve is a commonly used statistical tool for describing the performance of diagnostic tests.

The ROC curve of a perfect test follows the left and upper borders of the graph. The better the test, the closer the ROC curve is to the upper left corner of the plot. If the curve is nearly a straight diagonal line, the assay's true-positive rate is similar to its false-positive rate; such a test is useless and has no discriminatory value. By describing the entire set of accuracy parameters (pairs of SN and 1−SP values) of nonbinary diagnostic tests, meaningful comparisons of these tests become feasible. Another advantage of the ROC curve is that it transforms test characteristics to a common scale, facilitating comparison of tests with different measurement scales. Furthermore, ROC curves are useful when deciding threshold values to use in clinical practice.

The area under the ROC curve is a widely used summary measure. An area of 1.0 indicates a perfect test, whereas an

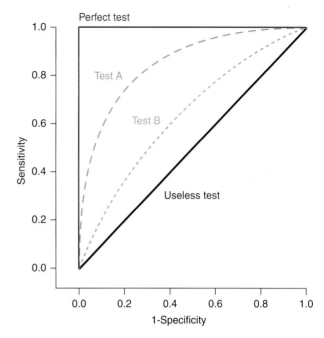

Figure 3 Receiver Operating Characteristic Curves. Test A has better performance than test B. Curves for perfect and useless tests also are shown.

area of 0.5 indicates a useless test. The standard error of the area under the curve can be estimated and used to conduct hypothesis testing.

- In a perfect test, the receiver operating characteristic (ROC) curve follows the left and upper borders of the graph and has an area under the curve of 1.0.
- In a useless test, the area under the ROC curve is 0.5.

Meta-analysis

Assume that researchers wanted to determine whether statins lower the risk of heart disease in patients with a family history of heart disease. A search of the literature yielded 3 studies that showed the following RRs: 0.70, 0.80, and 1.50. This means that statins reduced the risk of heart disease by 30% and 20%, respectively, in the first 2 studies and increased the risk by 50% in the third study. If all studies were of good quality and used good methodology, which should be believed? What is the true effect of statins?

The averaged RRs ([0.70+0.80+1.50]/3) is 1.00, which suggests that statins have no effect on the risk of heart disease. Obviously, this approach is problematic because it does not incorporate any element of precision (ie, we do not know how confident we are in the estimates of the 3 RRs). For example, what if the third study (showing increased risk of heart disease with statin use) was a study of only 10 patients and the first 2 studies were of 10,000 patients each? Because of random error committed during population sampling, the smaller study with a small number of events is more likely to generate a large standard error and variance, a wide CI, and potentially erroneous results. We are less confident that the results from the small study represent the true effect of statins. Therefore, larger studies with a greater number of events should have more influence than a smaller study when a common RR is being estimated from the individual RRs.

When study results are added quantitatively to estimate the **pooled effect** in a meta-analysis, each study finding is weighted by its precision. Precision is the opposite of variance; thus, in a meta-analysis, studies are weighted by the inverse of their variance. To calculate a common effect across the studies, multiply the effect obtained from each study (eg, the RR) by the inverse of its variance; sum the products of multiplications; and divide the result by the sum of the weights. With this approach, larger studies with more events are more influential than smaller studies with fewer events. In the statin example above, giving more weight to the first 2 studies makes the meta-analytic result (the pooled RR) closer to the original RRs of 0.70 and 0.80 instead of the unweighted RR of 1.0.

In meta-analyses, the process of choosing studies for inclusion must be comprehensive, systematic, and follow explicit inclusion and exclusion criteria. For example, if only 3 of 10 studies are selected to evaluate the effects of statins on heart disease, the results likely will not represent the whole body of evidence (results will be biased). In **systematic reviews**, measures are taken to protect studies from bias (eg, the review is conducted by a blinded pair of authors), and authors usually adhere to an explicit review strategy with reproducible results.

Meta-analysis results usually are presented in a forest plot. Figure 4 is a forest plot summarizing the results of 4 fictional studies (I-IV). A square represents the point estimate from each study (eg, the RR) and the lines through the squares represent 95% CIs from each study. The diamond represents the summary effect (pooled estimate), and the width of the diamond represents the 95% CI of the pooled estimate. Note that the results of studies I, III, and IV are not statistically significant because the 95% CI of the RR includes the value 1.0; however, the overall combined effect is statistically significant. By including a larger sample size and a greater number of events, the analysis has gained precision.

- In a meta-analysis, studies are weighted by their precision. Larger studies with more events are more influential than smaller studies with fewer events.
- The process of choosing studies for inclusion in a meta-analysis must be comprehensive, systematic, explicit, reproducible, and unbiased.

Fixed-Effect and Random-Effects Models

Two methods may be used in a meta-analysis to generate a single, pooled estimate. The **fixed-effect model** is based on the assumption that treatment confers one underlying true effect and that differences between studies are attributable to random error (chance). Essentially, if studies were infinitely large, they would all show the same result. Consequently, when studies are weighted to generate the pooled estimate, only within-study variation (study variance) is taken into account.

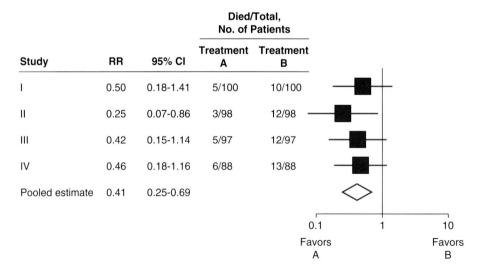

Figure 4 Meta-analysis of 4 Studies (Forest Plot). The square represents relative risk (RR) and the line represents the 95% confidence interval (CI). The diamond shows the summary effect (pooled estimate) of all studies with its 95% CI. A log scale is used when the treatment effect is expressed as RR (or odds ratio) to make the data distribution more symmetric.

The **random-effects model** assumes that treatment may confer multiple, different effects. These effects are distributed in a particular manner (usually the normal distribution) and have a mean value. The difference in effects across studies has 2 causes: within-study variation (study variance) and between-study variation (true differences in how the studies were performed [termed **heterogeneity**]). Heterogeneity could be due to differences in study design, inclusion criteria, patients, intervention, outcome definition or measurement, etc. The weight of each study in the fixed-effect model is the inverse of the study variance; in contrast, study weight in the random-effects model is the inverse of the sum of within-study variance and between-study variance. Therefore, pooled estimates obtained with the random-effects model, when heterogeneity level is high, will have larger variance (ie, more conservative [wide] CIs and larger P values), and the results are less likely to be statistically significant compared with the fixed-effect model. If heterogeneity level is low, both models will give similar results.

In most medical research, the random-effects model is more appropriate because studies tend to have heterogeneous populations, interventions, outcomes, and other known and unknown factors. Nevertheless, the fixed-effect model can be appropriate when studies are very similar (eg, a researcher repeated a study with a similar protocol) or when small studies have large treatment effects that might be spurious (the fixed-effect model decreases the relative weight of small studies).

- In the fixed-effect model, treatment is assumed to have one true effect. When studies are weighted to generate the pooled estimate, only within-study variation (study variance) is taken into account.
- In the random-effects model, treatment is assumed to have multiple effects, and the model accounts for study variance and heterogeneity.
- Pooled estimates from a random-effects model will have larger variance than those from a fixed-effect model.

Assessing Heterogeneity

Several statistical methods are used to assess heterogeneity; the most common 2 are the Cochran Q and the I^2 test. The **Cochran Q** is a yes/no test with a null hypothesis that there is no underlying between-study heterogeneity; it generates a probability based on the χ^2 distribution (P value). The **I^2 test** represents the proportion of variability that is not attributable to chance (ie, random error); its value ranges from 0% to 100%. The I^2 test helps assess the magnitude of heterogeneity, rather than giving only a yes/no answer.

Figure 5 shows a meta-analysis based on studies with very high heterogeneity (I^2 statistic=82%). The point estimates from the individual studies are far from each other and the CIs do not all overlap; even without knowing the I^2 statistic, the heterogeneity level is obviously high. In addition, note that the fixed-effect model and random-effects model show different results (wider CI in the random-effects model). In contrast, the studies in Figure 4 have no significant heterogeneity (I^2 statistic=0%). The point estimates of individual studies are almost identical, the CIs overlap, and both models would give similar results; these characteristics are consistent with low heterogeneity.

Study	RR	95% CI	Died/Total, No. of Patients Treatment A	Died/Total, No. of Patients Treatment B	
I	0.50	0.18-1.41	5/100	10/100	
II	2.50	1.36-4.59	30/98	12/98	
III	0.42	0.15-1.14	5/97	12/97	
IV	2.69	1.53-4.73	35/88	13/88	
Fixed effect	1.69	1.18-2.95			
Random effects	1.19	0.48-2.95			

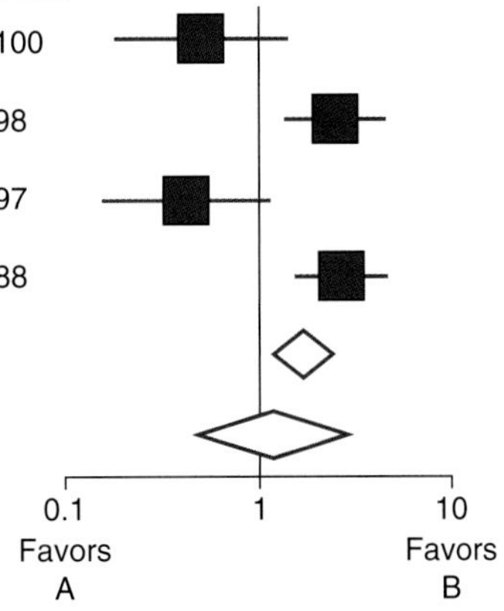

Figure 5 Meta-analysis of 4 Studies With Significant Heterogeneity (Forest Plot). CI denotes confidence interval; RR, relative risk. Log scale is used when the treatment effect is expressed as RR (or odds ratio) to make the data distribution more symmetric.

Example 3. Heterogeneity in meta-analysis.

The results of studies evaluating the effect of statins on the risk of heart disease are pooled. The RR is 0.80 (95% CI, 0.40-1.30). Because the CI includes the value 1.0, the analysis suggests that statins do not significantly reduce risk. The I^2 statistic is 80%, indicating that 80% of the heterogeneity between studies is not due to chance.

Age as a subgroup effect is explored by separately analyzing studies with older patients and studies with younger patients. The RR for older patients is 0.60 (95% CI, 0.50-0.90); for younger patients, the RR is 1.10 (95% CI, 0.91-1.60). The CIs do not overlap, and a statistical test for differences between the 2 RRs (termed interaction test) shows significance (P<.05). This means that the effect of statins on lowering the risk of heart disease is different according to age (more effective in older patients).

Tests for heterogeneity often are underpowered and may not detect considerable heterogeneity when it actually exists. Readers of meta-analyses need to evaluate the similarity of the studies being pooled (in terms of patients, interventions, outcomes, and study design). If clinical or statistical heterogeneity is suspected, it may be inappropriate to pool these studies for a meta-analysis; such results should be presented qualitatively. Alternatively, results could be pooled, but subgroup interactions should be explored to explain heterogeneity. Nevertheless, tests for subgroup interactions produce lower quality evidence and result in fundamentally observational conclusions, even if the original studies were randomized. Findings of subgroup interactions are more reliable when the following conditions are met: 1) subgroups are determined a priori, before data are analyzed; 2) the subgroup effect is biologically plausible; 3) the subgroup effect is sizable; 4) the interaction test is statistically significant; and 5) the interaction is noted within the studies (rather than only between the studies).

- Cochran Q is a yes/no test that asks whether studies are heterogenous, whereas the I^2 test can assess the magnitude of heterogeneity.
- Tests for heterogeneity often are underpowered and may not detect considerable heterogeneity when it actually exists.
- If heterogeneity is suspected, results can still be pooled, but subgroup interactions should be explored.

Agreement

Researchers commonly must make a judgment call about a clinical matter (eg, whether a patient has depression, whether a chest radiograph has abnormal findings, etc).

Such decisions often are made by 2 independent observers, and the agreement between them is statistically estimated. High levels of agreement indicate higher **reliability** of the measurement process, but it does not necessarily indicate better **validity** because the 2 observers can both be wrong.

Agreement is assessed in different ways, depending on the number of observers and the type of observations (dichotomous or continuous variables). The most common measure of agreement is the chance-adjusted agreement or **kappa (κ) statistic**, used when 2 observers make decisions with at least 2 categories. The calculation of this statistic adjusts the actual agreement between the 2 observers (observed agreement) by the agreement that can occur by chance (expected agreement). It is calculated with the following formula:

$$\kappa = \frac{\text{Observed agreement} - \text{expected agreement}}{1 - \text{expected agreement}}$$

The numerator quantifies the amount of agreement that is not due to chance, and the denominator indicates the maximal possible amount of agreement that is not due to chance. The κ statistic ranges in value from −1 to 1, where −1 indicates maximal disagreement, 0 indicates agreement similar to chance, and 1 indicates maximal agreement. The values for interpreting the κ statistic have been arbitrarily selected, but values of 0.2 to 0.4, 0.4 to 0.6, 0.6 to 0.8 and >0.8 generally are considered to correspond to minimal, fair, good, and excellent agreement, respectively.

One limitation of the κ statistic is that it underestimates agreement when the distribution of answers is extreme (when the probability of agreement by chance would be high). In the example shown in Table 7, if most patients did have depression and only very few did not, κ could be low, even if the observed agreement was high. The CI for κ can be calculated using normal approximation methods.

- The κ statistic is a common measure of agreement between 2 observers. It compares the actual agreement between observers with the agreement that can occur by chance.
- The κ statistic ranges in value from −1 to 1, where 1 indicates maximal agreement.

Bayesian Statistics

Overview

In the world of statistics, there are 2 major philosophies—frequentist and Bayesian statistics. Everything presented up to this point is consistent with frequentist statistics. Bayesian statistics, named after mathematician Thomas Bayes, dates back to as early as 1763. The basic idea of Bayesian analysis is straightforward and intuitive: it is the

Table 7 Calculation of the Kappa (κ) Statistic.

Two psychiatrists are determining whether a sample of patients have depression.

Psychiatrist 2	Psychiatrist 1		
	Depression	No Depression	Total
Depression	$a=50$	$b=4$	$a+b=54$
No depression	$c=6$	$d=40$	$c+d=46$
Total	$a+c=56$	$b+d=44$	$a+b+c+d=100$

Observed agreement: $\dfrac{a+d}{a+b+c+d}=0.90$

Value of cell (a) as expected[a] by chance: $a_e=\dfrac{(a+b)(a+c)}{a+b+c+d}=30.24$

Value of cell (d) as expected[a] by chance: $d_e=\dfrac{(b+d)(c+d)}{a+b+c+d}=20.24$

Expected agreement: $\dfrac{a_e+d_e}{a+b+c+d}=0.50$

κ statistic: $\dfrac{\text{Observed agreement}-\text{expected agreement}}{1-\text{expected agreement}}$

$=\dfrac{0.90-0.50}{1-0.50}=0.80$

[a] The expected value of a cell in a 2×2 contingency table is calculated by multiplying the row and column marginals (totals) and dividing by the grand total (similar to the process used to calculate the χ^2 statistic).

process of updating the knowledge or belief investigators have about a parameter of interest. For example, DLRs incorporate knowledge gained from a diagnostic test to formulate posttest odds of having a disease.

Although Bayesian statistics have probably existed longer than frequentist statistics, the latter methods seem more popular than Bayesian methods and are more dominant in health sciences research. The intensive computing required by many of the Bayesian methods is one reason that their use was limited before the revolution of computer techniques. However, the development of balanced and rigorous strategies of applying Bayesian methods and the increasingly efficient computing techniques of recent years have made Bayesian methods more common in the medical literature.

The **Bayes theorem**, the foundation of Bayesian statistics, fundamentally is a simple and uncontroversial statement of probability. Mathematically, it is expressed with the following formula:

$$p(b\,|\,a)=\frac{p(a\,|\,b)}{p(a)}\times p(b)$$

In this formula, $p(b\,|\,a)$ represents the probability of event b happening if event a has occurred (conditional probability of b given a), and $p(b)$ is the probability of event b

happening regardless of event a occurring. The multiplication operation of the original probability of event b occurring transforms it to the new probability, $p(b\,|\,a)$, which takes into account the occurrence of event a.

- Bayesian analysis is the process of updating the knowledge or belief investigators have about a parameter of interest.

Example 4. Updating survival probability
   The overall 5-year survival rate of a certain cancer is 60%. Of new diagnoses, 70% are usually for early stage disease. In addition, past research shows that 80% of survivors had early stage diagnosis. What is the probability of survival of someone who just received a diagnosis of early stage cancer?
   By using the Bayes theorem and assigning values $p(b)=0.6$, $p(a)=0.7$, $p(a\,|\,b)=0.8$, the updated probability of survival is as follows:

$$p(b\,|\,a)=\frac{0.8}{0.7}\times0.6=0.69$$

Prior Distributions

The Bayesian approach matches an essential characteristic of scientific research—learning from experience. Before conducting a clinical trial to assess the treatment effect of a new regimen, investigators will examine the existing preliminary or historical data to formulate an opinion concerning the plausibility of possible values of the treatment effect. These possible values are termed **prior distribution**. After patients are treated in the trial, the collected data can be described statistically with a likelihood function. By combining the prior beliefs about the treatment effect with the newly collected data, investigators can update their knowledge of the treatment effect. The updated knowledge upon which inference is based is termed **posterior distribution**.

The application of Bayes theorem in Bayesian analyses is expressed as follows: posterior distribution ∝ likelihood × prior distribution, where ∝ denotes "proportional to," and the posterior and prior distributions and likelihood usually take parametric distribution forms.

Formulating the prior distributions is a challenging task of Bayesian analysis. This unavoidably subjective process is one reason the Bayesian method is controversial. The prior distribution can be elicited from experts or derived from historical or other sources of data (eg, the results of previous similar studies). The process of choosing the prior distribution can introduce bias on multiple levels: 1) biased selection of experts or data sources; 2) biased opinions of individual experts; 3) bias in the elicitation process itself. When multiple external data sources exist, the derivation of the prior distribution is affected by homogeneity across sources and potential systematic biases. Different methods have been developed under various assumptions to formulate the prior distributions on the basis of multiple external data.

In many situations, a noninformative or reference prior distribution is chosen because of the scarcity of available information or because investigators want the information contained in the likelihood to dominate the posterior distribution. In those cases, a uniform distribution over the range of interest or a normal distribution with tremendous variance is chosen to indicate that all possible values of the parameter of interest are equally plausible. This ensures that the prior distribution has minimal influence on the posterior distribution. When a uniform prior distribution is used, the Bayesian analysis and an analogous frequentist analysis may produce essentially identical conclusions. Sensitivity analysis assessing the impact of different choices of prior distributions has a crucial role in Bayesian analysis, no matter how the prior distributions are formulated.

- The prior distribution, based on existing preliminary or historical data, is updated on the basis of data collected in a trial to form the posterior distribution (updated knowledge of the treatment effect).
- The prior distribution can be biased by data sources, expert opinions, and the elicitation process. In some cases, a noninformative reference prior distribution is used.

SUGGESTED READING

Guyatt G, Meade MO, Rennie D, Cook DJ (eds). Users' guides to the medical literature: essentials of evidence-based clinical practice. 2nd ed. New York: McGraw-Hill Medical; c2008.

Jekel JF, Katz DL, Elmore JG, Wild D. Epidemiology, biostatistics and preventive medicine. 3rd ed. Philadelphia (PA): Saunders/Elsevier; c2007.

Pagano M, Gauvreau K. Principles of biostatistics. 2nd ed. Pacific Grove (CA): Duxbury; c2000.

Pepe MS. The statistical evaluation of medical tests for classification and prediction. New York: Oxford University Press; c2008.

Rosner B. Fundamentals of biostatistics. 6th ed. Belmont (CA): Thomson-Brooks/Cole; c2006.

Spiegelhalter DJ, Abrams KR, Myles JP. Bayesian approaches to clinical trials and health care evaluation. Hoboken (NJ): Wiley; c2004.

Questions and Answers

Questions

1. Investigators randomized patients to receive a statin or placebo and wanted to compare the proportion of patients who had a heart attack in each group. What is the appropriate statistical test?
   a. χ^2 Analysis
   b. Student t test
   c. Time-to-event analysis
   d. Logistic regression
   e. Linear regression

2. Investigators gave a group of patients medication to raise their white blood cell count. Which statistical test is appropriate to compare the number of white cells before and after taking the medication?
   a. Fisher exact test
   b. Logistic regression
   c. Paired t test
   d. Linear regression
   e. χ^2 Analysis

3. What is the appropriate statistical test to assess the effect of age, sex, socioeconomic class, and race on survival after a heart attack?
   a. Fisher exact test
   b. Logistic regression
   c. Paired t test
   d. Linear regression
   e. χ^2 Analysis

4. What is the appropriate statistical test to determine the effect of a pregnant woman's prenatal weight on the birth weight of the newborn?
   a. Fisher exact test
   b. Logistic regression
   c. Paired t test
   d. Linear regression
   e. χ^2 Analysis

5. What is the appropriate statistical test to compare the age of patients who responded to 3 different antibiotics?
   a. Fisher exact test
   b. Analysis of variance
   c. Paired t test
   d. Linear regression
   e. χ^2 Analysis

6. A study showed that the risk of death from a heart attack is 6% and that this risk decreases to 3% for patients who were taking aspirin at the time of presentation. All the following statements about the effect of aspirin on death are correct *except*:
   a. The relative risk is 0.50.
   b. The relative risk reduction is 0.50.
   c. The absolute risk reduction is 0.03.
   d. Because risk is halved by aspirin use, these results are statistically significant.
   e. The confidence interval for the relative risk would be narrower if more deaths were observed during the study.

7. After an initial history and examination, a patient who presented with shortness of breath was shown to have a 70% probability of a pulmonary embolism. A ventilation-perfusion scan showed positive results. The scan has a diagnostic likelihood ratio for a positive test of 5.0. What is the probability that this patient has a pulmonary embolism?
   a. 70%
   b. 75%
   c. 82%
   d. 92%
   e. 99%

8. All the following statements about diagnosis are correct *except*:
   a. A test with high sensitivity is useful in excluding a disease.
   b. If prevalence of a disease in the population is high, the positive predictive value of a test increases.
   c. A good diagnostic test will have both a high diagnostic likelihood ratio for a positive test and a high diagnostic likelihood ratio for a negative test.
   d. A good diagnostic test will have a receiver operating characteristic curve in the left upper corner.
   e. The diagnostic likelihood ratio for a positive test equals the sensitivity/(1–specificity).

Answers

1. **Answer a.**
The χ^2 analysis is best for comparing 2 proportions from independent samples.

2. **Answer c.**
The paired *t* test is best for comparing 2 dependent, continuous variables. The variables are dependent because the preintervention and postintervention values of each patient are compared.

3. **Answer b.**
Logistic regression is the best test to control for numerous variables. In this example, investigators want to determine the effect of several explanatory variables (some are categorical and some are continuous) on a dichotomous outcome or response variable.

4. **Answer d.**
Linear regression analysis is the best method to determine the effect of one continuous variable on another continuous variable.

5. **Answer b.**
Analysis of variance is the appropriate test because it enables the comparison of 3 groups (defined by a categorical variable, ie, the antibiotic taken) in terms of association with a continuous outcome variable (ie, age).

6. **Answer d.**
The relative risk is 0.03/0.06=0.50. The relative risk reduction is 1−0.50=0.50. The risk difference is 0.06−0.03=0.03. No information is provided regarding the precision of these estimates; hence, it is inaccurate to state that results are statistically significant. The confidence interval will become narrower as the number of events increase.

7. **Answer d.**
Pretest probability=0.70. Pretest odds=0.70/(1−0.70)=2.33. Posttest odds=2.33×5=11.65. Posttest probability=11.65/(1+11.65)=0.92.

8. **Answer c.**
A test with high sensitivity is usually associated with low false-negative rate; hence, it will be a good test to exclude a disease. The increase in prevalence leads to increased positive predictive value. A good diagnostic test should have a high diagnostic likelihood ratio for a positive test and a low diagnostic likelihood ratio for a negative test. A good diagnostic test will also have a receiver operating characteristic curve in the left upper corner. The calculation for the diagnostic likelihood ratio for a positive test is correct as shown.

3

EPIDEMIOLOGY 1: BASIC CONCEPTS

Cindy Kermott, MD, MPH

Epidemiology is a method of studying the cause, distribution, and determinants of disease. It also can be used to investigate conditions that contribute to or protect against the "6 D's" of outcome measurement in human populations: death, disease, discomfort, disability, dissatisfaction, or destitution. Furthermore, it applies study results to the prevention, promotion, preservation, protection, and control of health problems in these populations and hence is an important foundation of public health.

As a method of investigation, epidemiology uses descriptive and analytic methods and draws on statistical tools to describe the data, evaluate hypotheses, and apply causal theory. **Descriptive epidemiology** involves characterization of data and investigation of the frequency, patterns, trends, and distributions of relevant factors. An example of descriptive data, collected by the Centers for Disease Control and Prevention (CDC), is shown in Table 1. **Analytic epidemiology** involves using methods that identify and quantify associations among factors, conducting hypothesis testing, and exploring causal relationships.

Unlike experimental research, which tends to confirm or refute hypotheses, epidemiology is observational, hypothesis-generating research. Epidemiology is especially useful in circumstances in which certain knowledge can be attained only through observation. In addition, epidemiology often explores associations and correlations to determine whether a causative relationship exists. If causal or modifying relationships are identified, interventions can be used to avert downstream adverse consequences.

More recently, epidemiology has been described as a core function of preventive medicine and public health, and it is a career chosen by many physicians. Some of the responsibilities of an epidemiologist are described in Box 1.

- Descriptive and analytic methods are used in epidemiologic investigations. Statistical tools are used to describe data, evaluate hypotheses, and apply causal theory.
- Epidemiologic research can be used to determine whether a causative relationship exists between a disease and its associated factors.

Key Historical Events That Shaped Epidemiology

James Lind, a Scottish naval surgeon in the 1700s, observed that sailors would become sick from scurvy after 4 to 6 weeks at sea. Further, cases most commonly occurred from April through June. Initially, he hypothesized that the weather or air was the source of disease. He continued to observe other details and compared the healthy with the affected. When he systematically observed and then experimented with the sailors' diet, he noted that those eating oranges and lemons remained healthy.

Benjamin Jesty, an English farmer and dairyman in the mid 1700s, noticed that his milkmaids who previously had acquired cowpox never got ill with smallpox. On the basis of this observation, he resolved to infect his family with cowpox with a procedure that was later known as vaccination. All naturally occurring smallpox was subsequently eradicated worldwide by 1977.

Table 1 Leading Causes of Death in US Adults, 1900 vs 2004

1900		2004	
Cause	%	Cause	%
Pneumonia and influenza	11.8	Heart disease	26.0
Tuberculosis	11.3	Cancer	23.1
Diarrhea, enteritis, ulcerations of the intestines	8.3	Cerebrovascular disease	5.7
Heart diseases	8.0	Chronic lower respiratory tract diseases	5.1
Intracranial lesions of vascular origin	6.2	Accidents	5.0
		Diabetes mellitus	3.0
Nephritis	5.2	Alzheimer disease	3.0
Accidents	4.2	Influenza or pneumonia	2.3
Cancer	3.7	Nephritis, nephrotic syndrome, nephrosis	1.9
Senility	2.9		
Diptheria	2.3	Septicemia	1.4
All other	36.1	All other	23.6

Data from Leading Causes of Death, 1900-1998 [Internet]. Centers for Disease Control and Prevention [cited 19 Aug 2009]. Available from: http://www.cdc.gov/nchs/data/dvs/lead1900_98.pdf. Data also from LCWK9 [Internet]. Centers for Disease Control and Prevention [cited 19 Aug 2009]. Available from: http://www.cdc.gov/nchs/data/dvs/LCWK9_2006.pdf.

Box 1 Responsibilities of Epidemiologists

Identify risk factors for disease, injury, or death

Describe the natural history (untreated course) of disease

Identify individuals and populations at greatest risk

Identify where a public health problem is greatest

Monitor diseases and other health-related events over time

Evaluate the efficacy and effectiveness of prevention and treatment programs

Aid in planning and decision-making for establishment of health programs and resource prioritization

Assist in administering public health programs

Communicate public health information

Be a resource person (eg, information expert)

Ignaz Semmelweis, an Austrian-Hungarian physician and medical director of the Viennese Maternity Hospital in the mid 1800s, noted that a clinic under his direction had greater numbers of maternal deaths due to childbed fever, a uterine infection that characteristically arose within 24 to 36 hours after childbirth. Through dedicated observation, he noted that many women who died had undergone pelvic examination by medical students who had come directly from the mortuary after conducting autopsies. Handwashing decreased the childbed fever mortality rate from 12.1% to 1.3% in 1848. At the time, it had been accepted that disease arose spontaneously, but Semmelweis's discovery suggested that an infective material could cause disease.

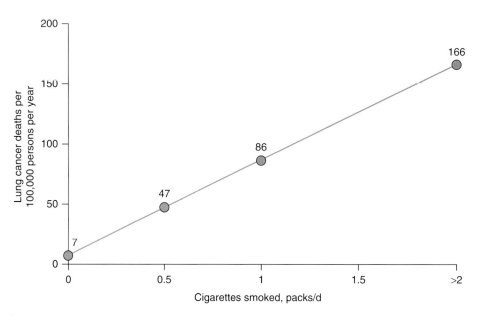

Figure 1 Dose-response Relationship Between Cigarette Smoking and Lung Cancer Death. (Adapted from Jekel et al [2007]. Used with permission.)

John Snow, an English physician and anesthesiologist, noted that nearly all deaths from **cholera** occurred a short distance from a community water source, the Broad Street pump in London. He was the first to compile descriptive statistics on cases, including location and time to death once infected. He plotted the flow of the public underground aquifer systems, as well as other data, and ultimately was able to show a cause-and-effect association. With these data, he convinced the authorities to close the Broad Street pump, and by doing so, he effectively stopped the epidemic. This was before the causative agent for cholera, *Vibrio cholerae*, had been identified.

Causality

The original work of Dr. Robert Koch, a German physician of the late 1800s, focused on the tubercle bacillus and other pathogens and showed their roles as causative agents of disease. On the basis of his observational and experimental studies, he set forth guidelines that were widely applicable to identifying causal relationships. These guidelines, now known as **Koch's postulates**, are used when determining whether a disease is caused by a single agent. The guidelines are as follows: 1) the parasite occurs in every case of the disease in question and under circumstances that can account for the pathologic changes and clinical courses of the disease; 2) it occurs in no other disease as a fortuitous and nonpathogenic parasite; and 3) after being fully isolated from the body and repeatedly grown in pure culture, it can induce the disease anew.

Causality criteria were first established by Sir Austin Bradford Hill in 1965 to assess causality of disease and outbreaks (Box 2). An argument for causality is the strongest when most of the causality criteria are met.

Theoretical Models of Causation and Factors That Influence Disease

Common causes of disease include allergies, chemicals, congenital problems, inherited traits, iatrogenic causes, idiopathic causes, infection, inflammation, metabolism, nutrition, physical agents, psychological problems, trauma, tumors, and vascular problems. Epidemiologists use a number of models to understand disease causation and explore the relationship between disease and associated factors, including those that may be protective.

The classic epidemiologic model, especially useful in describing communicable disease, is the **epidemiologic triangle** (Figure 2). It illustrates the relationships among a host, an agent, and the environment with regard to disease causation. A change in any of the 3 components initiates the disease process. For example, exposure of a nonimmunized patient (host) to an influenza virus (agent) may result in influenza infection. Prevention of disease relies on

Box 2 Causality Criteria

1. Consistency
   The same factor appears repeatedly in different circumstances and always in association with disease.

2. Strength of association
   Stronger associations between exposure and outcome increase the likelihood of a causal relationship.

3. Specificity
   Only 1 factor is consistently implicated.

4. Temporal factors
   Exposure must precede disease development.

5. Coherence of explanation (congruence)
   The association fits within the existing knowledge paradigm, and observations make logical sense.

6. Biologic plausibility
   The mechanism must be consistent with current understanding of the biologic processes (eg, the relationship between a pathogen's virility, dose response, and host susceptibility should be plausible).

7. Experiment
   Substantial evidence from a controlled research experiment supports a causal association. Blinding and randomization effectively control bias and the effects of confounders, respectively.

8. Analogy
   The knowledge gained from other causal associations can be transferred if the associations are similar in nature.

9. Dose-response
   Increasing exposure increases the risk of disease (Figure 1), although a threshold exposure level may be needed before a disease is acquired. However, the absence of a dose-response relationship does not exclude causality.

preventing exposure to the agent, enhancing host attributes that resist disease, and minimizing environmental factors that can affect health and disease progression.

The specific cause of a health-related event or disease cannot always be described in terms of simple interactions between a host, agent, and environment; causes often are multiple and heterogenous (eg, consider the causes of

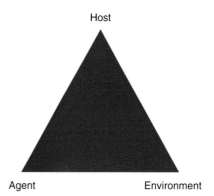

Figure 2 Epidemiologic Triangle.

coronary artery disease). A **web of causation** is a commonly used epidemiologic model that explains disease, disability, or health events with multiple, interconnected causes. Figure 3 shows a web of causation for lead poisoning in a community.

- Causality criteria are used to assess causality of disease and outbreaks.
- An epidemiologic triangle illustrates the relationships among a host, an agent, and the environment with regard to disease causation.

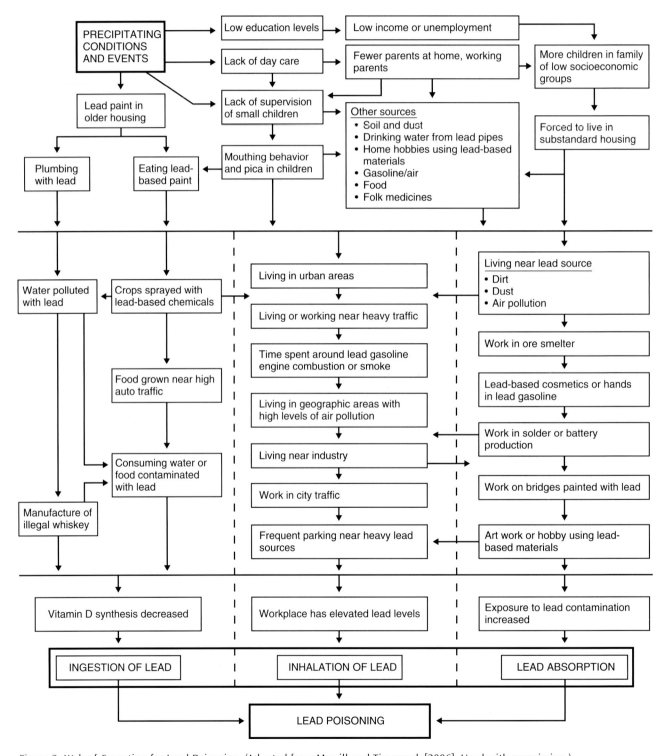

Figure 3   Web of Causation for Lead Poisoning. (Adapted from Merrill and Timmreck [2006]. Used with permission.)

- A web of causation is used to explain disease, disability, or a health event with multiple, interconnected causes.

Data Sources

A critical component of epidemiologic studies is acquisition of population-level data. Some data are collected routinely by health care organizations and government agencies. For example, a vital record is established by documenting major life events. The federal government collates data, obtained at the local and state level, pertaining to births, deaths (including fetal deaths and causes of death), marriages, and divorces in the United States. However, these records have many potential sources of error such as unreported births and deaths, inaccurate death certificate diagnoses, and inaccurate demographic and clinical data.

Data from hospitals include those pertaining to daily admissions and visits to the emergency department. The primary indications for the visit (ie, the chief concerns) are available for emergency department visits. Discharge diagnoses are usually available in the form of an *International Classification of Diseases, Ninth Revision* (ICD-9) billing code; these typically describe signs and symptoms, but they may also indicate a specific disease.

Hospital morbidity information provides an opportunity to study a unique set of occurrences relevant to hospital settings. These include nosocomial infections, iatrogenic conditions, and adverse medication reactions. However, one weakness of hospital records is the potential for inconsistent disease reporting. Morbidity data from hospitals do not necessarily indicate disease prevalence in a community because not all people seek medical care when ill and others may travel great distances to seek care at different facilities. Furthermore, health insurance policies may limit some patients' access to certain facilities, and others may have no access at all.

Medical care insurance carriers and other third-party payers (eg, Medicare, Medicaid, Veterans Administration) also have collected administrative and other clinical data that can be used for studying epidemiologic trends. They are also useful in the study of other matters of public health interest, including patterns of use and cost-effective management methods.

Data from physician practices consist of reported patient symptoms and signs and clinical examination findings. The medical record, if electronic, can be searched, although differential diagnoses and excluded diagnoses often are included in the text. ICD-9 billing codes can indicate symptoms, signs, and suspected diagnoses, but they do not always indicate the final (confirmed) diagnosis. Available corroborating data such as laboratory test findings might be used to establish a higher confidence level about a diagnostic entity. ICD-9 codes may be grouped into syndromic categories, balancing sensitivity and specificity with the ultimate goal of maximal diagnostic or biosurveillance capture.

Managed care programs, larger health maintenance organizations, preferred provider organizations, and independent practice associations generally are prevention-oriented and active in cost analysis and control. They routinely maintain good medical records and document morbidity and mortality data that can be used for health policy research. However, these data are limited because they may not be representative of the health status of an entire community.

- Epidemiologic data can be collected by government agencies, hospitals, medical insurance carriers, third-party payers, physician practices, and managed care programs.
- Each data collection system has potential weaknesses such as introduced errors, incomplete records, limited access, and nonrepresentative populations.

Registries, the US Census, and Surveys

Registries are listings of all occurrences of a disease or condition within a defined region. These listings contain detailed information for the purpose of identifying patients for long-term follow-up and for further analysis by specific laboratory or investigational epidemiologic methods. A registry can be developed by creating a record with demographic and other identifying data, the diagnosis of concern, frequency of occurrence, survival, treatment or follow-up, and other unique details that are pertinent to the condition. This registration creates a databank from which studies can be conducted. A number of prominent databases, based on the population of stable communities, have acquired decades of data. Two of the most notable epidemiologic databases are the Rochester Epidemiology Project of Olmsted County, Minnesota, and the Framingham Heart Study in Massachusetts.

In the United States, the federal government undertakes a population **census** every decade (all years ending with a 0) that is effective on April 1. Findings are available on the Internet (http://www.census.gov) and include information on births, deaths, disability, fertility, and other subjects.

Surveys, a comprehensive measure of health status and potentially influential factors, can contribute to a larger health perspective. For example, many environmental factors that contribute to health can be investigated—seat belts, air and water quality, crime, and the built environment. Surveys may have limited usefulness if the response rate is poor, and survey answers may be affected by recall bias. The **National Health Survey** was established by the US Congress in 1956 to record information about the health status of the American population on an ongoing basis. The US Department of Health and Human Services has directed the CDC to monitor the nation's health through dedicated reporting. The survey is coordinated by the National Center for Health Statistics. Surveys are a major source of nationwide information on common illnesses, injury, disability, functional deficits, and use of health care services. This knowledge allows the government to target resources and enact policies with the goal of maintaining the health and safety of the population. Some of the key national health surveys are shown in Table 2.

- Registries are detailed listings of all occurrences of a disease or condition within a defined region.
- In the United States, a government-based population census occurs every decade.
- Nationwide surveys comprehensively measure health status and factors that potentially influence health.

Surveillance Systems

Surveillance is defined as an ongoing and systematic process of collecting, analyzing, interpreting, and disseminating health data. Each surveillance system has a population of interest; this population typically shares certain factors such as geographic region, exposure, occupation, institution, or disease. Personal information from subjects is required to obtain follow-up information, to provide necessary services, and to identify subjects for subsequent, detailed investigations. When a surveillance system is developed, the overall objectives of surveillance and the logistics of obtaining and maintaining such a system must be considered. A typical cycle of surveillance is as shown in Figure 4.

In the United States, the CDC is the federal agency responsible for surveillance of most types of acute infectious diseases. They also conduct outbreak investigations if requested by a state or if the outbreak crosses a number of state lines (the federal government has jurisdiction over matters of interstate commerce and its implications).

Case-defining is an essential step in the development of a surveillance system, and definitions must balance the needs for sensitivity, specificity, and feasibility. Case definitions vary among surveillance systems, and thus ascertainment rates also may vary. For diseases with a long latency period, case definition becomes even more complicated. Behavioral data are often self-reported, and illegal

Table 2 National Health Surveys

Survey	Subjects	Details
National Health Interview Survey	Individuals within households	Questioned about limitation of daily activities, acute and chronic disease conditions, and physician or hospital visits
National Health and Nutrition Examination Survey	Randomly selected individuals from the general population	Undergo health screenings and physical examinations in 3-year cycles
		Mobile units used for data collection
		Augments information gathered in the National Health Interview Survey
National Hospital Discharge Survey	Individuals discharged from hospitals	. . .
National Notifiable Disease Surveillance System	Individuals within US consuls overseas, states, municipal authorities (reporting mandated only at the state level)	Data are collected by the Centers for Disease Control and Prevention
		Summary reports (*Morbidity and Mortality Report, Summary of Notifiable Disease in the United States*) are generated annually
National Nursing Home Survey	Individuals in long-term care facilities	Provides basic information about nursing homes and their residents and staff; institutions are certified by Medicare or Medicaid or have a state license to operate as a nursing home
National Ambulatory Medical Care Survey	Patients seen in hospital emergency and outpatient departments; treating physicians are not federal employees, they are office-based physicians primarily engaged in direct patient care	Identify patient, physician, and visit characteristics for various acute and chronic diseases
National Survey of Family Growth	Sample of households across the United States	Family planning and fertility
Survey Linked to Vital Records	Individuals with a vital record—birth, death, marriage, divorce	Augments the National Vital Statistics System

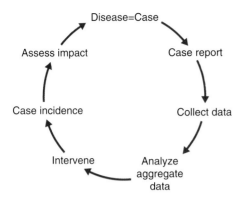

Figure 4 Surveillance Cycle.

behaviors may be underreported as a result. Similarly, exposures are often self-reported and may be affected by bias.

In **active surveillance**, organizations initiate procedures to obtain information. For example, in the Behavioral Risk Factor Surveillance System, periodic surveys are undertaken by state health departments, in cooperation with the CDC. A random sample of the population is interviewed over the telephone about various behaviors that may affect health. Health behaviors have included exercise, smoking, dietary intake, alcohol consumption, use of seat belts, and medical care use.

For **passive surveillance**, the organization that analyzes data relies on the initiative of other organizations to collect and report the data. For example, in the case of reportable diseases, each state has the authority to determine which diseases should be designated as notifiable. However, the Council of State and Territorial Epidemiologists establishes the entities that are nationally reportable (Box 3), and individual state health departments voluntarily report this information to the CDC. This information is tabulated by the CDC and published in the *Morbidity and Mortality Weekly Report* and also in an annual summary.

- Surveillance is defined as an ongoing and systematic collection, analysis, interpretation, and dissemination of health data.
- Case definitions must balance the needs for sensitivity, specificity, and feasibility.
- Surveillance can be performed actively or passively.

Investigation of an Outbreak: Epidemiology in Action

An **outbreak** is a localized cluster of illness, exposures, or events; these occur at an unusually increased frequency when compared with baseline surveillance data. Bioterrorism acts, crime, and infectious diseases can occur in outbreaks.

An **endemic** disease or condition prevails within a community or region and is constantly present without substantial variation. Such a disease is in equilibrium with regard to forces that promote and deter its occurrence. In contrast, an **epidemic** is a cluster of cases in a wider geographic region, and a **pandemic** is a sudden surge of cases that occur extensively over a vast region. When an outbreak occurs, it is important to realize that the disease equilibrium has somehow been disrupted, and the goal of an outbreak investigation is to discover what has changed. By taking corrective actions, the balance may be restored and the epidemic controlled.

One of the first steps of an investigation is to **establish the existence of an outbreak**. This usually is done by comparing the current number of cases with the number from the previous few weeks or months or from a similar period during the previous few years. After baseline surveillance data are obtained, time trends (prevalence and incidence) may be considered evidence of an outbreak. It is important to determine whether the trend could be explained by changes in case detection, reporting, or both. Often, when a real or suspected outbreak is announced, the consequently increased index of suspicion by reporters leads to an observed increase in case detection. In addition to verifying the existence of an outbreak, the public health physician or epidemiologist must verify the diagnosis to ensure that the problem has been reported accurately and that the increase in cases is not attributable to diagnostic errors.

The next step of an outbreak investigation is to **establish a case definition**. Case definitions for disease typically combine laboratory criteria and clinical signs or reported symptoms. Case definition criteria establish the reporting standard for data collection and ensure that cases are consistently diagnosed, regardless of where, when, or who identified them. For example, the Arizona Department of Health Services suggests that case definitions include "the clinical information about the disease, characteristics about the people who are affected, information about the location or place, [and] a specification of time during which the outbreak occurred." Early in an investigation, a case definition that includes "confirmed," "probable," and "possible" cases of the disease or condition allows investigators to identify as many cases as possible. Later, as a clearer understanding of the outbreak emerges, the case definition may be altered to eliminate subjects classified as possibly having the disease. This change keeps the epidemiologist from having to return to interviewees for additional data.

Knowing **patient behavioral and health factors** (person), **timing of symptom onset** (time), and **geographic location** (place) is the next step when assessing the outbreak. These data may be useful when developing causal hypotheses. The **epidemic curve**, the time course of an epidemic, can be shown with a graph of the number of cases and their date of onset (Figure 5). This visual representation is used

Box 3 Nationally Notifiable Infectious Diseases in the United States

AIDS	Pertussis
Anthrax	Plague (*Yersinia pestis*)
Arboviral neuroinvasive and nonneuroinvasive diseases	Poliomyelitis, paralytic
Botulism	Poliovirus infection, nonparalytic
Brucellosis	Psittacosis
Chancroid	Q fever
Chlamydia trachomatis, genital infections	Rabies—animal, human
Cholera	Rocky Mountain spotted fever
Coccidioidomycosis	Rubella, including congenital syndrome
Cryptosporidiosis	Salmonellosis
Cyclosporiasis	Severe acute respiratory syndrome–associated coronavirus (SARS-CoV) disease
Diphtheria	
Ehrlichiosis or anaplasmosis	Shiga toxin–producing *Escherichia coli*
Giardiasis	Shigellosis
Gonorrhea	Smallpox
Haemophilus influenzae, invasive disease	Streptococcal disease, invasive, Group A
Hansen disease (leprosy)	Streptococcal toxic-shock syndrome
Hantavirus pulmonary syndrome	*Streptococcus pneumoniae*—drug-resistant, invasive disease; non–drug-resistant, invasive disease, in children younger than 5 years
Hemolytic uremic syndrome, postdiarrheal	
Hepatitis—acute, viral (A, B, C); chronic (B, C)	Syphilis
Human immunodeficiency virus infection	Tetanus
Influenza-associated pediatric mortality	Toxic-shock syndrome (non-Streptococcal)
Legionellosis	Trichinellosis (trichinosis)
Listeriosis	Tuberculosis
Lyme disease	Tularemia
Malaria	Typhoid fever
Measles	Vancomycin-resistant *Staphylococcus aureus*; intermediate *Staphylococcus aureus*
Meningococcal disease	
Mumps	Varicella
Novel influenza A virus infections	Vibriosis
	Yellow fever

Adapted from Nationally Notifiable Infectious Diseases, United States 2009 [Internet]. Atlanta (GA): Centers for Disease Control and Prevention; [cited 19 Aug 2009]. Available from: http://www.cdc.gov/ncphi/disss/nndss/phs/infdis2009.htm.

to estimate when a specific event occurred in the course of the epidemic. In addition, it may be possible to estimate a probable period of exposure before disease onset; this can help determine whether an outbreak resulted from a common-source exposure, from person-to-person spread, or both.

An epidemic curve with a steep upward slope and a gradual downward slope (such as that shown in Figure 5) is indicative of a **single-source epidemic**, in which all cases occur within 1 incubation period. If the duration of exposure is prolonged, the epidemic curve has a plateau instead of a peak and is termed a **continuous, common-source epidemic**. A series of progressively taller peaks, one incubation period apart, indicates person-to-person spread and is termed a **propagated epidemic**.

The next step of an outbreak investigation entails **testing the hypothesis for causation** to evaluate its credibility. Depending on the nature of the outbreak, cohort or case-control studies commonly are used. Cohort studies compare groups of people with or without exposure to suspected risk factors. Case-control studies examine the frequency of exposure among cases compared with controls;

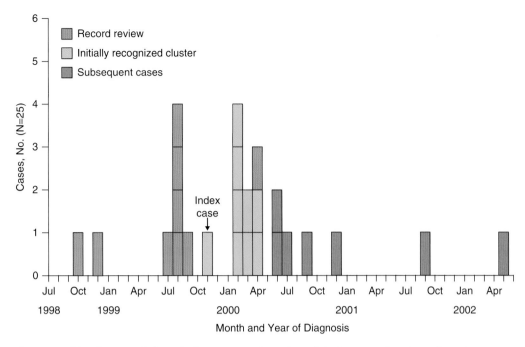

Figure 5 Epidemic Curve. Tuberculosis cases were investigated during an outbreak at a homeless shelter in North Carolina. (Adapted from McElroy PD, Southwick KL, Fortenberry ER, Levine EC, Diem LA, Woodley CL, et al. Outbreak of tuberculosis among homeless persons coinfected with human immunodeficiency virus. Clin Infect Dis. 2003 May 15;36[10]:1305-12. Used with permission.)

conventionally, a 2×2 table is used for comparison. An odds ratio (odds that a case is exposed divided by the odds that a control is exposed) can be calculated and used to explore exposure-disease relationships. More details about these investigative methods are described in Chapters 2 and 4.

When analytic epidemiologic studies do not confirm the hypothesis, **reconsideration or refinement of the hypothesis** may be necessary. To look for common links, visiting affected patients and seeing their homes may help find other possible sources (eg, food products) of the outbreak. From a public health perspective, the most important aspect of outbreak management is to **take control measures**. These are often enacted before the source of the outbreak or the route of spread is ascertained. Common types of control measures include sanitation, containment, quarantine, and prophylaxis. In addition, early diagnosis and treatment is recommended, and disease vectors should be controlled if pertinent and known (eg, *Ixodes* tick for Lyme disease). Finally, **communication of findings** through oral briefings and written reports is important to promote prevention and control measures.

- An outbreak investigation begins by establishing the existence of an outbreak.
- After the case definition is established, factors such as person, time, and place are used to develop causal

hypotheses. The hypotheses are tested to evaluate credibility, and reconsideration or refinement of the hypotheses may be necessary.
- Control measures may be taken before the outbreak source or route of spread is ascertained. Prevention and control measures must be communicated.

Ethical and Legal Aspects of Epidemiologic Studies

Human Subjects Review

Although clinical research has and continues to produce myriad benefits to society, multiple abuses have occurred historically. The Nuremberg war crime trials of the mid 1940s highlighted abuse of concentration camp prisoners as human research subjects in biomedical experiments. As a result, a code of standards was drafted to assure that research involving human subjects would be conducted ethically. These standards, now known as the Nuremberg code (Box 4), was the first of many ethics codes that followed.

Unfortunately, around the same time as the development of the Nuremberg code, the **Tuskegee Syphilis Study** was being conducted in the United States. It would later be shown to have violated many principles described in the

Box 4 Key Principles of the Nuremburg Code

1. Consent of human subjects must be voluntary.

2. The nature of the experiment should be one that yields fruitful results for the good of society, results that are unprocurable by other methods or means.

3. The experiment should be designed after considering results of animal studies and the natural history of the disease or other problem under study so that the anticipated results will justify performance of the experiment.

4. The experiment should be conducted in a manner that avoids all unnecessary physical and mental suffering and injury.

5. No experiment should be conducted when there is an a priori reason to believe that death or disabling injury will occur.

6. The degree of risk to be taken should never exceed that determined by the humanitarian importance of the problem to be solved by the experiment.

7. Subjects must be protected against even remote possibilities of injury, disability, or death.

8. The experiment should be conducted only by scientifically qualified persons.

9. During the course of the experiment, the human subject should be at liberty to end the experiment.

10. The experiment should be terminated when the scientist has probable cause to believe that continuation is likely to result in injury, disability, or death to the subject.

Box 5 Ethical Principles and Application of the Belmont Report

Ethical principles

1. Respect for persons
   Individuals should be treated as autonomous agents. Those with diminished autonomy (eg, immature, incapacitated, or otherwise vulnerable) are entitled to protection. Subjects should enter research voluntarily and with adequate information.

2. Beneficence
   Individuals should be protected from harm during research. All efforts to secure their well-being should be established, with harms minimized.

3. Justice
   Equitable distribution is observed among participants, with respect to the benefits of research and bearing its burdens.

Application

1. Informed consent
   Research subjects are given the opportunity to choose to participate on a volunteer basis (ie, free from coercion and undue influence) via a consent process that involves information and comprehension.

2. Assessment of risks and benefits
   Risk involves both chance (probability) and severity (magnitude) of an adverse event. Benefit is defined as positive value with respect to health or welfare. The investigator must ensure that the study design is based on a thorough review of all relevant data and consideration of alternative methods of obtaining the desired results. The review committee must determine whether the risks inherent in the study are justified on the basis of a favorable risk-benefit assessment (ie, a "favorable ratio" of risks and benefits, as determined by a systematic assessment, must be apparent).

3. Selection of subjects
   Fair procedures and outcomes in the selection of subjects must be used. Individual justice requires offering risky and beneficial research opportunities to all groups.

Nuremberg code, although the latter had not yet been developed when the study was taking place. Individuals enrolled in the study were not required to give informed consent and were not informed of their diagnoses or the availability of penicillin as a treatment. Instead, subjects were told they had "bad blood" and, in return for participating, received free medical treatment, rides to the clinic, meals, and burial insurance in case of death.

Public recognition of these events ultimately led to establishment of the National Human Investigation Board, the required establishment of institutional review boards (IRBs), and the 1979 **Belmont Report**. The Belmont Report, drafted by the US Department of Health, Education and Welfare (now the Department of Health and Human Services), attempted to identify principles relevant to human subject research that would provide an analytic framework to guide the resolution of ethical problems (Box 5).

In the early 1980s, revised regulations pertaining to the conduct of research involving human subjects were published. This document, Title 45 Code of Federal Regulations, Protection of Human Subjects (45 CFR 46), embodied and codified the ethical principles described by the Belmont Report. It describes the minimal ethical and legal obligations of investigators and institutions conducting or supporting federally funded research involving human subjects.

Institutional Review Boards

IRBs are committees charged by the US government to protect the rights and welfare of human subjects involved in research. The use of IRBs began in the National Institutes of Health, when a 1966 memorandum required investigators receiving funding from public health grants to have their research reviewed by a committee of institutional associates. Each IRB is charged with reviewing all research proposals and has the authority to approve, require modifications in, or disapprove any research activity covered by the 45 CFR 46 code.

To maintain participant trust and confidentiality, the physical security of data is considered an essential ethical responsibility. The 1996 **Health Insurance Portability and Accountability Act** (HIPAA) applies to health information collected or maintained by health care providers who engage in certain electronic transactions or participate in specific health plans and health care clearinghouses.

The US Department of Health and Human Services has issued the "Standards for Privacy of Individually Identifiable Health Information," which applies to entities covered by HIPAA. Within the Department, the Office for Civil Rights is responsible for implementing and enforcing the privacy regulation.

Master data sets used in clinical research often contain personal, identifying information. Procedures to protect the security of these data sets include limited access, physical security, and use of passwords in computerized data systems. A working data set, a subset of the master set, is often deidentified before release to a research investigator to ensure security, although a unique, randomly generated code for each participant may be added for reidentification purposes. A **deidentified data set** must be stripped of the 18 personal identifiers defined by HIPAA (Box 6). Note that the unique reidentifying code is allowed in deidentified data sets.

- The Nuremberg code was the first set of standards drafted to assure that research involving human subjects would be conducted ethically.
- Institutional review boards (IRBs) review all research proposals and may approve, require modifications in,

Box 6 Eighteen Elements to Deidentify Data Sets[a]

1. Names
2. Geographical subdivisions smaller than a state
3. All elements of dates (except year) directly relating to an individual (including birth, death, admission, discharge)
4. Telephone numbers
5. Fax numbers
6. Electronic mail addresses
7. Social security numbers
8. Medical record numbers
9. Health plan beneficiary numbers
10. Account numbers
11. Certificate or license numbers
12. Vehicle identifiers (including license plates and serial numbers)
13. Device identifiers and serial numbers
14. Web universal resource locations
15. Internet protocol address numbers
16. Biometric identifiers (including fingerprints and voice prints)
17. Full face photographic or comparable images
18. Any other unique identifying number, characteristic, or code

[a] All elements must be removed in a deidentified data set.
Adapted from the Health Insurance Portability and Accountability Act. 42 USC § 201 (1996).

or disapprove any research activity covered by Title 45 Code of Federal Regulations, Protection of Human Subjects.

- In the United States, the Health Insurance Portability and Accountability Act (HIPAA) defines federal protections for personal health information.

SELECTED READING

Green LW, Ottoson JM. Community health. 7th ed. St. Louis: Mosby; c1994.

Jekel JF, Katz DL, Elmore JG, Wild D. Epidemiology, biostatistics and preventive medicine. 3rd ed. Philadelphia (PA): Saunders/Elsevier; c2007.

Merrill RM, Timmreck TC. Introduction to epidemiology. 4th ed. Sudbury (MA): Jones and Bartlett Publishers; c2006.

Rothman KJ, Greenland S. Modern epidemiology. Philadelphia (PA): Lippincott-Raven; c1998.

Thacker SB, Berkelman RL. Public health surveillance in the United States. Epidemiol Rev. 1988;10:164-90.

Timmreck TC. An introduction to epidemiology. Sudbury (MA): Jones and Bartlett Publishers; c2002.

Questions and Answers

Questions

1. An association was observed between the length of time an individual stayed in a hotel and the likelihood of illness. Only those individuals who ate at a restaurant across the street from the hotel were affected, and the likelihood increased with the portion of rice contained in the meal. Which causal criterion is best represented in this scenario?
   a. Dose-response
   b. Analogy
   c. Consistency
   d. Experiment
   e. None of the above

2. Which group has the authority to disapprove any research activity covered by Title 45 Code of Federal Regulations, Protection of Human Subjects (45 CFR 46)?
   a. Agency for Health Care Research and Quality
   b. Centers for Disease Control and Prevention
   c. Institutional review board
   d. State health department
   e. Medicare

3. All individuals with a unique congenital heart disorder have a record created that contains demographic and other identifying data, treatment and follow-up information, and length of survival. This collection of records is placed in a databank. Which data source does this best represent?
   a. Reportable diseases
   b. Vital record
   c. Morbidity
   d. Registry
   e. Survival data

4. Of the 3 ethical principles relevant to research involving human subjects, which is *not* part of the Belmont Report?
   a. Justice
   b. Informed consent
   c. Beneficence
   d. Respect for persons
   e. None of the above

5. Citizens are randomly selected from the general population in 3-year cycles to undergo examinations and health screenings in which national survey?
  a. National Health and Nutrition Examination Survey
  b. National Ambulatory Medical Care Survey
  c. National Health Interview Survey
  d. Survey Linked to Vital Records
  e. National Health Survey

6. The most important aspect of an outbreak investigation is to begin administering control measures, often before the source of the outbreak or the route of spread is ascertained. Which of the following is consistent with this goal?
  a. Containment
  b. Case definition
  c. Hypothesis testing
  d. Characterizing the outbreak by person, time, and place
  e. Case control

Answers

1. **Answer a.**

   Because increasing exposure increased the risk of disease, this is an example of the dose-response causal criterion. When the same factor appears repeatedly in different circumstances and is always associated with disease, it meets the causal criterion of consistency. Although absent in this example, substantial supporting evidence from a controlled research experiment also would lend weight to causality.

2. **Answer c.**

   Institutional review boards (IRBs) are committees charged by the US government with protecting the rights and welfare of human subjects involved in research. IRBs review all research proposals and have the authority to approve, require modifications in, or disapprove any research activity covered by the 45 CFR 46 code.

3. **Answer d.**

   The data source described is consistent with a registry. Reportable diseases are established by the Council of State and Territorial Epidemiologists; they are reported voluntarily by state health departments to the Centers for Disease Control and Prevention. Vital records documenting major life events (births, deaths, marriages, divorces) are obtained by local and state government. Hospital morbidity records include nosocomial infections, iatrogenic conditions, adverse medication reactions, and other occurrences relevant to hospital settings.

4. **Answer b.**

   The Belmont Report attempted to identify principles relevant to human subjects research that would provide an analytic framework to guide the resolution of ethical problems. These principles include respect for persons, beneficence, and justice.

5. **Answer a.**

   Through the National Health and Nutrition Examination Survey, individuals are selected randomly and undergo health screenings and physical examinations in 3-year cycles. This survey is conducted to augment the information gathered by the National Health Interview Survey.

6. **Answer a.**

   Common types of control measures include sanitation, containment, quarantine, and prophylaxis. In addition, early diagnosis and treatment is recommended, and disease vectors should be controlled if pertinent and known.

4

EPIDEMIOLOGY 2: STUDY DESIGN

Muktar H. Aliyu, MBBS, DrPH

The usefulness of evidence arising from scientific research is influenced by several factors, and foremost among these factors is the design of the epidemiologic study from which the findings are drawn. In evidence-based medicine, the quality of scientific evidence is often graded on the basis of the type of study design (eg, by using the United States Preventive Services Task Force rating system) and includes appraisal of the methods by which studies of exposure and outcomes are planned and implemented. Several factors must be considered when designing a scientific study, including the hypothesis being tested, study cost, time frame, subject characteristics, choice of variables or measurements, and ethical concerns.

In this chapter, the different types of study designs commonly encountered in clinical research, common measures of morbidity and mortality in epidemiology, and errors (random and systematic) that may threaten conclusions derived from inferences arising from epidemiologic studies are discussed.

Types of Study Designs

Most epidemiologic studies can be broadly categorized as observational, experimental, or quasiexperimental.

Observational Studies

In **observational studies**, the investigator has a passive role and does not manipulate the exposure of interest. Observational studies can be further subclassified as descriptive or analytic studies.

Descriptive studies characterize the distribution of diseases and health-related factors in terms of time, place, and person, with the purpose of establishing identifiable, disease-specific attributes. The main objective of descriptive studies is to formulate hypotheses that can be further evaluated with analytic studies.

A **case report** is a detailed summary of a clinical encounter with a single patient, usually one with an uncommon or previously unrecognized disease. A **case series** summarizes a group of patients with similar diagnoses and similar treatment. Case reports and case series often provide the first clues about the emergence of a new disease or the etiologic basis for rare conditions.

Cross-sectional studies are the most common type of study design. They provide an instantaneous view of a population sample at a single time point. One example of a cross-sectional study is the US National Health Interview Survey, a household survey of civilian, noninstitutionalized persons in the United States. Survey data are used to monitor trends in illness and disability, to evaluate federal health programs, and to track progress toward national health goals. One weakness of cross-sectional studies is that information about exposure and outcome are collected concurrently. Because only prevalent cases are considered, temporal relationships (and thus causes of disease) are difficult to establish.

Analytic studies quantitatively explore the relationship between variables in an attempt to answer research questions.

Analytic studies provide information on the existence and the strength of an association; they therefore are used to test hypotheses. The major types of analytic studies are cohort, case-control, and ecologic studies.

In **cohort studies**, the cohort is assembled before the outcome of interest develops; patients are monitored over time to determine outcome status. Cohort studies can be either prospective or retrospective, depending on when the study is initiated. In a **prospective cohort study**, the study begins before the outcome occurs. For example, a prospective cohort study of the association between green tea consumption and risk of colorectal cancer could be conducted by assembling a large cohort of Chinese women and collecting data during 2 to 3 years of follow-up. However, a major problem with prospective cohort studies is the potential for attrition, when study participants are lost to follow-up. In a **retrospective cohort study**, the investigator reviews patient records to determine exposure status and then follows patients over time, through their records, to determine outcome. Retrospective cohort studies are commonly performed in occupational studies. They are cheaper, quicker, and easier to conduct than prospective cohort studies. For example, London et al used a retrospective cohort design to determine whether early mobilization of patients with blunt, solid-organ injuries was associated with delayed bleeding requiring laparotomy.

Data for the study were obtained from trauma registry records.

Case-control studies involve the retrospective comparison of individuals with a specific outcome (**cases**) and those without the outcome (**controls**) and examine the probability of exposure to risk factors of interest. In case-control studies, the controls must resemble cases in every way, except for not having the outcome of interest. For example, a study could compare miners with mesothelioma (cases) and miners without mesothelioma (controls) and evaluate their exposure to asbestos dust. Case-control studies are suitable for the study of rare diseases and can be used to evaluate multiple exposures. They are quicker and cheaper to conduct than cohort studies. However, like cross-sectional studies, temporal associations are difficult to establish in case-control studies. In addition, case-control studies are prone to specific types of selection and information biases (discussed later in this chapter). Figure 1 provides a graphical representation of retrospective cohort, prospective cohort, and case-control study designs.

Nested case-control and **case-cohort studies** are hybrid designs that combine features of case-control and cohort studies. In both study designs, cases and controls are selected from the same defined source cohort and monitored to assess outcome. In case-cohort studies, controls are selected randomly from the total cohort at baseline,

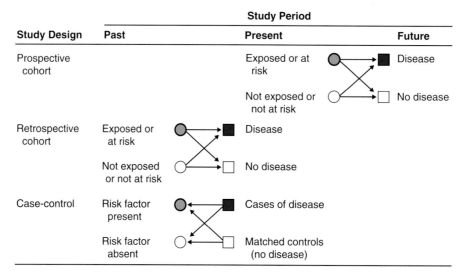

Figure 1 Common Study Designs: Prospective Cohort, Retrospective Cohort, and Case-Control. Shaded circles denote persons who are exposed to the risk factor or are at risk of outcome development (prospective and retrospective design), or they represent individuals for whom the risk factor is present (case-control design). White circles denote persons not exposed to the risk factor and not at risk of developing the outcome (prospective and retrospective design), or they represent individuals for whom the risk factor is absent (case-control design). Shaded squares denote persons with the outcome or cases of disease. White squares denote controls or persons without the outcome or disease.

before any cases are identified (ie, before disease development). In nested case-control studies, controls are selected from the group of at-risk members of a cohort and are matched to each case as the cases occur (termed **incidence density sampling**). An example of a nested case-control study is a recent study by Bertone-Johnson et al. In that study, cases were 1,057 women aged 27 to 44 years, free of premenstrual syndrome (PMS) at baseline, who had development of PMS over 10 years. The control group included 1,968 women reporting no diagnosis of PMS during the same period. Both cases and controls were drawn from a cohort of eligible women participating in the prospective Nurses' Health Study II. The study showed that cigarette smoking in adolescence and early adulthood may be associated with an increased risk of moderate-to-severe PMS.

In contrast to case-control and cohort studies, in which the unit of observation is the individual, **ecologic studies** analyze and compare aggregate or summary data from groups. The unit of observation in ecologic studies is often a geographically defined population (eg, counties, states, or countries). An example of an ecologic study is an assessment of the association between the geographic distribution of the incidence of inflammatory bowel disease in Manitoba, Canada, and the sociodemographic characteristics of the study population. **Ecologic fallacy** is the tendency to ascribe differences arising from summary or aggregate data to the level of the individual, thereby leading to flawed conclusions.

Experimental Studies

Experimental studies differ from observational studies in that the condition under which the study is conducted is controlled by the investigator. These studies commonly assign treatments through **randomization**, the random allocation of subjects to experimental (intervention) and control arms. The researcher manipulates study events to ascertain the effect of planned interventions in the 2 groups.

Two major categories of randomized clinical studies are clinical trials and community trials. **Clinical trials** are a powerful tool in the evaluation of new therapeutic agents or procedures. Usually, participants and investigators are **blinded** or **masked** (unaware of group assignment). In addition, the validity of findings from clinical trials is enhanced because individuals are analyzed on the basis of the **intent to treat** (original randomized group assignment), even if it changes during the course of the study. **Community trials** involve the allocation of groups, rather than individual participants, to experimental and control groups. They typically are used to test the efficacy of primary preventive measures (eg, vaccines) or community-wide public health measures (eg, water fluoridation).

In **quasi-experimental studies**, random allocation of subjects to different groups does not occur. Such studies often are performed when randomization is impractical or unethical. Quasi-experimental studies are more prone to selection bias and confounding than experimental studies. Therefore, the internal validity of conclusions derived from quasi-experimental studies (ie, the confidence associated with inferences made on the basis of study findings) is considered inferior to that of true experimental studies. Most quasi-experimental studies involve assessments before and after an intervention (eg, the effect of a new computerized data entry system on rate of medication errors in a community hospital). Table 1 summarizes the advantages and disadvantages of cross-sectional, cohort, case-control, ecologic, and experimental study designs.

Recent advances in statistical methods have given rise to **meta-analysis**, a new type of epidemiologic study design. Results of individual studies with related research hypotheses are combined systematically to produce a summary estimate of effect. The advantage of this method is the enhanced power and statistical precision generated by the greater sample size. However, the validity of a meta-analysis depends on the quality of the source studies and the comprehensiveness of the literature search used to find them. Publication bias (discussed later in this chapter) is a distinct possibility in meta-analysis, and care must be exercised to ensure that this bias does not distort conclusions. Meta-analysis is a valuable tool in studies of cost effectiveness and is widely used in making clinical and policy decisions.

- Descriptive studies characterize the distribution of diseases and health-related factors and are used to formulate hypotheses. Analytic studies are used to test hypotheses.
- In a prospective cohort study, patients are enrolled before the outcome occurs. In a retrospective cohort study, patient records are reviewed to determine exposure status and outcome.
- Case-control studies retrospectively compare individuals with or without a specific outcome and consider the probability of exposure to risk factors of interest. Nested case-control and case-cohort studies combine features of case-control and cohort studies.
- Ecologic studies analyze and compare aggregate or summary data from groups.
- Clinical trials and community trials randomly assign subjects or groups of subjects to receive a treatment or control intervention.
- In quasi-experimental studies, random allocation of subjects to different groups does not occur because of feasibility or ethical concerns.
- In meta-analysis, results of individual studies with related research hypotheses are combined systematically to produce a summary estimate of effect.

Table 1 Advantages and Disadvantages of Different Epidemiologic Study Designs

Study Design	Advantages	Disadvantages
Cross-sectional study	Low cost	Examines relevant cases only
	Easy to conduct	Cannot calculate risk (no incident cases)
		Temporal association cannot be determined
Cohort study	Incidence can be calculated; provides direct estimates of absolute risk	Large sample size often is required
	Temporal relationships can be determined	Prospective studies are relatively expensive
		Prospective studies require a longer follow-up period
	Several outcomes can be assessed	Loss to follow-up is not unusual
	Good for rare exposures	Internal validity may be compromised by events in the participants' environment or changes within subjects over time (history and maturation effects)
	Retrospective studies are quick and inexpensive	
Case-control study	Efficient; fewer subjects needed	Can study only 1 outcome
	May evaluate multiple exposures	Recall bias; relies on memory
	Good for rare diseases	Selection of appropriate control group may be difficult
	Yields results relatively quickly	No incident cases; can only estimate relative risk (odds ratio)
	Minimal risk to cases	
Ecologic study	Economical	Causality is difficult to establish
	Easy to conduct	Ecologic fallacy is a major drawback
Randomized clinical trials	Optimal research study design	Expensive
	Randomization and blinding assure high internal validity	Low external validity
		Blinding may not be practical
		Ethical considerations may apply

Adapted from Varkey P, Hagen PT. Principles of biostatistics and epidemiology in clinical preventive medicine. In: Lang RS, Hensrud DD, editors. Clinical preventive medicine. United States of America: AMA Press; c2004: p.15. Used with permission.

Measures of Morbidity and Mortality

Rates, Ratios, and Proportions

Measures of morbidity and mortality provide quantitative estimates of the frequency of disease or death in the population. Such estimates are represented by rates, ratios, and proportions. A **rate** measures the occurrence of a particular event in a population at risk during a specified period. **Crude rates** are actual observed rates based on the entire population, whereas **specific rates** apply to particular subgroups characterized by a common feature. **Adjusted rates** are crude rates that are modified to account for the effects of other characteristics (eg, age) to facilitate valid comparisons of populations. Generally, rates are the most accurate measures of risk. A **ratio** denotes a comparison of size of 2 quantities (the numerator is not included in the denominator). **Proportions** are measures in which the numerator is always part of the denominator.

Measures of Morbidity

The frequency that a disease occurs in a population can be described broadly in terms of incidence and prevalence.

Cumulative incidence or **risk** is the probability of a new event (eg, disease, death, injury) occurring during a specified period in a defined population. Cumulative incidence is calculated by dividing the number of new cases of the event (eg, persons with flu-like symptoms) by the number of persons initially at risk of outcome development (eg, all persons exposed to the index case), per some constant multiplier (usually 1,000). Cumulative incidence is especially useful in disease outbreak investigations.

An **attack rate** is a type of cumulative incidence that is commonly used to quantify the number of persons affected by a disease outbreak among persons at risk. **Incidence density** or **incidence rate** measures the rapidity with which new cases of a disease occur. Incidence density considers the net time of observation (person-time) of individuals at risk of disease development in the population. Incidence density is a more accurate measure of disease occurrence, especially if the follow-up period is lengthy or if events recur in an individual.

A **prevalence rate** is the total number of individuals who experience the event at a point in time (or during a defined period) divided by the population at risk of developing the event at a point in time or during a defined period, per some constant multiplier. Depending on the

Table 2 Formulas for Common Measures of Morbidity in Epidemiologic Studies

Measure	Formula
Cumulative incidence per 1,000	$\dfrac{\text{No. of new cases}}{\text{Persons at risk}} \times 1{,}000$
Attack rate	$\dfrac{\text{No. of new cases}}{\text{Persons at risk}} \times 100$
Incidence rate[a]	$\dfrac{\text{No. of new cases}}{\text{Total person-time}}$
Prevalence per 1,000 (particular point in time or during a specified period)	$\dfrac{\text{No. of cases of a disease}}{\text{No. of persons in the population}} \times 1{,}000$
Prevalence (assume steady state; incidence and duration stable)	Incidence × duration

[a] Total person-time is defined as the cumulative time spent by each individual at risk in the population.

time frame being considered (a particular point in time vs a specified period), prevalence rates can be classified as a **point prevalence rate** or a **period prevalence rate**. The product of incidence of disease multiplied by duration of disease may also be used to determine **prevalence**, provided that incidence and duration both remain stable over time. Formulas for calculating common measures of morbidity are shown in the Table 2.

Measures of Mortality

All changes in human population size, composition, and distribution are governed by the interplay of 3 demographic processes: fertility, mortality, and migration. **Mortality** rates of a population are characterized by the life expectancy of age-sex subgroups within the population. **Life expectancy** at a given age is the average number of years a person of that age is expected to live, given the age-specific death rate that is prevalent in the population at that time. Life expectancy at birth is a good indicator of the level of human development of a country. A **population pyramid** is a graphical representation of the age-sex structure of a population. The shape of the population pyramid denotes the rate of growth of the population. A rapid-growth ("young") population produces a shape with a broad base and tapering tip (triangular), whereas a slow-growth ("aging") population has a bulge in the middle and a relatively narrow base (rectangular). A country with a decreasing or zero-growth population shows a progressively shrinking base. Figure 2 shows population pyramids for rapid growth, slow growth, and decreased or zero growth.

The crude, specific, and adjusted mortality rates commonly encountered in epidemiologic studies are described in Table 3. Crude death rates are strongly influenced by the age composition of populations and are therefore not ideal indices to use when comparing mortality rates of populations with differing age distributions.

Standardization is a process by which populations that differ in terms of certain important characteristics are made comparable so that valid assessments can be made. Standardization can be performed directly or indirectly.

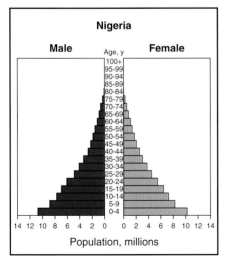
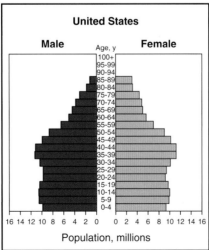
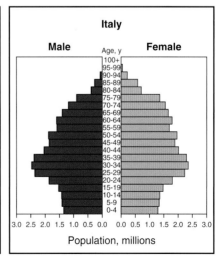

Figure 2 Population Pyramids. The figure shows examples of rapid growth (*left*, Nigeria), slow growth (*center*, United States), and zero or decreased growth (*right*, Italy) from the year 2000. (From US Census Bureau, Population Division, International Data Base [cited 31 Oct 2008]. Available from: http://www.census.gov/ipc/www/idb/country.php.)

Table 3 Definitions of Crude, Specific, and Adjusted Mortality Rates and Ratios Commonly Used in Epidemiologic Studies

Rate or Ratio	Numerator	Denominator	Usual Multiplier
Crude birth rate	Total number of live births during a specified period	Midyear population from which births occur	1,000
Crude death rate	Total number of deaths during a specified period	Midyear population from which deaths occur	1,000
Age-specific death rate	Deaths of persons in particular age group during a specified period	Midyear population from which deaths occur	1,000
Cause-specific death rate	Number of deaths due to a particular cause during a specified period	Midyear population from which deaths occur	100,000
Infant mortality rate	Number of deaths among infants aged <365 d during a specified period	Number of live births in the same period	1,000
Neonatal mortality rate	Number of deaths among infants aged <28 d during a specified period	Number of live births in the same period	1,000
Fetal death rate	Number of fetal deaths (≥20 wk gestation)	Total number of births (live and still)	1,000
Maternal mortality rate	Number of pregnancy-related maternal deaths during a specified period	Number of live births in the same period	100,000
Perinatal mortality rate	Number of stillbirths and deaths in infants aged <7 d	Total number of births (live and still)	1,000
Postneonatal mortality rate	Number of deaths of infants aged 28-365 d	Number of live births in the same year	1,000
Proportionate mortality rate	Number of deaths due to specific disease during a specified period	Total number of deaths from all causes in the same period	100
Standardized mortality ratio	Number of observed deaths	Number of expected deaths	100
Case-fatality ratio	Number of deaths due to specific disease during a specified period	Number of persons receiving diagnosis of the disease during the same period	100

Consider the example of populations that differ in age. For **direct standardization**, age-specific death rates of the populations being compared are applied to a standard population to yield the expected number of deaths for each age group. These expected deaths are summed and then divided by the total number of deaths in the standard population to obtain standardized (age-adjusted) death rates for each population. The standard population is often the larger population from which the compared populations are being drawn (eg, the US population). **Indirect standardization** is used if age-specific death rates for the populations being studied are not available. In this case, the expected number of deaths in the study population is calculated by applying age-specific death rates from a standard population to each age group of the study population. The **standardized mortality ratio** is calculated by dividing the total number of observed deaths in the study population by the number of expected deaths in the population; it is considered a measure of the **excess mortality risk** in the study population relative to the standard population.

A ratio of the number of deaths attributable to a specific cause to the total number of deaths in the population is termed the **proportional mortality ratio**. Proportional mortality ratios lack information on risk of death, and caution should be exercised when comparing ratios from different populations, especially if populations differ in terms of the relative contribution of other causes of death.

A concept similar to life expectancy is the **years of potential life lost** (YPLL), an indicator of premature death. YPLL represent the number of years an individual would have lived, given the prevailing average life expectancy of the population at that point in time. YPLL emphasizes deaths that occur during the most productive years of life, and it is commonly used to prioritize funding for public health programs. In the United States, unintentional injuries remain the leading cause of YPLL before age 65.

Measures of Disability

The definition of **disability** varies, depending on the organization defining the term and on the purpose for which it is intended to be used. The World Health Organization defines disability as ". . .any restriction or lack (resulting from an impairment) of ability to perform an activity in the manner or within the range considered normal for a human being." The Americans with Disabilities Act defines an individual with a disability as "a person who has a physical or mental impairment that substantially limits one or more major life activities, a person who has a history or record of such an impairment, or a person who is perceived by others as having such an impairment." Regardless of which definition of disability is used, measures of disability are valuable adjuncts to indicators of mortality and morbidity.

Measures of disability can be broadly classified into event-type indicators and person-type indicators. **Event-type indicators** measure the effect of acute and chronic illness on the occurrence of specific events. Examples of event-type indicators include work-loss or school-loss days, bed-disability days, and days of restricted activity. **Person-type indicators** describe the extent of limitations imposed by a disability on an individual. Person-type indicators include measures of limitation of the ability to perform basic activities of daily living (eg, eating, bathing, dressing) and measures of mobility limitation (eg, confinement to bed, need for assistance to ambulate inside or outside the home).

A composite measure of premature mortality and disability is the **disability-adjusted life year** (DALY); it is a popular indicator of the overall burden of disease in a defined population. DALYs extend the concept of YPLL to include equivalent years of healthy (nondisabled) life lost because of disability. DALYs are computed as the sum of the present value of future years of life lost through premature death and the present value of future years of life after adjusting for the average severity of any mental or physical disability caused by a disease or injury. DALYs are used as a decision-making tool and provide an evidence base for prioritizing public health problems.

- Rates are the most accurate measures of risk.
- Infant mortality rate is a key indicator of the health status of a community or population.
- Population dynamics are governed by the interplay of fertility, mortality, and migration.
- Proportional mortality ratios lack information on risk of death and can lead to spurious results if used to compare 2 or more populations.
- In the United States, unintentional injuries are the leading cause of years of potential life lost (YPLL) before age 65 years.
- The disability-adjusted life year (DALY) is a composite measure of premature mortality and disability.

Validity and Bias in Research

A complete understanding of study design cannot be achieved without a review of validity and bias in research. Regardless of how rigorously a research study is designed, the legitimacy of its conclusions depends on **internal validity**, the extent to which study findings can be attributable only to the exposure under investigation. Legitimacy also is affected by **external validity**, whether findings can be generalized to the population or setting from which the study sample was drawn.

Bias is any systematic error that occurs in the design or conduct of scientific research. **Lack of precision** or **random error** is variation in study findings that can be explained by chance. Precision depends on sample size, whereas bias is influenced by the participant selection process, methods of information collection, and appropriateness of analytic procedures. Bias is commonly classified into 3 broad categories: selection bias, information bias, and confounding. Note that the classification scheme is quite arbitrary and that the categories are not exclusive.

Selection Bias

Selection bias arises when a systematic error in ascertainment of study participants leads to spurious associations between exposure and outcome. **Incidence-prevalence bias** or **Neyman survival bias** is a type of selection bias that occurs when the risk factor is associated with prognostic factors or is itself a prognostic determinant. For example, if individuals with more severe disease are more likely to be missed during subject ascertainment, survivors could be disproportionately represented by individuals with lower frequency of exposure.

Selection bias in cohort studies commonly relates to differential losses during follow-up. Individuals who are lost to follow-up may differ from those who remain in the study with regard to the probability of having the outcome of interest. In hospital-based, case-control studies, **Berkson selection bias** may occur when an association between exposure and a disease or between 2 exposures is more likely in hospitalized patients than in controls drawn from the general population. Similarly, the **healthy-worker effect** may be observed in occupational studies when employed persons have lower death rates or less disease than a sample drawn from the general population.

Publication bias is a type of selection bias associated with a systematic tendency to publish certain studies and not others, thereby resulting in a biased sample of all studies. Whether a study is eventually published is influenced by multiple factors such as study size and design, nature of findings, quality, funding, and prestige. Small investigations and studies that do not suggest differences in outcome frequently are not submitted for publication or are rejected if submitted. The presence and extent of publication bias commonly is assessed with a **funnel diagram** (Figure 3), a plot of effect size versus study sample size (or some other measure of precision such as standard error). Publication bias is indicated by an asymmetric funnel shape. The lower left region of the plot, where smaller and negative publications would appear, is devoid of studies.

Information Bias

Information bias arises from errors in measurement during data collection and leads to misclassification of exposure or outcome status of study participants. **Differential misclassification** can occur when 1) the proportion of subjects misclassified with regard to exposure depends on disease status or 2) the proportion of subjects misclassified with regard to disease depends on exposure status. Differential misclassification can either underestimate or exaggerate the true effect. **Nondifferential misclassification** occurs when study participants are misclassified at random (ie, when misclassification of exposure is independent of disease status or when misclassification of disease does not depend on exposure status). Nondifferential misclassification of exposure is associated with more predictable results (underestimation of effect size, termed **bias toward the null**).

A major problem with case-control studies is **recall bias**, the imprecise recollection of past exposure by cases, which often leads to differential misclassification. For example, mothers of children with congenital malformations may be more likely to recall specific behaviors in pregnancy than control subjects with healthy babies. **Interviewer bias** can occur when an interviewer consciously or unconsciously elicits inaccurate information from study participants that supports preconceived notions. In the case of

observer bias, prior knowledge of exposure status by the assessor can influence conclusions. Observer bias can be avoided in clinical trials by blinding observers to participant status. In contrast, participants in observation studies can change their behavior in response to being observed, a phenomenon termed the **Hawthorne effect**. Like interviewer and observer bias, **measurement bias** can result from incorrect measurements during baseline or follow-up assessments.

Regression bias is caused by the tendency for extreme values to revert toward the mean with repeated measurements (termed **statistical regression** or **regression toward the mean**). Regression bias, which underestimates the true effect of an association, is more likely to occur when participants are included in a study because of their extreme conditions or scores. In such a situation, subsequent measurements will result in values that are by chance closer to the average.

Lead-time bias mostly is encountered in screening tests. The survival advantage in screened persons is inflated because a screening test only advances the time of diagnosis. The calculation of survival from the time an early diagnosis is made results in biased conclusions (Figure 4). **Length bias** refers to the higher likelihood of a screening test detecting an indolent condition with a longer preclinical phase than a rapidly progressive disease with a shorter time course (or worse prognosis).

- Generalizability is synonymous with external validity.
- Lack of systematic error corresponds to internal validity.
- Absence of random error is synonymous with precision.

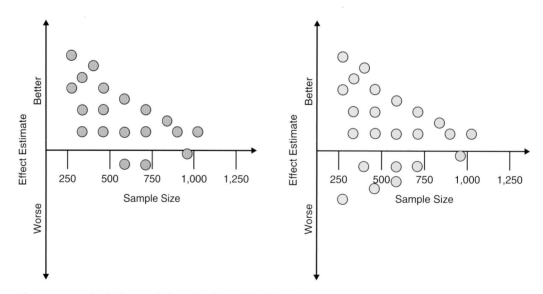

Figure 3 Hypothetical Funnel Plots Showing Publication Bias. *Left*, Publication bias is evident because the lower left region of the funnel plot is devoid of studies. *Right*, The distribution of studies indicates publication bias is not present.

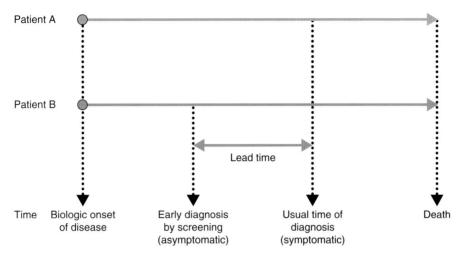

Figure 4 Lead-Time Bias. Patient B appears to have longer survival than patient A only because the diagnosis occurred earlier in the course of disease.

- Nondifferential misclassification of exposure is associated with bias toward the null, whereas in differential misclassification, findings can underestimate or exaggerate the true effect.

Confounding and Control of Confounding

Confounding is a distortion of the association between an exposure and an outcome that is caused by a failure to account for the extraneous influence of 1 or more additional variables (**confounders**). A variable must satisfy 3 criteria to be considered a confounder: 1) it is an independent risk factor for the outcome of interest; 2) it is noncausally or causally associated with the exposure of interest; and 3) it is not an intermediary in the causal pathway. An example of confounding is the role of cigarette smoking in the initial association of alcohol intake and lung cancer. In this scenario, smoking is an independent risk factor for lung cancer, in addition to being associated with alcohol use.

Control of confounding can be performed in the **design stage** or **analysis stage** of a study. As a study is designed and conducted, confounding can be managed through matching, restriction, or randomization. During analysis, confounding can be adjusted by using multivariate techniques or stratification.

Matching is the process of selecting cases and controls to ensure that they are similar with respect to confounding factors. Matching can be performed in pairs or in groups. Caution should be exercised to avoid matching exposure status and not overmatching variables that are closely associated with exposure. This may result in similar distributions of the variable of interest between groups being compared, which causes the effect size to be underestimated.

Restriction is a process of controlling confounding by excluding potential study subjects on the basis of predefined characteristics. Only subjects with the same or similar values for a potential confounder are included in the study. For instance, if participant age is a potential confounder, only subjects within a prespecified age range are enrolled in the study. Restriction may potentially limit the generalizability of study findings. Restriction also assumes that important sources of confounding can be identified before the study begins, but this often is not the case.

Randomization is a process of randomly allocating study participants into groups to receive a preventive or therapeutic intervention (experimental group) or to not receive the intervention (control group). Randomization reduces selection bias in allocation of treatment. Whereas matching and restriction can control for only the known potential confounders, randomization ensures that groups are similar in terms of known and unknown (potential) confounders.

Multivariate analysis applies statistical regression techniques to simultaneously control for several confounding variables. Each potential confounder is included in the regression model, and the separate effect of each variable on the outcome is independently assessed.

Stratification involves the cross-tabulation of data on exposure and disease into nonoverlapping groups defined by 1 or more potential confounders. The effect of the potential confounding variable can then be assessed within each stratum. If confounding is present, the association between the exposure and outcome variables after stratification will be the same within each stratum of the confounder. Stratification is a straightforward and logical method of controlling confounding. The drawback of stratification is that it is difficult to implement when several variables need to be considered simultaneously to control confounding. Such a scenario requires a large number of strata and leads to imprecise results because of sparseness of data.

- Randomization protects against selection bias and minimizes the effect of known and unknown sources of confounding.
- Confounding can be controlled in the analysis phase of a study through stratification or by mathematical modeling.
- Overmatching can underestimate a true association.
- Multivariate regression isolates the effect of a variable from other potentially confounding variables and is the preferred method of simultaneously adjusting for the effects of many potential confounders.

Effect Modification

Stratification analysis is a useful tool for describing the phenomenon of effect modification (interaction). **Effect modification** occurs when the strength of the association between 2 variables varies according to the level of a third variable. Unlike confounding, in which the true association between the exposure of interest and the outcome is obscured, in effect modification, the effect modifier alters the magnitude or direction of the relationship. Figure 5 illustrates effect modification as it pertains to the association between infants born small for their gestational age and maternal alcohol consumption and tobacco use during pregnancy. If effect modification is present, stratum-specific risks estimates (eg, odds ratios, relative risks) will vary by level of the effect modifier. In contrast, if confounding is present, the adjusted risk estimate will differ from the crude effect estimate by at least 15%.

Confounding and interaction generally are discrete events, although the same variable can be both a confounder and an effect modifier. Confounding should always be identified and controlled to assure internal validity. In contrast, effect modification does not violate the internal validity of a study; it should therefore be described but does not need to be eliminated.

- In confounding, the pooled, adjusted effect estimate will be significantly different from the crude estimate, whereas in effect modification, the stratum-specific effect estimates will vary in magnitude or direction (or both) by the level of the effect modifier.

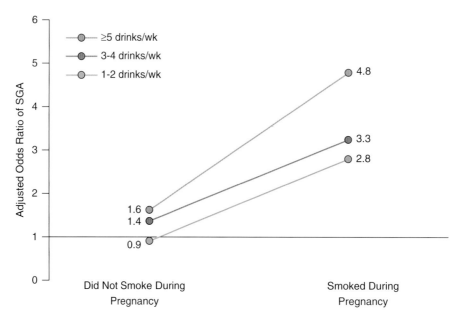

Figure 5 Effect Modification. The adjusted odds ratios of delivering an infant that is small for gestational age (SGA) varies by level of maternal alcohol consumption and tobacco use during pregnancy. Odds ratios were adjusted for maternal race, obesity, gestational weight gain, parity, marital status, maternal education level, adequacy of prenatal care, fetal sex, and year of birth. (Data from Aliyu MH, Wilson RE, Zoorab R, Brown K, Alio AP, Clayton H, et al. Prenatal alcohol consumption and fetal growth restriction: potentiation effect by concomitant smoking. Nicotine Tob Res 2009;11[1]:36-43.)

SUGGESTED READING

Bertone-Johnson ER, Hankinson SE, Johnson SR, Manson JE. Cigarette smoking and the development of premenstrual syndrome. Am J Epidemiol. 2008 Oct 15;168(8):938-45. Epub 2008 Aug 13.

Fletcher RH, Fletcher SW. Clinical epidemiology: the essentials. 4th ed. Philadelphia (PA): Lippincott Williams & Wilkins; c2005.

Gordis L. Epidemiology. 3rd ed. Philadelphia (PA): Elsevier/Saunders; c2004.

Greenberg RS, Daniels SR, Flanders WD, Eley JW, Boring JR III. Medical epidemiology. 4th ed. New York: Lange Medical Books/McGraw-Hill; c2005.

A guide to disability rights laws [Internet]. US Department of Justice, Americans with Disabilities Act [2005 September; cited 31 Oct 2008]. Available from: http://www.ada.gov/cguide.htm.

Hebel RJ, McCarter RJ. Study guide to epidemiology and biostatistics. 6th ed. Sudbury (MA): Jones and Bartlett Publishers; c2006.

Jekel JF, Katz DL, Elmore JG, Wild DMG. Epidemiology, biostatistics and preventive medicine. 3rd ed. Philadelphia (PA): Saunders/Elsevier; c2007.

Last JM, ed. A dictionary of epidemiology. 4th ed. New York: Oxford University Press; c2001.

London JA, Parry L, Galante J, Battistella F. Safety of early mobilization of patients with blunt solid organ injuries. Arch Surg. 2008 Oct;143(10):972-6.

Szklo M, Nieto JF. Epidemiology: beyond the basics. 2nd ed. Boston (MA): Jones and Bartlett Publishers; c2007.

Torrence ME. Understanding epidemiology. St. Louis: Mosby; c1997.

World Health Organization. International classification of impairments, disabilities, and handicaps: a manual of classification relating to the consequences of disease. Geneva (Switzerland): World Health Organization, c1980.

Questions and Answers

Questions

1. In a study initiated in 1980, a group of 5,000 women of childbearing age was asked about transdermal estradiol use. The occurrence of cases of cervical cancer was then studied in this group from 2000 through 2007. What study design best describes this investigation?
   a. Cross-sectional study
   b. Case-control study
   c. Prospective cohort study
   d. Retrospective cohort study

2. In a hypothetical study of the association between cholelithiasis and alcohol intake, the odds ratio of having gallstones (comparing persons who drink alcohol with individuals who do not) is calculated to be 0.86 for men and 0.74 for women. The most appropriate interpretation of these results is which of the following?
   a. The effect of alcohol is confounded by sex
   b. The effect of alcohol is modified by sex
   c. The effect of sex is confounded by alcohol
   d. Sex is both a confounder and an effect modifier of the effect of alcohol

3. What is one approach to avoiding bias caused by the phenomenon of regression toward the mean?
   a. Use a single measurement instead of repeated measurements for physiologic parameters that do not fluctuate
   b. Use a single measurement instead of repeated measurements for physiologic parameters that fluctuate
   c. Use an average of repeated measurements instead of a single measurement for physiologic parameters that fluctuate
   d. Use an average of repeated measurements instead of a single measurement for physiologic parameters that do not fluctuate

4. In a case-control study of hospitalized patients, controls were not representative of the distribution of exposure in the source population from which the cases were drawn. What type of bias is this?
   a. Neyman survival bias
   b. Berkson bias
   c. Recall bias
   d. Publication bias

5. A screening program is designed for the early detection of endometrial cancer after a large clinical study showed promising results. The survival time from diagnosis in postmenopausal women whose endometrial cancer was detected by screening was 4 months longer than the survival time of women who did not undergo screening and presented with postmenopausal vaginal bleeding. This difference in survival is most likely due to what effect?
   a. Length bias
   b. Healthy-worker effect
   c. Lead-time bias
   d. Observer bias

6. To determine the effectiveness of dietary counseling on nutrition behavior, a group of subjects with weight management problems had their eating habits videotaped during a 3-week period after the counseling sessions. This study is likely to be particularly prone to what type of bias?
   a. Hawthorne effect
   b. Interviewer bias
   c. Berkson bias
   d. Regression bias

Answers

1. Answer c.

In a prospective cohort study, all subjects in a source population are classified on the basis of exposure status and are monitored over time to ascertain outcome (eg, disease status). Cohort studies can therefore determine temporal relationships and provide direct estimates of risk.

2. Answer b.

The odds ratio for men having gallstones associated with alcohol consumption is different from that of women. Sex therefore modifies the relationship between alcohol and cholelithiasis.

3. Answer c.

"Regression toward the mean" is a statistical term used to describe the shift toward the mean of extreme values that occurs with repeated assessments. To guard against measurement errors associated with this phenomenon, use of an average value (derived from repeated measurements) is preferred over single measurements for physiologic parameters that vary.

4. Answer b.

Berkson bias occurs when both exposure and disease affect procedures used to select study participants. For example, a hospital-based case-control study may find a spurious association between 2 diseases or between an exposure and a disease because the reason for hospitalization may be related to the exposure being studied.

5. Answer c.

Screening may appear to help people live longer because of falsely improved survival rates, even if early treatment is no more effective than treatment at the time of clinical diagnosis. Lead-time bias can be avoided by comparing age-specific mortality rates instead of survival rates for screened and unscreened persons.

6. Answer a.

Changes in the behavior of study participants could result from their awareness of being studied and not because of experimental manipulation. This type of bias was coined from studies of workers at the Hawthorne plant of the Western Electric company in Illinois, whereby improvements in job productivity were attributed to workers systematically altering their behavior when they were being observed.

5

BEHAVIORAL MEDICINE AND SUBSTANCE ABUSE

Warren G. Thompson, MD

The goal of preventive medicine is to prevent premature death and disability. The successful practitioner of preventive medicine must be skilled at facilitating behavior change in patients because behaviors such as smoking, sedentary lifestyle, poor nutrition, alcohol misuse, and illegal drug use are the leading causes of premature death and disability in the United States. This chapter focuses on the key knowledge and skills necessary for physicians to stimulate changes in patient behavior.

Promoting Behavior Change

Role of the Physician

The **leading health indicators,** as described in Healthy People 2010, reflect major public health concerns in the United States; they were selected on the basis of their importance, their ability to motivate action, and the availability of data to measure progress (Box 1). As is evident, most of these indicators can be influenced through behavioral change. The indicators are intended to help improve understanding of the importance of health promotion and disease prevention and to encourage wide participation in improving health in the next decade.

To facilitate changes in patient behavior, effective preventive medicine physicians determine the patient's perspective about the nature of the problem, including how it should be evaluated and treated. They are enthusiastic and knowledgeable. They allow patients to tell their story and listen well, especially early in the interview. They are

empathetic and encourage the patient to elaborate on emotion; they do not interrupt or redirect when the patient mentions an emotional issue. They do not say "I understand" before the patient has had a chance to explain a difficult situation (saying "that must be difficult" would be better). They provide hope for patients making behavior change and help the patient overcome guilt or shame by teaching patients to consider prior failures in behavior as learning opportunities. They counter barriers to change (eg, if the patient says, "I'll gain weight if I quit smoking," the physician replies, "You can prevent weight gain by starting an exercise program and developing a good eating plan").

Box 1 Leading Health Indicators in the United States

1. Physical activity

2. Overweight and obesity

3. Tobacco use

4. Substance abuse

5. Responsible sexual behavior

6. Mental health

7. Injury and violence

8. Environmental quality

9. Immunization

10. Access to health care

Adapted from Healthy People [Internet]. Rockville (MD): Office of Disease Prevention and Health Promotion, U.S. Department of Health and Human Services; What are the leading health indicators? [cited 17 June 2009]. Available from: http://www.healthypeople.gov/LHI/lhiwhat.htm.

Teaching patients about the pathophysiology of disease and stating consequences are not effective techniques for behavior change. In contrast, encouraging and engaging the patient's involvement in managing their illness can be helpful. Although flexibility in the methods used to achieve goals is essential, practitioners should be firm about the importance of achieving those goals.

Methods and Models of Behavior Change

The Stanford University Faculty Development Program in Preventive Medicine described an excellent **6-step method for behavior change** that was drawn from several experts in the field; this has been modified and expanded here (Box 2). Steps 4 and 6 provide practical ideas for assisting patients; an application of these steps in the context of weight loss is shown in Table 1.

A number of models attempt to explain behavior change; these include the health belief model, the theory of planned behavior, the motivational interviewing model, the transtheoretical model of behavior change, and the PRECEDE/PROCEED model. These models have many overlapping features.

The **health belief model** states that patients will change behavior if they have the following beliefs: 1) they are susceptible to consequences if they do not change behavior; 2) the consequences of not changing behavior are sufficiently severe to warrant change; and 3) the benefits of change are greater than the risks, costs, and barriers to change. Additional factors subsequently have been added, including self-efficacy

---

Box 2 Model for Health Care Provider–Assisted Patient Behavior Change

Step 1. Identify the problem

1. Appraise risk

2. Explicitly state problem and associated outcomes

3. Assess knowledge, beliefs, and barriers. Ask the patient:

   a. What do you know about X?

   b. Do you think changing X is necessary?

   c. Have you ever tried to change X in the past? What happened?

   d. Do you think you can change X now?

   e. What are some barriers you may have when changing X?

Step 2. Build commitment and confidence

1. Develop a trusting doctor-patient relationship by listening and showing empathy (praise, respond to emotion)

2. Provide counterarguments to belief barriers

3. Stimulate patient involvement

4. Negotiate and contract with the patient to change behavior (negotiate on position, not principle)

Step 3. Increase patient self-awareness

1. Instruct patient to keep a diary or log

2. Provide checklists

Step 4. Develop and implement the action plan

1. Improve knowledge and restructure environment

   a. Provide new information on the consequences of behavior and the benefits of change

   b. Restructure the cognitive environment

      i. Instill belief in ability to change (if patients think they will fail, they fail)

      ii. Teach the patient to use distraction and to avoid dwelling on tempting thoughts

Step 4. Develop and implement the action plan (cont.)

   c. Restructure the physical environment (suggest ways of avoiding temptation)

2. Modify behavior

   a. Teach and practice behavioral skills; monitor the progress

   b. Ask patient to put weekly goals in writing; troubleshoot at the end of the week

3. Establish incentives

   a. Ask patient to design short-term rewards (or punishment) for desirable (or undesirable) behavior

4. Establish social support

   a. Help the patient elicit social support for change

   b. Suggest role models

Step 5. Evaluate the action plan

1. Determine what changes (if any) took place and why

2. Encourage follow-up visits for behavior change

3. Support success; build confidence

4. Develop strategies to overcome identified problems

Step 6. Maintain change

1. Identify situations that lead to relapse

   a. Internal predictors (eg, stress, depression)

   b. External predictors (eg, peer pressure, alcohol)

2. Develop and rehearse strategies to prevent relapse

   a. Establish plans to avoid relapse triggers and/or to alter and adapt behavior to those triggers

   b. Work with patient to reduce stress and depression

3. Continue rewards and social support for maintenance

4. Provide long-term follow-up

Adapted from Stanford Program on Faculty Development in Preventive Medicine, 1986-1995. Available from: http://www.stanford.edu/group/SFDP/progsfdc.html.

Table 1 Behavior-Changing Techniques for Weight Loss

Weight Loss Technique	Example	Suggestions for Patients
Self-monitoring	Record calories ingested	Consider using a hand-held, computerized, calorie-tracking device.
		Record consumption whenever eating, not at the end of the day or week.
	Record exercise	Set realistic goals (eg, time or distance walked).
Environmental modification: the physical environment	Set a goal of permanently changing eating habits (not following short-term diets)	Reduce calories by eating fewer high-fat foods and eating more fruits, vegetables, and fiber.
		Keep fruit accessible and visible.
		Avoid fruit juice and other sugary beverages.
		Consult with a dietitian.
	Be mindful in the grocery store	Buy fruits and vegetables.
		Avoid problem foods that are very tempting.
	Reduce consumption of food outside the home	Choose wisely in restaurants (share meals, skip dessert).
		Bring food to work instead of eating at cafeterias and snacking.
		Minimize consumption of fast foods.
	Increase physical activity	Set aside time for daily walks.
		Walk when using the telephone at home or work.
		Park farther away from destination (or walk or bike instead of drive).
		Exercise with a partner.
		Use stairs instead of the elevator.
		Know that physical activity is the most important predictor of weight-loss maintenance.
		Consult with a trainer or exercise therapist (if feasible).
Environmental modification: the thinking pattern	Create an environment in which self-control can succeed	Avoid temptation instead of trying to resist (if possible).
		Use distraction (go for a walk after dinner instead of snacking).
		Reframe temptations (focus on less pleasant aspects of the temptation instead of the desirable aspects).
	Plan ahead for high-risk times	Know that most people do not adhere to an eating plan upon returning home after work and before bedtime.
		Establish an alternative behavior ("If faced with temptation X, I will do behavior Y").
	Set clear and attainable short-term goals that are needed to reach the long-term goal	Set specific, reasonable, and proximal goals ("I will walk 20 min, 5 d/wk, during the next 2 weeks").
		If goals are attained, set new goals.
		If goals are not attained, determine the reasons for failure. If the strategy was correct but the plan was not executed, try again. If the strategy was faulty, develop a new strategy.
	Avoid dwelling on guilt	Know that guilt is not an effective modifier of long-term behavior (can have counterproductive effects).
Self-efficacy	Focus on success, not failure	Expect setbacks. Do not allow setbacks to destroy belief in the ability to effect change.
		Focus on learning and implementing new strategies instead of dwelling on blame and guilt.
		Consult with a behavioral psychologist (if feasible)
Engage social supports	Solicit support from family and physician	Explain to family that their help is needed and appreciated.
		Anticipate needing help with temptation avoidance and exercise, which often requires change in other family members' eating and exercise habits.
		Physician should be generally optimistic but should avoid excessive optimism about how much weight a patient will lose
		Physician should teach patients to view lack of success as a learning opportunity to refine strategies.
		Physician should recommend frequent follow-up.

Adapted from Thompson WG, Cook DA, Clark MM, Bardia A, Levine JA. Treatment of obesity. Mayo Clin Proc. 2007;82(1):93-102. Used with permission of Mayo Foundation for Medical Education and Research.

(enhancing patient confidence about whether changes can be made) and cues to action from social networks and other outside influences. This model is most valuable for assessing motivation to change. It has less predictive power than other models to explain behavior.

The **theory of planned behavior** suggests that the best predictor of human behavior is intention. Intention is in turn influenced by attitudes toward the specific behavior, the perceived behavioral control (ability to perform a specific behavior), subjective beliefs of the normative expectations of others, and beliefs about factors that may impede or facilitate performance of the behavior. Generally, if attitude and the subjective norm are favorable and the patient perceives a high level of control, the intention to perform the behavior is strong (Figure 1).

The **model of motivational interviewing** is used to determine discrepancies between the patient's goals and actions, respond to resistance to behavior changes, and build self-efficacy to make the change. It is both client-centered and semi-directive, and it emphasizes empathy while being nonjudgmental, nonconfrontational, and non-adversarial. Table 2 shows the 4 principles on which the model is based.

The **transtheoretical model of behavior change** states that patients are usually in 1 of 5 stages of change: 1) precontemplation, 2) contemplation, 3) preparation, 4) action, or 5) maintenance. The model uses the principle of decisional balance to try to move patients from one stage to the next. The counselor is encouraged to use the stage of change to guide counseling techniques. For example, informing a patient of the dangers of smoking may be useful for a smoker in the precontemplation phase but would be of little benefit in a patient already in the action

Table 2 Model of Motivational Interviewing

Principle	Guidance for Counselors
Show empathy	Share with patients your understanding of the patient's perspective.
Develop patient's awareness of discrepancy	Help the patient appreciate the value of change by exploring discrepancies between life goals and the current day-to-day actions and behaviors
Respond to resistance	Accept the patient's reluctance to change as a natural (not pathological) condition
Support self-efficacy	Embrace patient autonomy and help the patient implement change successfully and confidently

phase who is motivated to stop. Although outcome data are mixed about whether this model helps clinicians in their efforts to help patients change behavior, it is currently the model most often applied.

The **PRECEDE/PROCEED model** is useful for behavior change on the individual and population levels. PRECEDE (predisposing, reinforcing, and enabling constructs in education, diagnosis, and evaluation) is a diagnostic and planning process for individual and public health programs. PROCEED (policy, regulatory, and organizational constructs in education and environmental development) focuses on implementation of the plans generated by the PRECEDE process.

As shown in Figure 2, the PRECEDE model argues that behavior depends on several factors: 1) demographic and

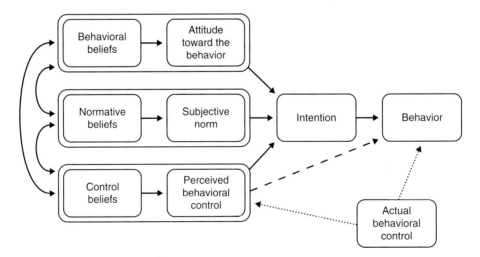

Figure 1 Conceptual Model for the Theory of Planned Behavior. (Adapted from Icek Aizen [Internet]. Amherst: University of Massachusetts. Theory of planned behavior diagram; [cited 30 Sept 2009]. Available from: http://people.umass.edu/aizen/tpb.diag.html. Used with permission.)

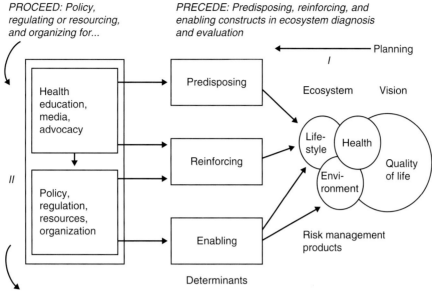

Figure 2 PRECEDE/PROCEED Model of Behavior Change. (Adapted from www.lgreen.net [Internet]. San Francisco [CA]: LWGreen@ comcast.net; 2003. The Precede-Proceed model of health programming and evaluation; [cited 27 Feb 2009], Available from: http://www.lgreen.net/precede.htm. Used with permission.)

socioeconomic characteristics (these can be predisposing or enabling factors that are not changed easily); 2) motivational factors (predisposing factors); 3) facilitators and barriers to change (enabling factors); and 4) rewards and penalties associated with the behavior (reinforcing factors). These last 3 factors should be addressed in the order shown (ie, if a patient believes that he or she should change behavior, then time should not be spent on persuasion or increasing motivation).

With a motivated patient, the behavioral change counselor should then proceed to enabling factors. Barriers to change may include inability to pay for treatment, adverse effects of treatment, and stress. The counselor should work with the patient to anticipate problems and develop strategies for overcoming them. Lastly, reinforcing factors should be assessed. Many patients have reinforcing factors such as unrealistic expectations (eg, 100-pound weight loss in 6 months) that need to be addressed. Social support from friends and family members is also a critical reinforcing factor.

The PRECEDE/PROCEED model is also a comprehensive model for community health. Phase 1 of PRECEDE involves determining the health care needs of the population. Next, the behavioral and environmental characteristics that facilitated development of those needs are elucidated. A plan is developed on the basis of an understanding of predisposing, enabling, and reinforcing factors that would best address the specific health care needs.

PROCEED involves the implementation and evaluation of that plan.

- The Stanford 6-step method for behavior change provides a framework for facilitating changes in patient behavior.
- The health belief model is best for assessing motivation to change.
- The theory of planned behavior predicts that changes in human behavior are based on intention.
- The model of motivational interviewing determines discrepancies between the patient's goals and actions, responds to resistance to behavior changes, and builds self-efficacy to make the change.
- The transtheoretical model of behavior change uses the principle of decisional balance to try to move patients from one stage of change to the next.
- The PRECEDE/PROCEED model is useful for managing behavior change on the individual and population levels.

Community-Level Influences of Behavior Change

Community and population health can be enhanced by recognizing the different levels of influence, namely intrapersonal, interpersonal, and organizational influences. More recently, attention is being paid to the importance of interpersonal influences through the study of **social networks**. Smoking cessation rates of individuals increase as more contacts in their social network quit smoking, and individuals gain weight as more contacts in their social network gain weight. Another example of social influence is an after-school program for teenagers that may not change attitudes but may reduce the opportunity to engage in risky behaviors. Organizational support for behavior change can be in the form of higher taxes on tobacco or alcohol, building recreational centers to enhance physical activity, cleaning up the environment (in one study, neighborhood deterioration was a better predictor of sexually transmitted disease than low education attainment), and using or regulating message delivery by the media.

Bringing about change at the population level may follow the principles of **diffusion of innovation**, as described by Everett Rogers. In this model, the social system comprises 5 adopter categories: 1) innovators, 2) early adopters, 3) early majority, 4) late majority, and 5) laggards. Innovators are important for change because they get the process started, but they are not very influential because too much uncertainty about the changed behavior still exists when they adopt the change. The early adopters are key to diffusing an innovation; this group tends to include the opinion leaders, and others usually solicit their advice about new innovations. This model of diffusion of innovation predicts whether innovations and change will be successful on a large scale.

How rapidly an innovation will be diffused depends on the characteristics of the innovation, how it is communicated, and the social system. The characteristics of innovation that determine its speed of adoption include its perceived relative advantage over current practice, compatibility with current practices and needs of the adopters, ease of use (simple vs complex), "trialability" (testable on a small scale), and observability (visibility of results).

The principles of this model can be useful for predicting behavior change or diffusion of best practices at the community or population level. For example, screening mammography has been widely adopted by physicians because it is perceived to detect early stage breast cancer, the test is easy for physicians to order, patient compliance is not burdensome, and results are visible in a short time. In contrast, smoking cessation counseling has been slower to diffuse because the results are not as visible (most people will not quit when advised to do so), the intervention is more complex than just ordering a test, and physician practices are not geared toward counseling.

- Intrapersonal, interpersonal, and organizational influences affect community and population health.
- Health changes at the population level may propagate in a manner predicted by the principles of diffusion of innovation.

Substance Abuse

Substance abuse is the harmful or hazardous use of psychoactive substances such as nicotine, alcohol, and illicit drugs. It accounts for a considerable amount of morbidity and mortality across the globe.

Tobacco Abuse

In the United States, tobacco abuse is responsible for 440,000 deaths annually and is the **leading preventable cause of death**. Tobacco abuse also accounts for 5 million deaths worldwide each year, partly because the prevalence of smoking among men in Eastern Europe and East Asia is 50% or higher. Nicotine does not cause as many behavioral consequences as other drugs of addiction, but it is just as addictive as these agents. Although nicotine addiction can be measured in several ways, the simplest method of determining the degree of addiction is to ask how soon after waking up does the patient have the first cigarette and to ask how many cigarettes are smoked per day.

The US Preventive Services Task Force (USPSTF) recommends that **all adults be screened and counseled to stop smoking**. Even brief advice doubles the likelihood that a patient will stop smoking. Unfortunately, approximately 50% of patients who smoke report that their physicians have never advised them to stop. Although a brief intervention is better than no intervention, longer counseling times often lead to better results. The "5 A's" for a brief intervention for smoking cessation are shown in Box 3. The principles of effective counseling for smoking cessation and prevention of relapse are outlined in Box 4. Of note, telephone quit lines have also been shown to improve smoking cessation rates.

The Cochrane meta-analysis of pharmacotherapy for smoking cessation estimates that **nicotine replacement products** and **medications** like bupropion, clonidine, and nortriptyline double the quit rate. The latter 2 medications are considered second-line agents because of the higher incidence of adverse effects. Varenicline triples the quit rate, but clinical experience with varenicline is less than that of the other medications, and the US Food and Drug Administration has recently added a warning to varenicline because of reports of increased agitation, depression, and suicidal ideation (although none were conclusively established to be due to the drug). A nicotine vaccine and rimonabant (a selective cannabinoid antagonist used for weight reduction in some countries) may be approved eventually in the United States for smoking cessation.

Combining nicotine replacement products such as a daily patch and a gum, lozenge, or spray as needed to curb cravings has some advantages, especially for heavy smokers. When combining nicotine replacement products, it should be remembered that the patch is the least addictive and should be stopped last. Studies have mixed results

Box 3 Brief Intervention to Facilitate Smoking Cessation (the 5 A's)

---

1. **Ask**—Physicians should ask their patients about tobacco use at each visit
2. **Advise**—Physicians should advise their tobacco-using patients to quit at each visit
3. **Assess**—Physicians should assess whether the patient is willing to stop smoking at the present time
4. **Assist**—Physicians should assist the patient in quitting
   a. If the patient is willing to quit, provide counseling and pharmacotherapy
   b. If the patient is not willing to quit:
      i. Provide the patient with information about the consequences of smoking and discuss the effects of passive smoking on the patient's family; if possible, personalize risks (eg, if the patient has back pain, point out that smoking decreases oxygen to lumbar disks and increases low back pain)
      ii. Point out discrepancies between patient goals (setting a good example for family, living a healthy life) and behavior; cessation rates are not increased by attempting to frighten the patient
5. **Arrange**—Physicians should arrange follow-up
   a. If the patient is willing to quit, schedule follow-up contact within 1 week by telephone or office visit
   b. If the patient is not willing to quit, assess tobacco dependence at the next clinic visit

---

Adapted from Agency for Healthcare Research and Quality [Internet]. Rockville (MD): AHRQ; revised May 2000. Helping smokers quit: a guide for clinicians [cited 8 Sept 2009]. Available from: http://www.ahrq.gov/clinic/tobacco/clinhlpsmksqt.htm.

regarding combining nicotine replacement with bupropion or nortriptyline. Nicotine replacement products should not be combined with varenicline because varenicline blocks the effect of nicotine on the brain.

Special Populations

There are 2 groups of patients for whom smoking cessation counseling is absolutely essential: **pregnant women** and **patients admitted to the coronary care unit**. With appropriate counseling, the quit rate of these groups is much higher than that of the general population.

The risks of smoking while pregnant are considerable (Box 5). The fetal nicotine level is approximately 15% higher than the maternal nicotine level, and high maternal carbon monoxide levels inhibit oxygen delivery to the fetus. The USPSTF recommends that pregnant women be screened for tobacco use and be provided with pregnancy-tailored counseling for tobacco users.

Two randomized trials of patients hospitalized with myocardial infarction have shown that as many as 60% will stop smoking after intensive counseling. A recent study of patients with acute coronary syndrome or cardiac failure admitted to the coronary care unit had a 2-year continuous abstinence rate of 33% in the therapy-intensive group

(patients received counseling [60 min/wk for 3 months] and free medication [including retreatment after relapse if necessary]) compared with a 9% abstinence rate in the control group (control treatment was 30 minutes of counseling and receipt of pamphlets). Furthermore, subsequent hospitalizations were reduced by 44% and mortality was reduced by 77% over 2 years. This was the first smoking cessation trial to show a significant reduction in total mortality after counseling.

Eighty percent of adult smokers begin smoking before age 18. Adolescents who smoke are 16 times more likely to drink heavily and 10 times more likely to use illicit drugs compared with nonsmoking adolescents. Furthermore, adolescents who smoke are 3 to 10 times more likely to have panic disorders and possibly other anxiety disorders (studies suggest smoking starts before the anxiety develops). Parental smoking is a strong predictor of adolescent smoking. Techniques described above may be used for counseling adolescents to quit use of tobacco.

Public Health Approaches for Addressing Tobacco Use

Public health approaches have had a marked effect on smoking cessation rates. **Restricting smoking in public places** to protect others from the risks of passive smoking has lowered smoking rates. Social networks are influential, and as more people quit smoking, such influences should serve to reduce smoking as well.

The United States has among the lowest taxes on tobacco products in the developed world. **Higher cigarette taxes** reduce consumption, especially among adolescents. Raising the price of cigarettes by 50% could reduce smoking rates by 12.5%. Raising the price of cigarettes by 10% could reduce adolescent smoking by 7%. Glantz and colleagues have shown that the California tobacco control program has saved the state $86 billion by lowering health care expenditures from 1989 to 2004. It also markedly reduced smoking rates.

- Tobacco abuse is the leading preventable cause of death in the United States.
- All patients who smoke should be counseled to quit. Pregnant women and patients admitted to the coronary care unit are very likely to quit with good counseling.
- Public health efforts (restricting smoking in public areas, raising cigarette taxes) have had a marked effect on improving smoking cessation rates.

Alcohol

Alcohol abuse is responsible for approximately 85,000 deaths annually, making it the **third-largest preventable cause of death** in the United States. (Obesity, the second-leading cause of death, is detailed in Chapter 9.) On average,

Box 4 Principles of Effective Counseling for Smoking Cessation and Prevention of Relapse

Prepare the patient for smoking cessation

1. Ask patient if he or she has tried to quit smoking previously; if yes, ask what happened

2. Determine barriers to smoking cessation

   a. "Too much stress": if the source of stress is temporary, it may be better to wait; if stress is ongoing, see Chapter 11 for guidelines on stress reduction

   b. "I've tried and I can't": most people who have quit successfully had previous unsuccessful attempts; people learn from experience

   c. "I'll gain weight": many people do not gain weight; exercise can help prevent weight changes

   d. "I'll just cut down": nicotine is a harmful drug and abstinence must be the goal; people who only decrease the number of cigarettes smoked often inhale more deeply when smoking and almost always revert to their former habits

3. Activate the patient—stimulate patient involvement

   a. Ask the patient to write down specific reasons to stop smoking

   b. Ask the patient to help determine how to overcome barriers (eg, plan alternatives to smoking when taking a break at work)

   c. Ask the patient to identify triggers for smoking (a cup of coffee, alcohol, stress, etc) and develop coping strategies

4. Negotiate, commit, and contract to change behavior

   a. Ask the patient to set a quit date

   b. Have the patient sign a contract agreeing to quit on a specific date

   c. Ask the patient to share this contract with family members

Help the patient stop smoking

1. Provide information on risks of passive smoking to family, benefits of stopping smoking, and nicotine replacement products and medications (eg, bupropion, varenicline, clonidine, nortriptyline)

2. Alter the cognitive environment

   a. Promote self-confidence and positive thinking

   b. Learn about what did and did not work in past attempts to quit

Help the patient stop smoking (cont.)

3. Modify the physical environment

   a. Avoid smoking cues

   b. Remove ashtrays and lighters

4. Social support

   a. Ideally, a spouse who smokes should also quit; if the spouse is unwilling, that person should avoid smoking in the presence of the patient

5. Establish rewards for success

   a. Use money formerly spent on cigarettes as a personal reward (eg, massage)

Prevent relapse

1. Advise the patient to get help if needed and to remember that nicotine is addictive

2. Advise the patient to avoid even one puff of a cigarette

   a. Failures often occur when an occasional cigarette is considered acceptable or when a patient "tests" himself

   b. If the patient can persevere through the first 2 weeks without a single cigarette, the chance of success is 50%; if the patient smokes in those first 2 weeks, failure is almost inevitable

3. Smoking cessation requires the patient to develop and rehearse strategies to deal with stress, boredom, and anger in alternative ways

4. Advise the patient to stay out of bars and to limit drinking

5. Advise the patient to practice saying no when around smokers

6. Advise the patient to increase use of nicotine replacements if feelings of anxiety, irritability, or craving occur or if the patient has trouble concentrating

7. What do former smokers say was helpful when quitting?

   a. Read *Out of the Ashes—Help for People Who Have Stopped Smoking* by Peter and Peggy Holmes

   b. Review reasons for wanting to quit

   c. Exercise

   d. Deep breathing

   e. Get rid of the thought of having another cigarette when it comes

   f. Reprogram—avoid triggers for smoking, substitute time spent smoking with an enjoyable activity

   g. Have someone to call when the urge to smoke arises

Adapted from Stanford Program on Faculty Development in Preventive Medicine, 1986-1995. Available from: http://www.stanford.edu/group/SFDP/progsfdc.html.

alcoholics die 10 to 15 years earlier than nonalcoholics. The most common causes of death for alcoholics are smoking-related diseases; particular for patients with head and neck cancers, the effects of smoking are exacerbated by alcohol. Most alcoholics do not have cirrhosis—heart disease and cancer are the leading causes of death in alcoholics, regardless of smoking status. Alcohol abuse is also one of the 10 leading causes of premature death worldwide. Eastern Europe and central Asia have the highest rates of alcohol-related problems.

Alcohol abuse results in $185 billion in direct and indirect costs annually in the United States. In addition, alcohol abuse frequently is associated with accidents, homicides, and suicides. More than three-quarters of all foster children

Box 5 Risks of Maternal Smoking During Pregnancy

1. Increased risk of umbilical vessel endothelial change

2. Increased risk of prematurity and low birth weight

3. Increased risk of fetal and perinatal mortality (estimated 4,600 infant deaths annually)

4. Increased risk of placenta previa and premature rupture of membranes

5. Increased risk of sudden infant death syndrome

6. Increased risk of conduct disorder and attention deficit disorder in male offspring (studies controlled for father's history)

7. Doubled risk of committing violent crime in male offspring with smoking 1 pack/d (studies controlled for father's history)

Box 6 The CAGE Questionnaire to Screen for Alcohol Disorders[a]

1. Have you ever felt you ought to *cut down* on your drinking?

2. Have people *annoyed* you by criticizing your drinking?

3. Have you ever felt bad or *guilty* about your drinking?

4. Have you ever had a drink first thing in the morning (*eye-opener*) to steady your nerves or to get rid of a hangover?

[a] If the patient answers "yes" to 3 or 4 questions, the likelihood ratio of having an alcohol disorder is 250, which virtually clinches the diagnosis. The likelihood ratio of 2 "yes" answers is 7; the likelihood ratio of 1 "yes" answer is 1.3; and the likelihood ratio of 0 "yes" answers is 0.2.

Adapted from Mayfield D, McLeod G, Hall P. The CAGE questionnaire: validation of a new alcoholism screening instrument. Am J Psychiatry. 1974 Oct;131(10):1121-3. Used with permission.

in the United States have alcohol- or drug-dependent parents. Fifty percent to 75% of domestic violence incidents involve alcohol, and 50% of violent crime is alcohol- or drug-related.

The National Longitudinal Alcohol Epidemiologic Survey reported that 44% of US adults are current drinkers, 22% are former drinkers, and 34% are lifetime abstainers. More than 8 million alcohol-dependent people live in the United States alone. The prevalence of alcohol abuse and dependence is 8.5% (3% in women). Hazardous drinking is observed in 15% of men and 5% of women. Binge drinking (defined as >4 drinks/occasion for men, >3 drinks/occasion for women) is responsible for a substantial proportion of alcohol-related morbidity and mortality. Sixty percent of men between 18 and 25 years of age binge drink.

All patients should be screened for alcohol problems because 1) alcohol abuse is common (affecting 10%-20% of the general medical outpatient population), 2) effective screening tests are available; without screening, the diagnosis is likely to be missed (50% to 90% of alcohol problems are missed in the office), 3) early identification can prevent development of physical and psychosocial problems in the patient, family, and society, and 4) effective treatments are available (especially if diagnosis is made early).

All women who are pregnant or trying to conceive should avoid alcohol. **Fetal alcohol syndrome** is the leading known cause of mental retardation (affects 1/1,000 births, which is >2,000 infants/year in the United States). Birth defects and neurodevelopmental problems are estimated to be 3 times higher with maternal alcohol consumption. Even small amounts of alcohol consumption during pregnancy can result in more behavioral problems when children are 6 or 7 years old. Moderate alcohol consumption while pregnant also results in a higher incidence of problem drinking at age 21 in male offspring, even after controlling for family history and other environmental factors.

Diagnosis of Alcohol-Related Disorders

The most common test used to screen for alcohol disorders is the **CAGE questionnaire** (Box 6; "CAGE" is a mnemonic based on the screening questions [cutting down, annoyance by criticism, guilty feeling, and eye-openers]). The CAGE questionnaire must be given face-to-face before questions on alcohol quantity or frequency are asked. It is less sensitive for the diagnosis of women and nonwhite patients. It is also not helpful for diagnosing hazardous drinking or binge drinking. It is important to pursue any affirmative answers to learn about the consequences of drinking for the patient. Other helpful questions may include "Have you ever had a drinking problem?"; "Do you use alcohol alone?" (for adolescents); and "Did your drinking increase after someone close to you died?" (for elderly patients). Laboratory tests (mean corpuscular volume, gamma glutamyl transferase, blood alcohol level) are not as sensitive as questionnaires or direct questions from the health care provider.

The best screening test for alcohol abuse and dependency is the **Alcohol Use Disorders Identification Test** (AUDIT) (Table 3). It can be given as a written test and has better sensitivity and specificity than the CAGE questionnaire for women, nonwhite patients, and populations with a lower prevalence of alcoholism. A score >5 should elicit further questions, and a score >8 should prompt concern about alcohol abuse or dependency. Alcohol-related problems can be categorized as alcohol dependence, alcohol abuse, and hazardous drinking (Box 7).

Management of Alcohol Abuse

Office visit interventions for alcohol abuse and dependence are as summarized in Box 8. The support group **Alcoholics Anonymous** (www.aa.org) should be recommended to all patients with alcohol abuse or dependence. Alcoholics Anonymous will provide a sponsor to those in need who serve as mentors to new members. Patients should be advised to attend at least 5 different group meetings to find

Table 3 Alcohol Use Disorders Identification Test (AUDIT)

Question	Score				
	0 Points	1 Point	2 Points	3 Points	4 Points
1. How often do you have a drink containing alcohol?	Never	Monthly or less	2-4 times a month	2-3 times a week	4 or more times a week
2. How many drinks containing alcohol do you have on a typical day when you are drinking?	1 or 2	3 or 4	5 or 6	7-9	10 or more
3. How often do you have 6 or more drinks on 1 occasion?	Never	Less than monthly	Monthly	Weekly	Daily or almost daily
4. How often during the past year have you found that you were not able to stop drinking once you had started?	Never	Less than monthly	Monthly	Weekly	Daily or almost daily
5. How often during the past year have you failed to do what was normally expected of you because of drinking?	Never	Less than monthly	Monthly	Weekly	Daily or almost daily
6. How often during the past year have you needed a first drink in the morning to get yourself going after a heavy drinking session?	Never	Less than monthly	Monthly	Weekly	Daily or almost daily
7. How often during the past year have you had a feeling of guilt or remorse after drinking?	Never	Less than monthly	Monthly	Weekly	Daily or almost daily
8. How often during the past year have you been unable to remember what happened the night before because you had been drinking?	Never	Less than monthly	Monthly	Weekly	Daily or almost daily
9. Have you or has someone else been injured as a result of your drinking?	No	. . .	Yes, but not in the past year	. . .	Yes, during the past year
10. Has a relative, friend, or doctor or other health care worker been concerned about your drinking or suggested you cut down?	No	. . .	Yes, but not in the past year	. . .	Yes, during the past year

Adapted from Saunders JB, Aasland OG, Babor TF, de la Fuente JR, Grant M. Development of the Alcohol Use Disorders Identification Test (AUDIT): WHO collaborative project on early detection of persons with harmful alcohol consumption—II. Addiction. 1993 Jun;88(6):791-804.

one with which they are compatible. Women should be advised to attend women-only meetings because the issues of female and male alcoholics typically differ. Patients need to attend regularly and for a sufficient duration (at least 2 years). Family should be advised to attend **Al-Anon**, a self-help group for family members of alcoholics.

Relapse is a major problem for patients with alcohol abuse or dependence. Forty percent of patients who have been sober for 2 years will relapse, but 5 years of sobriety is predictive of prolonged sobriety. Complete abstinence is just the first step in recovery. Critical additional steps to prevent relapse include 1) learning to say no to drinking in social situations, 2) handling heavy-drinking friends who try to undermine the patient's sobriety, 3) handling stress and being mindful of symptoms of anxiety, 4) avoiding boredom because the time previously spent drinking and recovering is now available, 5) learning to get along again with family and close friends because family problems often increase when drinking stops, and 6) identifying and developing coping strategies for situations that can trigger drinking.

When patients have the urge to drink, several techniques can be used to deal with the situation. These techniques include distraction (eg, performing an alternate, enjoyable activity), redirection of thoughts and not dwelling on drinking, reprogramming to avoid activities that trigger

drinking, and use of a social support network. As with smoking, the most common cause of relapse is a failure to develop and use coping strategies in a crisis.

Public Health Approaches to Address Alcohol-Related Disorders

Increased taxes on alcohol are associated with reduced alcohol consumption and reduced incidence of liver cirrhosis. Lowering the legal blood-alcohol limit while driving to 0.08% for adults and to 0.02% for those younger than 21 years has resulted in fewer fatal automobile accidents. Iceland has a high incidence of alcoholism but a low incidence of automobile accidents from alcohol because the civil penalties are quite severe.

- Alcohol abuse is the third-largest preventable cause of death in the United States, and it is associated with smoking-related diseases, accidents, homicides, and suicides.
- The CAGE questionnaire and the Alcohol Use Disorders Identification Test (AUDIT) are common screening tests for alcohol disorders.
- Groups such as Alcoholics Anonymous can provide support for patients struggling with sobriety and relapse.

Box 7 Diagnosis of Alcohol Dependence, Alcohol Abuse, or Hazardous Drinking

Diagnosis of alcohol dependence—patient meets at least 3 of the following criteria:

1. Continued drinking, despite physical or psychological consequences caused or exacerbated by alcohol

2. Neglect of other activities

3. Inordinate time spent drinking and recovering

4. Drinking more than intended or during a longer period than intended

5. Inability to control drinking

6. Tolerance (increased amounts needed for effect)

7. Withdrawal symptoms on cessation

8. Drinking to relieve or avoid withdrawal symptoms

Diagnosis of alcohol abuse—patient meets 2 of the following criteria within the past year and does not meet criteria for alcohol dependence:

1. Recurrent drinking resulted in failure to fulfill major obligations at work, school, or home

2. Recurrent drinking in situations in which it is physically hazardous

3. Recurrent alcohol-related legal problems

4. Continued use despite persistent or recurrent alcohol-related social or interpersonal problems

Diagnosis of hazardous drinking—patient meets any one of the following criteria and does not meet criteria for alcohol dependence or abuse:

1. More than 7 drinks/wk or 3 drinks per occasion for all women and men older than 65 years

2. More than 14 drinks/wk or 4 drinks per occasion for men younger than 65 years

3. Any use of alcohol by children or teenagers, personal or family history of alcohol dependence, breastfeeding or pregnant women, before or during situations requiring attention or skill (eg, driving)

Data from Task Force on DSM-IV and Work groups for the DSM-IV Text Revision of the American Psychiatric Association. Diagnostic and statistical manual of mental disorders, DSM-IV-TR. 4th ed. Washington, DC: American Psychiatric Association; c2000.

- Public health measures such as increased alcohol taxes or severe civil penalties are associated with reduced alcohol consumption.

Illegal Drugs

Illegal drugs are **among the 10 leading preventable causes of premature death and disability** in the United States and other developed countries. Much of the economic burden of illegal drug use is attributable to crime and incarceration; human immunodeficiency virus and AIDS associated with drug use accounts for 10% of the total cost. Although early recognition and treatment can reduce drug use in the short term, more studies are needed to demonstrate long-term benefit.

Box 8 Brief Interventions for Alcohol Abuse and Dependence

1. Present the diagnosis to the patient

    a. Use explicit evidence; emphasize consequences the patient has suffered as a result of alcohol abuse

    b. Be empathetic and nonjudgmental

    c. Avoid arguments about diagnosis

    d. Avoid using the word "alcoholic"

2. Indicate that the patient is responsible for change

    a. Listen to patient's goals

    b. Point out discrepancies between goals and actions

3. Determine the patient's readiness for change

    a. If the patient does not believe there is a problem

        i. Suggest bringing a family member to the next appointment

        ii. Suggest a 2-week trial of abstinence

    b. If the patient is thinking about change

        i. Give pamphlets about the problem

        ii. Suggest an abstinence trial

    c. If the patient is ready to change

        i. Reinforce and praise the decision

        ii. Remind the patient that the most common error is to underestimate the help needed to quit

        iii. Give support options (eg, Alcoholics Anonymous [www.aa.org], Substance Abuse Treatment Facility Locator [findtreatment.samhsa.gov], Self-Management and Recovery Training [www.smartrecovery.org], The Self-Help Sourcebook Online [www.mentalhelp.net/selfhelp])

        iv. Consider pharmacotherapy

Data from Samet JH, Rollnick S, Barnes H. Beyond CAGE: A brief clinical approach after detection of substance abuse. Arch Intern Med. 1996 Nov 11;156(20):2287-93.

Marijuana is the most commonly used illegal drug in the United States, with 6% of the population older than 12 years reporting use in the past month. An increasing body of evidence suggests that marijuana increases the risk of the development of schizophrenia. Heavy use also increases the risk of chronic lung diseases. Cocaine is used by less than 1% of the population, and heroin and methamphetamine are used by even fewer people; however, they are associated with considerable risk of addiction and undesirable health and societal outcomes.

A number of screening tests are available for illegal drug use, but their use in primary care settings has been insufficiently tested. Most tests are modeled after alcohol screening tests. The USPSTF indicates that the evidence is insufficient to recommend screening of any population for illegal drug use. However, the American Academy of Pediatrics and the Guidelines for Adolescent Preventive Services both recommend that adolescents be screened for

Box 9 Questions for Adolescent Substance Abuse (CRAFFT Questionnaire)[a]

1. Have you ever ridden in a *car* driven by someone (including yourself) who was high or had been using alcohol or drugs?

2. Do you use alcohol or drugs to *relax*, feel better about yourself, or fit in?

3. Do you ever use alcohol or drugs while you are *alone*?

4. Do you ever *forget* things you did while using alcohol or drugs?

5. Do your *family or friends* ever tell you that you should cut down on your drinking or drug use?

6. Have you ever gotten into *trouble* while you were using alcohol or drugs?

[a] Two or more affirmative answers should prompt further questioning.
Adapted from Knight JR, Sherritt L, Shrier LA, Harris SK, Change G. Validity of the CRAFFT substance abuse screening test among adolescent clinic patients. Arch Pediatr Adol Med 2002;156:607-14. Used with permission.

illegal drug use. The **CRAFFT questionnaire** is recommended for screening adolescents (Box 9; "CRAFFT" is a mnemonic based on the screening questions [ridden in a car, to relax, while alone, did forget, asked by family, get in trouble]).

Much of the treatment of illegal drug use is similar to that for alcohol abuse. Self-help groups include Narcotics Anonymous and Cocaine Anonymous. Behavioral interventions such as brief motivational counseling have been beneficial for marijuana use in short-term studies. Buprenorphine has been shown to help opiate abuse in short-term studies.

- Short-term benefits have been demonstrated for early recognition and treatment of illegal drug use.
- Screening tests and treatment for illegal drug use are similar to those for alcohol abuse.

SUGGESTED READING

The Agency for Health Care Policy and Research Smoking Cessation Clinical Practice Guideline. JAMA. 1996 Apr 24;275(16):1270-80.

Agency for Healthcare Research and Quality [Internet]. Rockville (MD): AHRQ; US Preventive Services Task Force, The Guide to Clinical Preventive Services, Recommendations of the United States Preventive Service Task Force; [cited Aug 2009]. Available from: www.ahrq.gov/CLINIC/USpstfix.htm.

Green LW, Kreuter MW. Health promotion planning: an educational and ecological approach. 3rd ed. Mountain View (CA): Mayfield Pub. Co.; c1999.

Holmes P, Holmes P. Out of the ashes: help for people who have stopped smoking. Minneapolis (MN): Deaconess Press; c1992.

Kotter JP. Leading change. Boston (MA): Harvard Business School Press; c1996.

Prochaska JO, Velicer WF. The transtheoretical model of health behavior change. Am J Health Promot. 1997 Sep-Oct;12(1):38-48.

Rogers EM. Diffusion of innovations. 3rd ed. New York (NY): Free Press; c1983.

Thompson WG, Lande RG, Kalapatapu RK. Alcoholism. e-medicine. Available from: http://emedicine.medscape.com/article/285913-overview.

Questions and Answers

Questions

1. When a patient is asked if he is interested in quitting smoking, he replies, "I haven't thought much about it; I like my cigarettes and just don't see why I should bother." The most appropriate response is:
   a. "I really think you should quit smoking. Would you like to work together to set a specific date on which you will quit?"
   b. "I recommend you quit smoking. Quitting will save you a lot of money in the end, will lower your risk of cancer and heart disease, and will decrease these same risks in your wife and children. I'd be happy to help if you change your mind."
   c. "I don't think that's a very smart choice. Smoking is killing you and your family. I'm going to schedule you to visit a nicotine dependence counselor."
   d. "Well, that's your choice. But in case you want it, here's a prescription for some nicotine gum."

2. A patient comes to her appointment saying she would like to stop smoking. Which is the best response to her request?
   a. "Let's work together to set a specific date on which you will quit."
   b. "Quitting smoking will save you a lot of money in the end and will lower your risk of heart disease."
   c. "That's great. Remember, if you relapse and start again, you run the risk of cancer, lung disease, and heart disease."
   d. "That's great. Remember, people who quit smoking often gain some weight."

3. Which of the following is true about combination therapy with nicotine patch and gum?
   a. Combining a nicotine patch with nicotine gum is contraindicated
   b. Nicotine patch dosing should be reduced if the patient starts using the gum regularly
   c. Evidence suggests that it is more effective than monotherapy for heavy smokers
   d. The patch should be stopped first, and then the gum can be slowly tapered off

4. What is the most accurate screening test for alcohol abuse?
   a. Mean corpuscular volume of red blood cells
   b. CAGE questionnaire (cutting down, annoyance by criticism, guilty feeling, and eye-openers)
   c. Gamma glutamyl transferase
   d. Alcohol Use Disorders Identification Test (AUDIT)
   e. Blood alcohol level

5. Which of the following statements is *incorrect* about Alcoholics Anonymous (AA)?
   a. Women should be encouraged to attend women-only meetings
   b. AA meetings are available in most locations and are free
   c. If a person has been to an AA meeting and not liked it, they should not be encouraged to try a different AA meeting
   d. Patients should be encouraged to attend meetings regularly and for an extended period of time
   e. AA will provide a sponsor to those in need who serve as mentors to new members

6. In the PRECEDE/PROCEED model of behavior change, social support is considered:
   a. A demographic factor
   b. A predisposing factor
   c. An enabling factor
   d. A reinforcing factor
   e. A community factor

Answers

1. **Answer b.**
This patient is in the precontemplation phase, and the goal should be to move the patient to contemplation. This patient needs to better understand the reasons for quitting. Setting a quit date or giving a prescription for nicotine gum is premature.

2. **Answer a.**
This patient is in the action phase. Rather than receiving more information on why she should stop smoking, she needs to set a quit date. The issue of weight gain does need to be addressed, but it should be discussed later to avoid discouraging the patient before she gets started. The physician could ask the patient what concerns she has about stopping and address weight gain if that is mentioned.

3. **Answer c.**
The patch and gum can be used concurrently. Generally, the gum is an adjunct to the patch. Addiction to the gum is more common than addiction to the patch, so the gum should be tapered and stopped before the patch is discontinued.

4. **Answer d.**
Laboratory tests have <50% sensitivity for the diagnosis of alcohol abuse. The CAGE questionnaire was previously the standard screening method; however, several studies have now shown the superiority of the AUDIT, particularly in populations with a lower prevalence of alcoholism and for the detection of binge drinking and hazardous drinking.

5. **Answer c.**
Patients should be encouraged to attend at least 5 different group meetings to find one with which they are compatible.

6. **Answer d.**
Social support is a crucial reinforcing factor. Demographic factors include age, sex, and other characteristics. Predisposing factors are motivational (eg, does the person believe change is necessary?; does he think he is able to do it?). Enabling factors are facilitators or barriers such as the cost of treatment. Community is not a separate factor in the model.

6

INFECTIOUS DISEASES

Salma Iftikhar, MD; Mary Jo Kasten, MD; and Zelalem Temesgen, MD

Infectious diseases account for 19% of all physician encounters and close to 130 million ambulatory care visits in the United States annually. Common infections include upper respiratory tract infection, urinary tract infection (UTI), sexually transmitted illness (STI), and enteric infections; these infections are the most frequent reasons for adult office visits. Common infectious diseases with public health significance are described in this chapter. Non–travel-related immunization is an important component of infectious disease prevention and is reviewed in Chapter 7.

Infectious Diarrhea

Infectious diarrhea is a major public health issue that accounts for nearly 28 million office visits and about 2 million hospitalizations annually in the United States. Diarrhea can be caused by direct invasion of the infecting organism or by a toxin produced by the organism. Syndromes can vary from diarrhea alone to diarrhea associated with vomiting, fever, and prostration.

Although recent antibiotic use or hospitalization can raise clinical suspicion for *Clostridium difficile* infection, the usual transmission of infectious diarrhea is through contaminated food or water. For example, *Escherichia coli* O157-H7 is suspected in patients with a history of consumption of undercooked ground beef or potentially contaminated fruits and vegetables. A recent history of travel is suggestive of *Salmonella*, *Campylobacter*, *Giardia*, or *Shigella* infection.

Viral enteritis is most common in children, but adults are not always immune. Outbreaks of viral diarrheal illness

such as Norwalk virus have occurred on cruise ships. Table 1 describes details of common diarrheal diseases and their treatment. Preventive measures for all diarrheal illness are described in Box 1.

- Infectious diarrhea is caused by direct invasion of the infecting organism or by a toxin produced by the organism.
- The usual method of transmission is through contaminated food or water.

Infective Endocarditis

Degenerative valvular disease, male sex, and age greater than 65 years are all risk factors for **native-valve** infective endocarditis. The most commonly affected valves are the mitral and aortic valves. Patients with mitral valve prolapse, bicuspid aortic valve, and aortic sclerosis are predisposed to infective endocarditis; patients with prosthetic valves are especially at risk. Common organisms that cause infective endocarditis include the viridans-group streptococci (30% to 40%), enterococci (15%), and coagulase-negative *Staphylococcus aureus* (25%). **Prosthetic-valve** infective endocarditis occurs more frequently in aortic valves than in mitral valves. *S aureus* and coagulase-negative *S aureus* typically are the causative agents.

A first-generation cephalosporin is the most commonly used antibiotic, but physicians should be mindful of antibiotic susceptibility patterns at their hospitals. For example, a high prevalence of infection by methicillin-resistant

Table 1 Common Diarrheal Illnesses

Causative Agent	Incubation Period	Mechanism of Transmission	Method of Confirming Diagnosis	Treatment
Escherichia coli O157:H7	1-8 d	Contaminated food (eg, under-cooked meat, raw fruit, milk)	Stool culture on special media	Supportive management only[a]
Shigella spp.	24-48 h	Person-to-person; contaminated food	Stool culture	Self limited; can use fluoroquinolones
Salmonella, non-*typhi*	1-3 d	Contaminated food (eg, unpas-teurized eggs, dairy products)	Stool culture	Self limited; in disseminated disease, use fluoroquinolones
Rotavirus	1-3 d	Fecally contaminated food	Stool immunoassay	Supportive management
Vibrio cholerae	1-3 d	Contaminated food and water[b]	Stool culture on special medium	Mainstay support is rehydration treatment (severe dehydration can occur within hours); tetracycline can shorten excretion
Clostridium difficile	1-7 d	Infection usually occurs after antibiotic use	*C difficile* toxin in stool	Oral metronidazole; oral vancomycin is preferred for severe disease
Cryptosporidium parvum[c]	1-7 d	Contaminated water; contaminated swimming pool	*Cryptosporidium* antigen test	Supportive management

[a] Can cause hemolytic uremic syndrome in children.
[b] Often associated with areas with poor sanitary conditions (eg, refugee camps) and areas in underdeveloped countries.
[c] Can cause severe illness in patients with acquired immune deficiency syndrome.

S aureus should prompt consideration of the use of vanco-mycin for perioperative prophylaxis. Recent changes in the American Heart Association guidelines suggest that only high-risk patients require prophylactic antibiotics with dental procedures (Box 2). No prophylaxis is required for genitourinary or gastroenterology procedures.

- Infective endocarditis can occur with native and prosthetic valves.
- Current guidelines suggest prophylactic antibiotics only for high-risk patients undergoing dental procedures.

Meningitis

The most common pathogens that cause bacterial meningitis are *Streptococcus pneumoniae*, *Haemophilus influenzae*,

Box 1 Preventive Measures for Diarrheal Illness

Avoid consuming undercooked meats, poultry, or seafood

Wash and peel fruits; avoid unpasteurized dairy products

Avoid consuming raw eggs

Drink bottled or boiled water during travel to developing countries or when contamination of the water supply is suspected

Avoid use of swimming pools if having diarrhea or when sanitization procedures are suspect

Use strict hand washing practices

Use alcohol hand sanitizers

Listeria monocytogenes, and *Neisseria meningitidis*. Less commonly, *E coli* and group B streptococcus are causative agents. **Community-acquired meningitis** is observed in patients with risk factors such as alcoholism, pneumonia, otitis media, sinusitis, diabetes mellitus, and cerebrospi-nal fluid (CSF) leaks. Clinical features include fever, altered mental status, and nuchal rigidity. CSF examination shows

Box 2 Cardiac Conditions Associated With the Highest Risk of Adverse Outcome From Endocarditis for Which Prophylaxis With Dental Procedures Is Reasonable

Prosthetic cardiac valve or prosthetic material used for cardiac valve repair

Previous infective endocarditis

Congenital heart disease[a]

 Unrepaired cyanotic CHD, including palliative shunts and conduits

 Completely repaired congenital heart defect with prosthetic material or device, whether placed by surgery or by catheter intervention, during the first 6 months after the procedure[b]

 Repaired CHD with residual defects that inhibit endothelialization at the site or adjacent to the site of a prosthetic patch or prosthetic device

Cardiac transplantation recipients with cardiac valvulopathy

Abbreviation: CHD, congenital heart disease.
[a] Except for the conditions listed above, antibiotic prophylaxis is no longer recommended for any other form of CHD.
[b] Prophylaxis is reasonable because endothelialization of prosthetic material occurs within 6 months after the procedure.
Adapted from Wilson et al (2007). Used with permission.

increased white cell count and decreased glucose (<40 mg/dL). Cultures are not always positive (positive in >70% of cases).

Treatment usually begins with a broad-spectrum antibiotic when meningitis is suspected. This should include coverage for *L monocytogenes*. Generally, high-dose ampicillin plus gentamicin can be used initially. Some studies have shown benefit with dexamethasone at the start of antibiotic treatment. It is administered intravenously (0.15 mg/kg), 15 minutes before the first dose of antibiotics, and every 6 hours thereafter for 2 to 4 days. Antibiotics can be tailored subsequent to the identification of the specific infectious organism.

Although **meningococcal meningitis** can occur in healthy individuals, it can be recurrent in individuals with terminal complement deficiency. It can present with complications such as Waterhouse-Friderichsen syndrome, which presents as disseminated intravascular coagulation and adrenal hemorrhage.

Immunization with either the polysaccharide or the conjugate vaccine is recommended for certain high-risk populations such as military recruits, Hajj pilgrims, asplenic patients, and patients with terminal complement deficiency. The vaccination is also recommended for postexposure prophylaxis and for prophylaxis during outbreaks. Close contacts should receive chemoprophylaxis with rifampin, cefotaxime, or ciprofloxacin. Chemoprophylaxis should also be given to nasopharyngeal carriers of *N meningitidis*.

- Recurrent meningococcal meningitis can occur in individuals with terminal complement deficiency.
- Immunization is recommended for certain high-risk populations.

Respiratory Infection

Respiratory infections account for greater than 35 million office and emergency department visits yearly and are a major cause of work days lost. Viruses cause most of these infections, but bacterial infections, including primary and secondary pneumonias, can be a clinically significant cause of morbidity.

Influenza

Influenza accounts for up to 20,000 deaths annually in the United States. Influenza **type A and B viruses** (orthomixoviruses) are the most common causes of influenza outbreaks, affecting 10% to 20% of the US population yearly. Diagnosis is established through polymerase chain reaction (PCR) assays of nasal swab samples or by culturing respiratory secretions. Elderly patients are at greater risk of death because of complications such as primary interstitial desquamative pneumonia or secondary bacterial pneumonia caused by *S pneumoniae*, *H influenzae*, or *S aureus*.

Influenza viruses are constantly changing, primarily through **antigenic drift**, a process in which a point mutation leads to variation in one of the influenza antigens. Immunity to key surface antigens, particularly the hemagglutinin and neuraminidase antigens, reduces the likelihood of infection and the seriousness of disease if it occurs. Changes in the virus caused by antigenic drift are usually mild, and substantial immunity usually exists to the new strain within a population with exposure to similar previous strains. **Antigenic shift**, the genetic reassortment between human and animal or avian strains, is a less common phenomenon but results in major changes in the virus. Immunity may be completely lacking, and the new virus has the potential to cause a pandemic. Influenza type B infects only humans and therefore is incapable of undergoing shift.

Prevention of influenza is best accomplished by **vaccination**. From November through January, use of an inactivated, trivalent vaccine (administered intramuscularly) or a live, attenuated-virus vaccine (administered intranasally) can provide immunity for several months. More details on influenza vaccination and chemoprophylaxis are provided in Chapter 7. Because virus transmission is through exposure to droplet nuclei, care should be taken to isolate symptomatic individuals; spread can also be limited by frequent hand washing and by avoiding the sharing of common household items, especially hand towels.

In 1997, a highly pathogenic influenza A subtype (H5N1) caused **avian influenza** outbreaks in poultry and, subsequently, the first described human infection. More human outbreaks have occurred since the initial report; the most recent outbreak in 2006 was largely restricted to Southeast Asia and had 232 confirmed human cases and 134 deaths. The infection results in rapid onset of symptoms and quick progression to respiratory failure. Diagnosis can be made by using a rapid antigen test; although PCR assays are more sensitive, they are less easily available. Treatment with oseltamivir or zanamivir should be administered, preferably within 48 hours of illness onset. Preventive measures include avoiding close contact with live poultry, proper hygiene when handling live poultry, and proper cooking of poultry products.

Severe Acute Respiratory Syndrome

Severe acute respiratory syndrome (SARS) was first described in 2002 in the Guangdong province of China. Infection is caused by a **coronavirus**, now named the SARS-associated coronavirus. The disease is highly contagious, and transmission is through **droplet exposure**. Infection is suspected clinically in individuals presenting with fever and a history of exposure through contact or travel to areas of documented transmission. Symptoms include fever, headache, dry cough, myalgias, and dyspnea. Patients may have rapid progression to respiratory failure and death.

Diagnosis is made through serum antibody and PCR assays. Infected individuals must be isolated, and standard infection control processes are used by individuals caring for the infected patient. Control measures include good hand hygiene and use of gown, gloves, mask, and eye protection. No specific treatment is available currently; symptomatic management is recommended. General respiratory disease prevention is recommended because the syndrome has not shown a tendency to spread. As of this writing, more than 1 year has passed since the last case was reported.

Bacterial Respiratory Infection

Bacterial respiratory infections include bronchitis, pharyngitis, sinusitis, otitis media, and pneumonia. Common agents of infection are *H influenzae*, group A streptococci, and *S pneumoniae*. Infection can be spread from person to person or can occur as a complication after viral infection in susceptible persons. Upper and lower respiratory tract infections are common complications of influenza; this underscores the importance of efforts toward prevention, early detection, and treatment of influenza. Another complication in the treatment of bacterial respiratory infections is the widespread use of antibiotics, which has resulted in resistant strains and greater difficulty in treatment.

Throat culture for rapid streptococcal antigen detection can be used for early identification of streptococcal pharyngitis. Treatment of streptococcal pharyngitis with penicillin, erythromycin, or cephalosporins is aimed at prevention of rheumatic fever and its complications. Treatment with antibiotics for 48 hours renders patients noninfectious and free to return to school or work. Individuals with repeated streptococcal pharyngitis should consider tonsillectomy, which often reduces recurrence. Prevention is by strict hand washing practices. Confinement of infected individuals may decrease person-to-person spread.

Acute Sinusitis

Acute sinusitis accounts for 25 million office visits per year. It is usually difficult to distinguish between viral and bacterial sinusitis. Treatment with antibiotics should be restricted to patients whose symptoms have lasted longer than a week and to those with facial pain, fever, and mucopurulent nasal discharge. Symptomatic treatment with decongestants and steam inhalation is recommended for most patients with acute sinusitis.

Pneumonia

In the United States, the mortality rate attributable to pneumococcal pneumonia is 150,000 to 600,000 cases per year and accounts for 12% to 60% of all pneumonia cases. Other agents known to cause pneumonia are *Klebsiella pneumoniae*, *H influenzae*, *Pseudomonas aeruginosa*, *Moraxella catarrhalis*, and *S aureus*. Atypical pneumonia is caused by *Legionella* spp, *Coxiella burnetii*, *Chlamydia psittaci*, *Chlamydia pneumoniae*, and *Francisella tularensis*.

However, a specific pathogen may not be identified in more than 50% of cases.

Community-acquired pneumonia is defined as an acute infection of the pulmonary parenchyma in a patient who has acquired the infection in the community rather than in the hospital (nosocomial pneumonia). It causes considerable morbidity and mortality. North American treatment guidelines for community-acquired pneumonia are shown in Table 2. **Nosocomial pneumonia** is a common reason for prolonged hospital stays.

Prevention of pneumonia is facilitated by applying strict hand washing techniques, following cough etiquette, and containing and disposing secretions quickly and efficiently. Pneumococcal vaccination is indicated in those older than 65 years; this subject is further reviewed in Chapter 7.

- Vaccination is the most effective preventive measure against influenza.
- Severe acute respiratory syndrome (SARS) can have rapid progression to respiratory failure and death; no specific treatment is available currently.
- Bacterial infections in the upper and lower respiratory tract are common complications of influenza.
- Good hand hygiene can limit the spread of many respiratory infections, including pneumonia.
- Widespread use of antibiotics has resulted in resistant bacterial strains and greater difficulty in treatment.

Table 2 North American Treatment Guidelines for Community-Acquired Pneumonia

Disease Severity[a]	Recommended Treatment
Mild (outpatient)	Macrolide or doxycycline, antipneumococcal fluoroquinolone
	OR
	High-dose amoxicillin (3 g/d) or high-dose amoxicillin-clavulanate (4 g/d) plus macrolide
Serious (hospitalized, non-ICU)	Ceftriaxone, cefotaxime, ampicillin-sulbactam, or ertapenem plus macrolide[b]
	OR
	Antipneumococcal fluoroquinolone alone
Severe (hospitalized, ICU)	(Ceftriaxone, cefotaxime, or ampicillin-sulbactam) plus IV azithromycin or IV fluoroquinolone

Abbreviations: ICU, intensive care unit; IV, intravenously administered.

[a] If *Pseudomonas* infection is a concern (eg, patient has structural lung disease such as bronchiectasis), treatment with an antipseudomonal agent (piperacillin-tazobactam, imipenem, meropenem, or cefepime) plus an antipseudomonal fluoroquinolone (ciprofloxacin or high-dose levofloxacin) is recommended.

[b] Doxycycline can be used if the macrolide is not tolerated.

Urinary Tract Infection

UTIs account for more than 8,000,000 visits per year to physicians in the United States (mostly for cystitis). UTI-related hospital admissions, primarily for pyelonephritis, are estimated at 100,000 per year (with an estimated cost exceeding $1 billion per year).

Microbial colonization of the urinary tract often occurs in institutionalized patients, patients with spinal cord injuries, and patients with chronic indwelling catheters. Causative organisms are most commonly *E coli*, *Staphylococcus saprophyticus* (a coagulase-negative staphylococcus), *Proteus mirabilis*, and *K pneumoniae*. Cultures and antibiotic sensitivity testing are required if an STI is suspected clinically or if the UTI is complicated with systemic symptoms or shows evidence of upper urinary tract involvement. Screening and treatment for patients with **asymptomatic bacteriuria** is not usually recommended, except for pregnant women and patients about to undergo transurethral procedures. For symptomatic UTI in pregnancy, urine cultures should always be obtained before treatment; cultures should be repeated 2 weeks after treatment.

Some women are prone to **recurrent UTI**; known risk factors include sexual activity, use of spermicidal gels, estrogen deficiency, diabetes mellitus, cystocele, incontinence, and impaired voiding. For patients who are prone to postcoital UTI, attention to hygiene, voiding before and after intercourse, and liberal fluid intake is usually enough to decrease the frequency of attacks.

Uncomplicated UTIs can be treated with increased fluid intake and a short course of antibiotics. Three-day treatment is favored because it is as effective as longer courses and is associated with fewer adverse effects. Any of the following antibiotic regimens are good options: 1) double-strength trimethoprim-sulfamethoxazole, twice daily for 3 days; 2) trimethoprim, 100 mg, twice daily for 3 days; or 3) nitrofurantoin, 100 mg, 3 times daily for 3 days. Ofloxacin and ciprofloxacin can also be used for treatment of UTIs, but these are relatively expensive and their use fuels concern about future quinolone resistance.

If symptoms persist or recur within 2 weeks, urine cultures should be repeated and antibiotic sensitivities checked; the patient should then be treated for 7 days with an effective agent. Prophylactic antibiotics can be considered for women with recurrent symptoms. Continuous prophylaxis has been advocated if 2 or more symptomatic UTIs occur during a 6-month period, despite documented eradication of infection. Effective prophylactic regimens include nitrofurantoin (50 mg, daily), trimethoprim-sulfamethoxazole (3 times weekly), or oral fluoroquinolone (daily or 3 times weekly). Postmenopausal women with frequent UTI may benefit from local (vaginal) estrogen. Probiotic agents, cranberry juice, and lactobacillus vaginal suppositories have shown mixed results in prophylaxis.

- Treatment of urinary tract infection (UTI) is not recommended unless the infection is symptomatic. Only pregnant women and patients about to undergo transurethral procedures should be screened and treated.
- Uncomplicated UTIs can be treated with increased fluid intake and a short, 3-day course of antibiotics.
- Continuous prophylaxis is advocated if 2 or more symptomatic UTIs occur during a 6-month period.

Tick-Borne Infection

Tick-borne infection is caused by transmission of microorganisms from their natural reservoirs through a tick bite. Ticks transmit the microorganisms during a blood meal when they regurgitate or defecate. The risk of infection is proportional to the density of ticks and the prevalence of infected ticks in the area. Infections transmitted by ticks include Rocky Mountain spotted fever, ehrlichiosis, Lyme disease, babesiosis, tularemia, tick-borne relapsing fever, leptospirosis, Q fever, and leishmaniasis.

Tick bites themselves are often asymptomatic; as many as 50% of patients with tick-borne infections do not recall a bite. The clinical manifestations of tick-borne infections are myriad and usually nonspecific. They range from fever, rash, joint pain, and neurologic symptoms. It is important to have a high index of clinical suspicion and to initiate appropriate diagnostic and therapeutic measures promptly for optimal outcome. Diagnostic tests for tick-borne infections are primarily serologic and PCR based.

Tick-borne infections are best prevented by avoiding exposure to vector ticks. When exposure is unavoidable, personal protective measures such as protective clothing, tick repellent (on skin and clothing), regular examination of the body for ticks, and prompt removal of attached ticks are important. After a tick bite has been recognized, the routine use of antimicrobial prophylaxis or serologic testing of asymptomatic patients in an attempt to prevent the development of disease is not recommended. In areas where the tick infection rate is at least 20%, a single dose of doxycycline can be prescribed for prevention of Lyme disease if the following conditions are met: 1) the tick is reliably identified as an adult or nymphal *Ixodes scapularis* tick, 2) the tick is estimated to have been attached for at least 36 hours, and 3) prophylaxis can be started within 72 hours of tick removal.

- The risk of infection is proportional to the density of ticks and the prevalence of infected ticks in the area.
- Tick bites themselves are often asymptomatic, and the clinical manifestations of tick-borne infections are myriad and usually nonspecific.
- Routine prophylaxis after a bite is not recommended. In some cases, a single dose of doxycycline can be prescribed for prevention of Lyme disease.

Tuberculosis

Primary tuberculosis (TB) usually occurs in children or immunocompromised individuals and is due to proliferation of mycobacteria. It can present as pneumonitis, with infiltrates or pleural effusion on chest radiographs. The more classic form of TB in adults is **reactivation TB**. This is increasing in prevalence in recent years because of AIDS and greater use of immunosuppressive medications. TB is the most common human immunodeficiency virus (HIV)–associated **opportunistic infection** (OI) in the world; it accounts for up to one-third of AIDS deaths worldwide. TB has an adverse effect on HIV progression. Similarly, HIV favors the acquisition of TB and accelerates the progression of TB from latent to active disease. The risk of reactivation of TB in patients with HIV is approximately 10% higher per year compared with a lifetime risk for reactivation in patients without HIV infection. Almost 26% of adult TB cases in the United States may be attributable to HIV infection.

Screening for latent TB infection is recommended for individuals with high risk of TB development, either through recent exposure or because of reactivation risk. A positive TB skin test should prompt chest radiography to exclude the diagnosis of active TB. **Prophylactic treatment** of latent TB is a 9-month course of isoniazid. Prophylaxis is indicated for patients with latent TB shown by a positive skin test (induration after exposure to purified protein derivative of *Mycobacterium tuberculosis*). Patients with induration smaller than 5 mm typically are children younger than 5 years, patients with HIV infection, and immunosuppressed patients with history of contact. An induration of 5 to 10 mm is observed in patients with HIV infection, organ transplant recipients, immunosuppressed patients, patients with recent contact with active TB, and patients with chest radiographs showing fibrotic changes (indicative of past infection). Induration larger than 10 mm is observed in recent TB skin test converters, HIV-negative injection drug users, high-risk persons (eg, health care providers), nursing home residents and caregivers, recent immigrants, children younger than 4 years, or persons exposed to high-risk or confirmed-active TB cases.

Bacille Calmette-Guèrin vaccination has been used in developing countries for prophylaxis against TB. However, it is not very effective; studies have shown an efficacy of 0% to 60%. It is typically understood that Bacille Calmette-Guèrin vaccine has minimal impact on TB skin test results. More recently, the blood test QuantiFERON TB Gold increasingly is used for ascertainment of diagnosis of latent TB.

Direct observed therapy can increase or guarantee patient compliance and reduce risk of resistance after intermittent dosing. Emergent multidrug-resistant strains are making treatment even more challenging, even as *Mycobacterium* TB resurges because of HIV, AIDS, and increasing immigrant populations. Patients with multidrug-resistant disease should be referred to experts for management. **Extensively drug-resistant (XDR) TB** has been recently reported from various parts of the world. XDR TB is defined as TB that is resistant to isoniazid, rifampin, any fluoroquinolone, and at least 1 of 3 injectable second-line drugs (capreomycin, kanamycin, and amikacin). HIV-infected persons are more likely to have TB development after they are infected, and with TB disease, they also have a higher risk of death.

- Tuberculosis (TB) presents as pneumonitis, with infiltrates or pleural effusion on chest radiographs.
- TB is the opportunistic infection most commonly associated with AIDS and accounts for up to one-third of AIDS deaths worldwide.
- Isoniazid generally is used for prophylactic treatment of patients with latent TB infection, but extensively drug-resistant TB (XDR TB) is now reported in many parts of the world.

Sexually Transmitted Illness

HIV is the STI that provokes the most fear and has caused the most serious illness and premature death during the past 4 decades. Many other STIs increase the risk of acquiring or transmitting HIV and can have serious long-term consequences such as infertility, delivery of an ill or stillborn infant, neurologic sequelae, cancer, and premature death.

Human Immunodeficiency Virus

Nearly 3 decades have passed since AIDS was first described. During this period, the relentless progression of HIV/AIDS from a handful of cases in select areas and populations to every region and country in the world has resulted in the continually increasing number of people affected by HIV. The latest report from the World Health Organization estimates that approximately 33 million people are living with HIV. More than 25 million have died of AIDS. More than 90% of all people living with HIV reside in developing countries where resources for diagnosis, prevention, and management of diseases are scarce.

HIV is a **lentivirus**, a member of the retrovirus family. Retroviridae are a large family of ubiquitous viruses that infect all classes of vertebrates. All retroviridae encode a unique **reverse transcriptase enzyme** that copies viral genetic information from RNA to DNA; this reverse-transcribed DNA is then integrated into the host cell genome. Two genetically distinct types of HIV have been identified, HIV-1 and HIV-2. HIV-1 is the predominant HIV type globally, whereas HIV-2 is found predominantly in Western Africa. HIV-1 is further classified into subtypes (ie, clades). In the United States, 98% of HIV is classified as HIV-1 clade B. Transmission is through a number of routes, including sexual, perinatal, parenteral inoculation (intravenous drug injection, occupational exposure), and through blood products (0.5 per 10,000) and donated organs.

The most commonly used screening test for HIV is the enzyme-linked immunosorbent assay (ELISA). A positive reaction should prompt a repeat of the screening test in duplicate. ELISA has high sensitivity and specificity (>99.97% for both) but has low predictive value in populations with a low prevalence of HIV. Therefore, positive results require verification and confirmation with an additional test. Western blots are most commonly used to confirm the diagnosis of HIV. More recently, rapid HIV tests can be performed using oral fluid, finger stick, or venipuncture sample, with sensitivities and specificities similar to those of ELISA. It does not require sophisticated laboratory equipment or highly trained technicians; results are available in minutes, making HIV testing feasible at the point of care (eg, emergency departments, STI clinics, physician offices, etc).

The introduction of **highly active antiretroviral therapy**, a treatment paradigm with concurrent use of 3 or more antiretroviral medications, has led to marked declines in HIV-associated morbidity and mortality. Currently, 22 antiretroviral medications are approved by the US Food and Drug Administration. They are classified into 6 categories on the basis of their mechanism of action: 1) nucleoside or nucleotide analogue reverse transcriptase inhibitors, 2) nonnucleoside analogue reverse transcriptase inhibitors, 3) protease inhibitors, 4) fusion inhibitors, 5) integrase inhibitors, and 6) chemokine receptor *CCR5* antagonists. Box 3 shows some of the medications in the various classes.

AIDS-defining clinical conditions, as established by the Centers for Disease Control and Prevention, are listed in Box 4. The US Department of Health and Human Services (DHHS) guidelines recommend antiretroviral therapy for all patients with a history of an AIDS-defining illness or severe symptoms of HIV infection, regardless of CD4+ T-cell count. The recommendation of when to start antiretroviral therapy in asymptomatic patients is more problematic; it is determined by the likelihood of the development of AIDS-defining illnesses or death.

Current DHHS guidelines recommend initiating antiretroviral therapy in patients with fewer than 350 CD4+ T-cells/mm³ who are otherwise asymptomatic. Although the incidence and prevalence of HIV-associated OIs and conditions have declined markedly, these infections and conditions continue to occur.

Several approaches are used to prevent OIs in patients infected with HIV. When the level of CD4+ T cells falls below the threshold for the respective OI, chemoprophylaxis should be started. If an OI occurs, specific treatment against the causative agents in conjunction with antiretroviral therapy is indicated. In most instances, treatment of

Box 3 Antiretroviral Medications

Nucleoside reverse transcriptase inhibitors

  Zidovudine

  Didanosine

  Stavudine

  Lamivudine

  Abacavir

  Tenofovir

  Emtricitabine

Nonnucleoside reverse transcriptase inhibitors

  Nevirapine

  Efavirenz

  Delavirdine

Protease inhibitors

  Saquinavir

  Indinavir

  Ritonavir

  Nelfinavir

  Lopinavir/ritonavir

  Atazanavir

  Fosamprenavir

  Tipranavir

  Darunavir

Fusion inhibitor

  Enfuvirtide

Integrase inhibitor

  Raltegravir

CCR5 inhibitor

  Maraviroc

the OI continues until immune reconstitution occurs and a sustained increase in CD4+ cells (usually cell counts >200 cells/mm³) is observed for a certain period. Indications for initiation of treatment and recommended therapeutic agents to prevent a first episode of OI (ie, primary prophylaxis) in HIV-infected adults and adolescents are shown in Table 3.

Prevention of HIV Infection

A number of approaches have been proposed and explored for preventing new HIV infections. **Behavioral strategies** generally promote changes in high-risk behavior for individuals and societies through various educational programs. Common strategies include delaying the first sexual experience for adolescents; decreasing the number of sex partners (including sex workers); engaging in safer sexual

Box 4 AIDS-Defining Clinical Conditions

Burkitt lymphoma, immunoblastic or primary brain

Candidiasis of bronchi, trachea, or lungs

Candidiasis, esophageal

Cervical cancer, invasive

Coccidioidomycosis, disseminated or extrapulmonary

Cryptococcosis, extrapulmonary

Cryptosporidiosis, chronic intestinal (for longer than 1 mo)

Cytomegalovirus disease (other than liver, spleen, or lymph nodes)

Encephalopathy (HIV-related)

Herpes simplex, chronic ulcers (for longer than 1 mo); or bronchitis, pneumonitis, or esophagitis

Histoplasmosis, disseminated or extrapulmonary

Isosporiasis, chronic intestinal (for longer than 1 mo)

Kaposi sarcoma

Leukoencephalopathy, progressive multifocal

Mycobacterium avium complex

Mycobacterium, other species, disseminated or extrapulmonary

Pneumocystis jiroveci pneumonia (formerly *Pneumocystis carinii*)

Pneumonia, recurrent

Salmonella septicemia, recurrent

Toxoplasmosis of the brain

Tuberculosis

Wasting syndrome due to HIV

Abbreviation: HIV, human immunodeficiency virus.
Adapted from the Centers for Disease Control and Prevention. 1993 revised classification system for HIV infection and expanded surveillance case definition for AIDS among adolescents and adults. MMWR 1992;41(RR-17).

practices (eg, condom use); decreasing substance use and improving access to treatment programs; increasing access to clean needles and syringes; avoiding needle sharing; increasing knowledge about how HIV is transmitted and how to protect oneself; reducing stigma of HIV infection; and encouraging HIV testing and disclosure of HIV serostatus between partners. **Biomedical strategies** attempt to reduce HIV transmission through biomedical and technological approaches. These approaches include control of STIs such as herpes simplex infections through prompt diagnosis and treatment; male circumcision; microbicides; prevention of mother-to-child transmission; and postexposure prophylaxis. The best results for preventing HIV infection are obtained when these strategies are used in combination with behavioral strategies.

STIs can facilitate the transmission of HIV, particularly infections that cause genital ulcerative lesions such as herpes simplex virus (HSV), syphilis, and chancroid.

Numerous studies have explored strategies of reducing HIV transmission by controlling STIs, but they unfortunately have not yielded consistent results. Four studies conducted in Africa had investigated whether improved diagnosis and treatment of chancroid, syphilis, gonorrhea, chlamydia, and trichomonas infection resulted in reductions in HIV incidence. Only 1 reported reduced incidence of HIV infection. Chronic HSV-2 suppression with valacyclovir has been reported to decrease genital HIV shedding in 2 randomized clinical trials. However, no impact on the risk of HIV transmission was observed in 2 studies that investigated the effect of acyclovir on HIV transmission in persons infected with HSV-2.

A consistent **association between male circumcision and reduced risk of HIV infection** has been noted in a number of observational studies. This association has been confirmed by the results of 3 randomized clinical trials conducted in HIV-uninfected men in South Africa, Kenya, and Uganda. Male circumcision appears to have an approximately 60% protective effect on HIV transmission in heterosexual men. A similar protective effect of circumcision on HIV transmission in female partners of circumcised men or in men who have sex with men has not yet been observed.

The effects of microbicidal gels and creams (placed in the vagina or rectum before sexual intercourse) have been assessed in randomized clinical trials, but none appear to prevent or reduce HIV transmission. Other candidate products are still undergoing evaluation.

Efforts toward developing an AIDS vaccine are ongoing, but researchers have faced enormous difficulties, including the lack of a full understanding of the correlate for protective immunity against HIV and the wide genetic diversity of HIV. Numerous trials of candidate vaccines have been conducted worldwide. Earlier trials focused on the HIV envelope protein gp120. More recently, vaccines designed to stimulate T-cell responses have garnered attention. Unfortunately, no vaccine trial has reported a positive result. In fact, the recently halted STEP study showed an increased likelihood of becoming HIV-positive after vaccination.

One of the early successes of antiretroviral therapy had been the dramatic decline in **perinatal transmission of HIV**. By implementing recommendations for universal prenatal HIV counseling and testing, antiretroviral prophylaxis, scheduled cesarean delivery, and avoidance of breastfeeding, the transmission rate of perinatal HIV infection has dramatically diminished to less than 2% in the United States. The Pediatric AIDS Clinical Trial Group Protocol 076 showed that zidovudine, administered to the mother during the antepartum and intrapartum periods and to the newborn for the first 6 weeks of life, reduces the perinatal transmission of HIV by two-thirds. HIV-positive women who receive antiretroviral treatment during the first trimester of pregnancy should continue the same therapy as long as it effectively suppresses viral replication.

Table 3 Primary Prophylaxis of Opportunistic Disease in Adults and Adolescents Infected With Human Immunodeficiency Virus[a]

Pathogen	Indication for Initiation of Prophylaxis	First Treatment Choice	Alternative Treatment
Hepatitis A virus	Antihepatitis A virus–negative and increased risk of chronic liver disease (B-III)	Hepatitis A vaccine, 2 doses (B-III)	. . .
Hepatitis B virus	Antihepatitis B core antigen–negative (B-II)	Hepatitis B vaccine, 3 doses (B-III)	. . .
Influenza virus	All patients annually (B-II)	Inactivated trivalent influenza virus vaccine	Oseltamivir or zanamavir
Mycobacterium avium complex	≥50 CD4+ cells/mm³ (A-I)	Azithromycin (A-I) OR Clarithromycin	Rifabutin (B-I) OR Rifabutin and azithromycin (C-I)
Mycobacterium tuberculosis	Contact with an active diseased person; tuberculin skin test reaction >5 mm; prior positive tuberculin skin test reaction without treatment	INH and pyridoxine for 9 mo (A-II)	Rifampicin (B-II) or rifabutin for 4 mo (C-III)
INH resistant	. . .	Rifampicin (A-III) for 4 mo OR Rifabutin (B-III) for 4 mo	. . .
Multidrug resistant	. . .	Choice of medication depends on results of susceptibility testing	. . .

Abbreviation: INH, isoniazid.

[a] Parenthetical text indicates the strength and quality of the recommendation. Strength of the recommendation is classified as follows: A, strong; B, usually offered; C, use is optional. Quality of the recommendation is classified as follows: I, evidence from ≥1 randomized and controlled trial; II, evidence from ≥1 controlled trial; III, opinion of experts.

Adapted from Knoll et al (2007). Used with permission.

However, efavirenz (a known teratogen) should be avoided during the first trimester. Otherwise, pregnant women with untreated HIV infection who meet standard adult antiretroviral treatment criteria for initiation of antiretroviral therapy should receive standard antiretroviral therapy. Those who do not require treatment for their own health should still receive standard antiretroviral therapy to prevent perinatal transmission, but delaying therapy until the second trimester can be considered.

Postexposure Prophylaxis

The risk of infection is a function of the type of exposure and the infectivity of the exposure source. The average risk of HIV transmission is approximately 0.3% after percutaneous exposure to infected blood and 0.09% after mucous membrane exposure. A retrospective case-control study of health care workers showed that zidovudine was associated with a 79% decrease in the risk of HIV transmission. After considering results of that study and those of animal studies and the Pediatric AIDS Clinical Trial Group, the US Public Health Service recommended prophylaxis for health care workers with **occupational exposure** to HIV.

Systems, including written protocols, should be in place to prompt reporting and facilitate management of exposed health care workers. For most HIV exposures, a 4-week regimen of 2 antiretroviral medications (zidovudine and lamivudine) is recommended. The addition of a third medication, usually a protease inhibitor, is recommended for exposures with an increased risk of transmission or when resistance to 1 of the recommended medications is known or suspected.

- Human immunodeficiency virus (HIV) transmission occurs through sexual and perinatal routes, parenteral inoculation, and through blood products and donated organs.
- Antiretroviral therapy, often with concurrent use of 3 or more antiretroviral medications, is recommended for all patients with a history of an AIDS-defining illness or severe symptoms of HIV infection. Treatment also is recommended for patients with fewer than 350 CD4+ T-cells/mm³ who are otherwise asymptomatic.
- The best approach for preventing HIV infection combines behavioral strategies (eg, changes in high-risk behavior) and biomedical strategies (eg, prompt

diagnosis and treatment; prevention of mother-to-child transmission).

Chlamydia

Chlamydia trachomatis infection is the **most common STI** in the United States. Although most infections are asymptomatic, affected patients may have urethritis, cervicitis, and pelvic inflammatory disease. Ectopic pregnancy and infertility are common sequelae. Condoms provide helpful protection against infection. Screening is simple with urine-based PCR tests. Risk factors include having multiple sex partners, a new partner, and unprotected intercourse. Screening women with high risk of infection and treating those affected decreases the incidence of pelvic inflammatory disease, ectopic pregnancy, and the overall prevalence of chlamydia in the targeted population. Box 5 shows indications for chlamydia screening.

Chlamydia infection of the urogenital tract can be diagnosed by swab specimens from the endocervix, vagina, or urethra, or by testing urine. Urine samples are easy to obtain and are often preferred because they can also be tested for gonorrhea. Rectal chlamydia infection can be diagnosed by testing a rectal swab specimen. Enzyme immunoassays, nucleic acid hybridization tests, and nucleic acid amplification testing can be performed with swab specimens. Nucleic acid amplification testing can also be performed with urine samples. Swab specimens can be cultured, but this is rarely done outside of research settings and forensic investigations because of expense. Recommended treatment for chlamydia is azithromycin (1 g, orally, single dose) or doxycycline (100 mg, orally, twice daily for 7 days).

Box 5 Indications for Chlamydia Screening

Men or women with symptoms suggestive of infection (for women, signs consistent with chlamydial infection during pelvic examination include discharge, cervical erythema, and cervical friability)

Women who present for an induced abortion

Girls admitted to a juvenile detention facility

All sexually active women younger than 20 y

Sexually active women aged 20 to 24 y who have more than 1 sex partner or a new partner in the past 3 mo

Sexually active women older than 24 y who have not used barrier contraceptives consistently and have more than 1 or a new sex partner in the past 3 mo

All pregnant women (women younger than 25 y and women with increased risk of infection should be screened at the first prenatal visit and retested during the third trimester)

Sex partners of a patient diagnosed with chlamydia infection in the previous 60 d

---

- Chlamydia is the most common sexually transmitted infection in the United States. Most cases are asymptomatic.
- Recommended treatment for chlamydia is azithromycin or doxycycline.

Chancroid

Chancroid, caused by *Haemophilus ducreyi*, is a common **genital ulcer disease** worldwide. Although the causative microorganism is extremely infectious, chancroid likely is underdiagnosed in the United States because of lack of clinical experience with the disease and difficulty culturing the organism. Diagnosis should be made on the basis of clinical findings. Infection with *Treponema pallidum* and HSV should be excluded as the cause of ulceration. If clinical evidence is consistent with chancroid, a **presumptive diagnosis** can be made. Some laboratories can perform PCR tests to confirm *H ducreyi* infection. All sex partners in the 10 days preceding signs of infection should be examined and treated for chancroid, even if they are asymptomatic.

Recommended treatments include azithromycin (1 g, orally, single dose), ceftriaxone (250 mg, intramuscularly, single dose), ciprofloxacin (500 mg, orally, twice daily for 3 days), or erythromycin base (500 mg, orally, 3 times per day for 7 days). Symptomatic improvement is expected in 3 days and objective improvement in 7 days. If no improvement is seen, the diagnosis should be reconsidered; furthermore, the possibility of coinfection with another STI such as HIV and the possibility of resistance to the antibiotic used should be explored. **Complete resolution** should occur in about 2 weeks unless the ulcer is very large or associated with fluctuant lymphadenopathy.

- Chancroid likely is underdiagnosed in the United States. However, a presumptive diagnosis can be made with sufficient clinical evidence.
- With appropriate antibiotic treatment, complete resolution should occur in about 2 weeks.

Genital Herpes

HSV is a common infection, with more than 500,000 new cases annually in the United States. Treatment does not eradicate the virus and has no definite effect on future recurrences or overall infectiousness. Daily antiviral therapy can prevent clinical recurrences and reduce viral shedding; however, even though individuals receiving suppressive treatment are less infectious, they can still transmit HSV. Condoms provide helpful protection against HSV infection. HSV-related genital ulcer disease increases the risk of acquiring HIV infection.

Diagnosis is established either by culturing HSV from lesions or by PCR tests for HSV DNA (the latter is a much more sensitive assay). Viral shedding is intermittent, so a negative test does not exclude HSV infection. HSV serologic testing is occasionally useful. Both HSV-1 and HSV-2 can cause genital disease, but HSV-2 is more common in genital disease and more prone to recurrence.

Treatment of genital HSV depends on the situation. For an initial episode in a nonimmunosuppressed patient, the following medications are useful: acyclovir (400 mg, 3 times daily for 7-10 days OR 200 mg, 5 times daily for 7-10 days); famciclovir (250 mg, 3 times daily for 7-10 days); or valacyclovir (1 g, twice daily for 7-10 days). For treatment of recurrent HSV episodes, a shorter course of acyclovir, famciclovir, or valacyclovir should be initiated during prodrome or the first day of outbreak. Severe disease requiring hospitalization, organ involvement, or central nervous system disease should be treated with intravenous acyclovir. Pregnant, seronegative women with an HSV-positive partner should abstain from intercourse and oral labial contact during the third trimester. Cesarean delivery is effective in preventing transmission of HSV to neonates and is recommended for women with evidence of active genital herpes at the time of delivery. However, it should be noted that most women who transmit HSV to their babies are asymptomatic at the time of delivery.

- Herpes simplex virus (HSV) is not curable, but daily antiviral therapy can prevent clinical recurrences and reduce viral shedding.
- Cesarean delivery is effective in preventing transmission of HSV to neonates.

Gonorrhea

Neisseria gonorrhoeae is a major cause of pelvic inflammatory disease, urethritis, and cervicitis. Condoms are effective physical barriers for men against *N gonorrhoeae*. Protection by condoms has not been well demonstrated for women. Notification of all sex partners in the past 60 days and treatment of partners are important and effective preventive measures. Reporting cases allows public health officials to concentrate preventive efforts where they are needed. Behavioral interventions primarily used to decrease the transmission of HIV have successfully decreased the incidence of gonorrhea.

Most men are symptomatic; however, **most women are asymptomatic or minimally symptomatic** and therefore may delay treatment. Women who are sexually active or pregnant and living in areas with a high prevalence of gonorrhea should be screened at the time of routine examinations. The bacteria can be transmitted to infants during birth and can result in blindness if untreated. PCR-based screening of urine samples obviates the need for a pelvic examination. Infected women should be rechecked for gonorrhea 3 to 5 months after treatment because reinfection rates are high.

Diagnosis of gonorrhea in men with symptomatic urethritis can be established by observing intracellular gram-negative diplococci in the urethral discharge. Gram stain is a very sensitive and specific assay for symptomatic men, but it is not sufficiently sensitive for asymptomatic men or for women. Diagnosis of gonorrhea at any site can be confirmed by appropriate cultures, which also allow antibiotic susceptibility testing. Nucleic hybridization can be performed using urine samples or swab specimens of endocervical or urethral discharge. Because the nucleic acid amplification test can detect both gonorrhea and chlamydia with a single urine specimen, it is a very convenient and frequently preferred testing method.

Uncomplicated gonorrhea of the urethra, cervix, or rectum should be treated with one of the following: ceftriaxone (125 mg, intramuscularly, single dose) or cefixime (400 mg, orally, single dose). Quinolones are no longer recommended because of increasing microbial resistance. Patients and partners should abstain from sex until treatment is complete.

- Gonorrhea often is minimally symptomatic or asymptomatic in women.
- Gram stain is not a reliable diagnostic assay for asymptomatic men and women; cultures and nucleic acid tests are more reliable.

Human Papillomavirus

Genital human papillomavirus (HPV) is the **most common viral STI** in the United States. Evidence strongly links certain strains of HPV to **cervical carcinoma** (strains HPV-16 and HPV-18 cause >70% of cervical cancers) and also suggests a role in vaginal, vulvar, anal, and penile squamous cell cancers. Genital HPV is transmitted through contact with infected lesions, mucosal surfaces, or fluids of subclinical lesions. Condoms markedly decrease the risk of acquiring HPV; however, HPV can be transmitted through contact with areas not covered by a condom.

Definitive diagnosis of HPV is made by detecting HPV nucleic acid; this assay often can be performed at the time of the Papanicolaou test. Because 90% of genital warts are caused by strains HPV-6 and HPV-11, warts are not an indication for HPV testing. Visible warts are diagnosed on the basis of their appearance, and nucleic acid testing is not needed. Genital warts should not prompt a cervical colposcopy or change in the frequency of Papanicolaou tests.

In the absence of warts or squamous intraepithelial lesions, no treatment is indicated. Genital HPV infection can resolve spontaneously, but no current therapy reliably eradicates infection. The primary goal of treating genital warts is removal for symptomatic and cosmetic reasons. No evidence indicates that removing warts decreases infectivity. Treatment options for external genital warts include patient-applied podofilox 0.5% gel or solution or imiquimod 5% cream. The physician can perform cryotherapy or laser surgery, apply podophyllin resin 10% to 25% in tincture of benzoin, trichloroacetic acid 80% to 90% or bichloroacetic acid 80% to 90%, or provide intralesional interferon therapy. No treatment is more effective than others.

HPV vaccine is recommended for females aged 9 to 26 years who have not been previously immunized against HPV. It is not helpful for women already infected with a disease-causing strain. More details are as described in Chapter 7.

- Human papillomavirus strains HPV-16 and HPV-18 cause at least 70% of cervical cancers. Strains HPV-6 and HPV-11 cause 90% of genital warts.
- No current therapy eradicates infection. The primary treatment goal of warts is removal. In the absence of warts or squamous intraepithelial lesions, no treatment is indicated.
- HPV vaccine is recommended for most females aged 9 to 26 years.

Syphilis

The prevalence and incidence of syphilis has decreased considerably in the United States during the past century. Syphilis, caused by *T pallidum* infection, increases the risk of HIV transmission by 3- to 5-fold. **Transmission risk is greatest during the first few months** of infection. Studies suggest that condom use decreases the risk of acquiring or transmitting syphilis, but condoms will not always prevent contact with infectious lesions.

Diagnosis of syphilis is usually made with serologic tests. Early stage syphilis can be definitively diagnosed by darkfield examination of tissue or exudate for spirochetes. **False-positive results** can occur with serologic tests; therefore, a treponemal test and a nontreponemal test must both have positive findings to make a presumptive diagnosis of syphilis. Treponemal tests include the fluorescent antibody absorbed test, *T pallidum* particle agglutination test, microhemagglutination assay, and enzyme immunoassay to *T pallidum* immunoglobulin (Ig) G or IgM antibodies. Treponemal tests will usually stay positive for life but can also be false-positive. Nontreponemal tests include the venereal disease research test and the rapid plasma reagin test. Nontreponemal tests usually correlate with disease activity but can be positive in other medical conditions.

No single test can be used to diagnose neurosyphilis. The venereal disease research laboratory test of CSF is very specific but insensitive. Some experts believe a negative fluorescent antibody absorbed test of CSF makes neurosyphilis very unlikely; however, this test has a notable false-positive rate. A CSF white blood cell count of >5 cells/mm^3 is sensitive but nonspecific for neurosyphilis.

Latent syphilis is infection without any evidence of disease. Early latent syphilis is diagnosed only when it is certain that infection occurred within the past 12 months. The Centers for Disease Control and Prevention recommends **prophylactic treatment** of all sexual contacts within the past 90 days of patients diagnosed with primary, secondary, or early latent syphilis. They further recommend testing of all sexual contacts within the past 3 months for primary syphilis, 6 months for secondary, and 12 months for early latent syphilis.

Parenteral penicillin G is the treatment of choice for all stages of syphilis. Pregnant women with a penicillin allergy should be desensitized against penicillin and treated with parenteral penicillin G to prevent congenital syphilis. Early latent, primary, and secondary syphilis in otherwise healthy adults can be treated with a single dose of intramuscular benzathine penicillin G (2.4 million units). Late latent syphilis, latent syphilis of unknown duration, tertiary syphilis with a gumma, or cardiovascular involvement without ocular involvement or neurosyphilis should be treated with 3 intramuscular doses of benzathine penicillin G (2.4 million units), 1 dose per week for 3 weeks.

All patients with evidence of neurologic or ophthalmologic symptoms, aortitis, other symptoms of active tertiary syphilis, or treatment failure should have a CSF examination. Some experts believe all HIV-infected patients with latent syphilis also should have a CSF examination. Neurosyphilis or syphilis with ocular involvement should be treated with aqueous crystalline penicillin G (18-24 million units daily by continuous infusion; or 3-4 million units every 3-4 hours for 10-14 days).

- Syphilis increases the risk of HIV transmission.
- Because of the rate of false-positive serologic test results, a presumptive diagnosis should be based on results of at least 2 tests.

Viral Hepatitis

Hepatitis A

Hepatitis A virus (HAV) is transmitted by fecal-oral contamination of food and water. It is prevalent in underdeveloped countries and in daycare settings. Men who have sex with men have a high risk of transmission. The incubation period is typically 3 weeks to 3 months. In children, the disease is usually mild (subclinical); adults may have fever and jaundice. The natural course of disease is typically benign, and the prognosis is excellent because there is **no risk of chronic liver disease**. Rarely, the patient may develop fulminant hepatic failure. Diagnosis often is made after considering the clinical history and detecting either IgM anti-HAV antibodies in serum within the first 6 months of infection or IgG anti-HAV antibodies after 6 months of infection.

The main preventive measure is the HAV vaccine. It is given to individuals traveling to HAV-endemic regions, intravenous drug users, men who have sex with men, and patients with chronic liver disease. Immune serum globulin and HAV vaccine should be administered prophylactically to household contacts or to those with known exposure to a contaminated source. Treatment is mostly supportive.

Hepatitis B

Hepatitis B is a DNA virus transmitted by sexual contact, parenterally, or perinatally from mother to fetus. The incubation period is 3 to 6 months. Hepatitis B infections can lead to **chronic liver disease** such as chronic hepatitis, cirrhosis, or liver failure. However, many hepatitis B infections can be subclinical. **Acute infections** may present with urticaria, arthralgias, malaise, and icterus. Jaundice lasts only a few weeks, and disease usually resolves within 6 months. Viral markers of hepatitis B have a specific pattern of expression and are used in clinical practice to differentiate between acute and chronic infection, as well as between infectiousness and immunity (Table 4).

Prophylaxis is with hepatitis immune globulin, which is indicated for household contacts and sexual contacts of infected persons. Hepatitis B vaccination is indicated in high-risk individuals, including infants and previously unvaccinated 10- to 12-year-old children. Health care workers, injection drug users, and individuals with multiple sexual contacts are at high risk and should be considered for immunization. Four treatment options for active hepatitis B have been approved by the US Food and Drug Administration. These treatments are interferon alfa, lamivudine, adefovir dipivoxil, and entecavir.

Hepatitis C

Hepatitis C virus (HCV) is an RNA virus. The most common route of infection is through blood transfusions and injection drug use. It is believed to **cause 40% of all chronic liver diseases**. It has a prolonged incubation period of up to several months. Patients may present with cryoglobulinemia or porphyria cutanea tarda. Antibodies to HCV indicate exposure but not immunity. Diagnosis is by detection of anti-HCV antibodies by ELISA. HCV RNA can be detected by PCR assays.

About 60% to 85% of cases ultimately have development of chronic hepatitis, as indicated by chronically elevated levels of alanine aminotransferase and aspartate aminotransferase. Approximately 20% to 30% of patients with chronic hepatitis C infection have development of cirrhosis. Patients with chronic hepatitis C infection are considered for liver transplantation.

- Hepatitis A usually has a benign clinical course and carries no risk of chronic liver disease.
- Hepatitis B infections can be subclinical but also can lead to chronic liver disease. Vaccination is indicated in high-risk individuals.
- Hepatitis C is believed to cause 40% of all chronic liver diseases. Patients may be considered for liver transplantation.

Travel Medicine

The most common preventable cause of death and hospitalization while traveling is accidents, including motor vehicle accidents, falls, and drowning. However, a complete travel medicine consultation needs to review not only general safety precautions but also infectious risks and prevention of deep vein thrombosis and altitude sickness. Many travel-related illnesses can be prevented with appropriate immunization. Table 5 summarizes recommended travel immunizations.

Table 4 Interpretation of Hepatitis B Serologic Patterns

HBsAg	Anti-HBs	IgM Anti-HBc	IgG Anti-HBc	HBeAg	Anti-HBe	HBV DNA, IU/mL	Interpretation
+	−	+	−	+	−	>20,000	Acute infection; occasionally "reactivation" of chronic hepatitis B
−	+	−	+	−	−/+	−	Prior infection with immunity
−	+	−	−	−	−	−	Vaccination with immunity
+	−	−	+	−	+	<20,000	Chronic hepatitis B inactive carrier
+	−	−	+	+	−	>20,000	HBeAg-positive chronic hepatitis B
+	−	−	+	−	+	>20,000	HBeAg-negative chronic hepatitis B

Abbreviations: Anti-HBc, hepatitis B core antibody; anti-HBe, hepatitis B e antibody; anti-HBs, hepatitis B surface antibody; HBeAg, hepatitis B e antigen; HBsAg, hepatitis B surface antigen; HBV, hepatitis B virus; Ig, immunoglobulin; IU, international units.
Adapted from Poterucha JJ. Gastroenterology and hepatology, part II. In: Ghosh AK, ed. Mayo Clinic Internal Medicine Review. 8th ed. Rochester (MN): Mayo Clinic Scientific Press and New York: Informa Healthcare USA; c2008. p. 299. Used with permission of Mayo Foundation for Medical Education and Research.

Table 5 Recommended Travel Immunizations

Vaccine	Ideal and Minimum Time Needed to Complete Vaccination Before Travel	Indications	Healthy Adults	Risk Groups	
				Pregnant Women	Immunocompromised Persons[a]
Hepatitis A	Ideal: 4 wk for short-term travel; 6 mo for expatriation. Minimum: day before departure	Nonimmune persons traveling to areas endemic for hepatitis A (Asia, Africa, Central and South America, Caribbean, East Europe, Russian Federation, and the Independent States). Check serologic findings before vaccination for immigrants returning to home country	Vaccinate	Vaccinate if risk exceeds any risk from vaccine (category C)	Vaccinate; if no seroconversion occurs after 4 wk in immunocompromised people, consider hepatitis A immunoglobulin before departure
Hepatitis B	Ideal: 6 mo. Minimum: complete 3 doses in 3 mo (0, 1, 2 mo) or 21 d (0, 7, 21 d) with a booster in 12 mo	Travelers who anticipate high-risk activities, people planning to travel for >4 wk, business personnel with multiple international trips annually	Vaccinate	Vaccinate	Vaccinate
Combined hepatitis A and hepatitis B	Ideal: 6 mo. Minimum: 21 d before departure, with a booster in 12 mo	Those meeting both hepatitis A and hepatitis B vaccine indications	Vaccinate	Vaccinate if risk exceeds any risk from vaccine (category C)	Vaccinate but check hepatitis A serologic findings before departure
Typhoid	Ideal: 4 wk. Minimum: 2 wk for protection	Travel to developing countries in Asia, Africa, and Latin America, especially if longer than 2-3 wk; or 1-wk travel to high-risk areas (eg, Indian subcontinent)	Vaccinate	Oral live vaccine is contraindicated; injectable vaccine is relatively contraindicated. Vaccinate if risk of disease is higher than vaccine risk	Oral live vaccine is contraindicated. Injectable vaccine may be used but may have lower efficacy

Disease	Timing	Indications			
Rabies	Ideal: 6 wk for full immunity Minimum: 21 d when 3 doses are accelerated	Long-term travelers to areas where rabies is a threat; or short-term travelers who are likely to have animal contact in enzootic areas	Vaccinate	Vaccinate only if risk is considered high	Vaccinate
Japanese encephalitis	Ideal: 2 mo Minimum for 3 doses: 24 d	Travel to endemic areas for >4 wk, especially rural areas	Vaccinate	Contraindicated	Vaccinate but efficacy may be low
Tick-borne virus (not available in United States)		Expatriates to endemic areas (eg, Eastern European countries, Independent States of Russia)	Vaccinate	Contraindicated	Vaccinate
Poliovirus	No specific time limit before travel if previously vaccinated; 3-12 mo if no previous primary series was given	Travelers to endemic areas—African and Asian countries only Due to near-worldwide eradication, recommendations are likely to change with continued eradication	Booster with inactivated poliovirus vaccine if primary series was completed >10 y ago Give primary series if primary series was not completed	Live oral vaccine contraindicated, but injectable poliovirus vaccine advised if risk is high	Live oral vaccine contraindicated but injectable poliovirus vaccine advised
Cholera (currently unavailable in United States)	4 wk	Health care delivery, missionary, or military workers in endemic and epidemic areas	Vaccinate for high-risk exposure as indicated	Contraindicated	Contraindicated

ª Immunocompromised persons include those receiving high-dose corticosteroids (20 mg/d for >3 wk), chemotherapy, or immunosuppressive regimens because of transplantation or other diseases, or persons with congenital or acquired immunodeficiency states, including human immunodeficiency virus or AIDS.

Adapted from Virk (2004). Used with permission.

Insects

Insect-borne diseases are not limited to developing countries but also occur in developed countries such as the United States. General insect precautions include covering exposed skin (long pants, long-sleeved shirts, socks), using an diethyltoluamide (DEET) insect repellant (adults should use a 25%-50% spray every 4-6 hours), treating clothing with the insecticide **permethrin** (and using permethrin-treated insect nets on the bed at night), and avoiding being outside from dusk to dawn, when insects are most active.

DEET should not be used with infants younger than 2 months, and lower concentrations should be applied more frequently for younger children. Concentrations of DEET higher than 50% are no more effective than concentrations between 35% and 50%. A spray is preferred because clothing, in addition to exposed skin, may be treated. DEET appears to be safe during pregnancy. Plant-derived repellents such as citronella and icaridin (at the currently available strength in the United States) provide very brief protection against insects and are therefore not recommended. Repellents with higher concentrations of icaridin, available in Europe, are an alternative to DEET repellents because they are well tolerated and provide longer protection.

Permethrin-treated bed nets should be used in sleeping quarters when the risk of being exposed to disease-carrying insects is high. Permethrin can also be sprayed on clothing, shoes, and tents in advance of a trip to provide additional protection against insect bites. This is strongly encouraged when the risk of bites is high. Ideally, one should avoid being outdoors during peak periods of insect activity.

Traveler's Diarrhea

Traveler's diarrhea is the most common travel-related infection. The usual cause is enterotoxigenic *E coli* infection, which generally results in a **self-limited** illness. The most important aspect of treatment is plenty of fluids to **avoid dehydration**. Pretravel advice should emphasize food and water guidelines (Box 6).

Antimotility medications such as loperamide and diphenoxylate hydrochloride are safe and helpful for adults with mild-to-moderate, nonbloody traveler's diarrhea that is not associated with systemic symptoms such as fever. However, antimotility medications potentially can make serious infectious diarrhea even worse. Many who travel to developing countries carry enough quinolone or azithromycin (plus an antimotility medication) to administer a short course of self-treatment in case of mild-to-moderate diarrhea. Quinolones are effective against most bacteria that cause traveler's diarrhea, but they are not recommended for children or pregnant women (azithromycin is safe and a reasonable option for these patients). Bismuth subsalicylate can also be used with antimotility

Box 6 Food and Water Consumption Guidelines for Travel

Consume bottled or boiled water; avoid ice

Eat only well-cooked, freshly prepared, steaming hot food (safest)

Avoid uncooked or undercooked meat or seafood

Avoid unpasteurized dairy products and juices

Peel or avoid fresh fruit and vegetables (peeling does not make food completely safe)

drugs for self-treatment of mild cases. It can also be recommended to travelers who want primary prophylaxis. Although **primary prophylaxis with antibiotics generally is not recommended**, it can be considered for immunocompromised travelers.

Malaria

Malaria is the most common travel-related infection that requires hospitalization. Malaria is transmitted by a nighttime-biting mosquito. Any traveler with fever in an endemic area should be tested for malaria. Malarial endemic areas include much of Africa, the Indian subcontinent, Southeast Asia, Central America, Hispaniola (Haiti and the Dominican Republic), the northern part of South America, and a few areas in the Middle East and Oceania. The estimated incidence rate of malaria among travelers to Western Africa is 24 cases per 1,000 travelers per month; in contrast, the rate among travelers to Central America is 0.1 cases per 1,000 travelers per month. Infection with *Plasmodium falciparum* tends to cause severe disease, particularly among nonimmune travelers.

Approximately one-half of imported malaria cases in the United States occurs among expatriates who return to malarial endemic areas to visit family and friends. Malaria is more common in those traveling to rural malarial endemic areas for a prolonged time and in those who do not follow insect precautions or use appropriate chemoprophylaxis. Malaria-related morbidity and mortality are highest in the very young and the very old, pregnant women, those not taking or taking inappropriate chemoprophylaxis, and persons for whom appropriate treatment is delayed.

Chloroquine, a antimalarial agent first used in the 1940s, remains effective for preventing malaria in Mexico, Hispaniola, Central America, and certain parts of China, the Philippines, and the Middle East. Chloroquine treatment is started 1 to 2 weeks before travel to the malarial endemic area, it is continued weekly while there and through 4 weeks after departure. The medication can be administered to children and pregnant women. Unfortunately, the drug can exacerbate psoriasis.

Mefloquine, doxycycline, and atovaquone–proguanil hydrochloride (available in a fixed-dose combination) are all effective medications in most parts of the world where malaria is resistant to chloroquine. The exception is along the Thai-Cambodia border and Thai-Myanmar border, where chloroquine- and mefloquine-resistant strains of *P falciparum* are prevalent; options for these areas are doxycycline or atovaquone-proguanil.

Doxycycline is very inexpensive and available worldwide. The medication is started 2 days before entering the malarial endemic area, and continued daily while there and through 4 weeks after departure. The major adverse effect of concern is the increased risk of severe sunburn. Doxycycline is contraindicated for pregnant women and young children.

Atovaquone-proguanil can be used for prophylaxis and is started 2 days before entering a malarial endemic area and continued daily while there and through 7 days after departure. Absorption improves if the medication is taken with food (and fewer gastrointestinal tract symptoms result). Atovaquone-proguanil is generally well tolerated, but for many travelers, particularly those on long trips, the expense is a major consideration. Additionally, atovaquone-proguanil is not currently recommended for pregnant women.

Rabies

Rabies is much more prevalent in developing countries than in the United States. All travelers should avoid contact with animals and should take any bite or scratch seriously. **Washing the bite or scratch with soap and water** is an important first step that decreases the risk of rabies. Most travelers will not have received the preexposure rabies vaccine series and need to seek emergent medical attention at a hospital that can provide both the rabies **immunoglobulin and vaccine**. The immunoglobulin is injected around the site of the injury and the vaccine is given in the opposite arm. The vaccine should be administered on the day of the exposure and on days 3, 7, 14, and 28 after exposure. Travelers in developing countries should be advised to return promptly to the United States and seek immediate follow-up care at a hospital with experience in postexposure rabies prevention.

- The most common preventable cause of injury and death while traveling is accidents.
- General precautions to prevent insect-borne disease include covering exposed skin, using DEET repellent, treating clothing and bed nets with permethrin, and avoiding being outside from dusk to dawn.
- Traveler's diarrhea, usually attributable to a self-limited *E coli* infection, often is transmitted through contaminated food and water. Treatment should focus on maintaining hydration.
- Travelers to malarial endemic areas should receive prophylactic treatment, usually with chloroquine.
- Rabies immunoglobulin and vaccine must be given rapidly (treatment must begin on the day of exposure).

SUGGESTED READING

CDC, Traveler's Health [Internet]. Atlanta: Centers for Disease Control and Prevention [cited 2008 Nov 19]. Available from: http://wwwn.cdc.gov/travel/.

Centers for Disease Control and Prevention. Updated U.S. Public Health Service guidelines for the management of occupational exposures to HIV and recommendations for postexposure prophylaxis. MMWR 2005;54(No. RR-9):1-11.

Centers for Disease Control and Prevention. Sexually transmitted diseases treatment guidelines, 2006. MMWR 2006;55(No. RR-11):1-94.

Centers for Disease Control and Prevention. Guidelines for prevention and treatment of opportunistic infections in HIV-infected adults and adolescents. MMWR 2009;58(No. RR-4):1-206.

Hill DR, Ericsson CD, Pearson RD, Keystone JS, Freedman DO, Kozarsky PE, et al. The practice of travel medicine: guidelines by the Infectious Diseases Society of America. CID 2006;43:1499-539.

Kasten MJ. HIV and sexually transmissible disease prevention. In: Lang RS, Hensrud DD, editors. Clinical preventive medicine. 2nd ed. United States of America: AMA Press; c2004. p. 596-7.

Knoll B, Lassmann B, Temesgen Z. Current status of HIV infection: a review for non-HIV-treating physicians. Int J Dermatol. 2007 Dec;46(12):1219-28.

Shoreland Inc. Travel and routine immunizations: a practical guide for the medical office. Shoreland Medical Marketing 2008.

Virk A. Travel: risks and prevention. In: Lang RS, Hensrud DD, editors. Clinical preventive medicine. 2nd ed. United States of America: AMA Press; c2004. p. 273-88.

Whitley RJ, Kimberlin DW, Roizman B. Herpes simplex viruses. Clin Infect Dis. 1998 Mar;26(3):541-53.

Wilson W, Taubert KA, Gewitz M, Lockhart PB, Baddour LM, Levison M, et al; American Heart Association Rheumatic Fever, Endocarditis, and Kawasaki Disease Committee; American Heart Association Council on Cardiovascular Disease in the Young; American Heart Association Council on Clinical Cardiology; American Heart Association Council on Cardiovascular Surgery and Anesthesia; Quality of Care and Outcomes Research Interdisciplinary Working Group. Prevention of infective endocarditis: guidelines from the American Heart Association: a guideline from the American Heart Association Rheumatic Fever, Endocarditis, and Kawasaki Disease Committee, Council on Cardiovascular Disease in the Young, and the Council on Clinical Cardiology, Council on Cardiovascular Surgery and Anesthesia, and the Quality of Care and Outcomes Research Interdisciplinary Working Group. Circulation. 2007 Oct 9;116(15):1736-54. Epub 2007 Apr 19. Erratum in: Circulation. 2007 Oct 9;116(15):e376-7.

Questions and Answers

Questions

1. A 62-year-old man asks for antibiotics before colonoscopy. He has had prophylactic treatment with amoxicillin before dental procedures for years. He has a grade 3/6 crescendo-decrescendo heart murmur and recently was told he has stable aortic stenosis. What is the next step?
   a. Cefazolin (1 g, intravenously) before procedure
   b. Amoxicillin (2 g, orally) before procedure
   c. Amoxicillin (2 g, orally) 1 hour before and 2 hours after procedure
   d. Advise him that no prophylaxis is needed
   e. Request a cardiology consultation

2. A 44-year-old homeless man presents with fever, cough, night sweats, and weight loss. He is positive for HIV, has crackles in both lung fields, and a chest radiograph shows bilateral lower lobe infiltrates. All the following are correct *except*:
   a. Evaluation should include sputum Gram stain and culture
   b. Sputum should be specifically stained and cultured for *Mycobacterium tuberculosis*
   c. Patient requires *Pneumocystis* pneumonia prophylaxis
   d. Patient requires antiretroviral treatment
   e. Infiltrates in lower lobes exclude the diagnosis of tuberculosis

3. A 35-year-old woman presents with persistent diarrhea after a recent trip to Morocco. She is otherwise healthy. On the second day of her trip, she had severe diarrhea and fever. After her return home 2 weeks ago, she was treated with ciprofloxacin for 7 days. When the diarrhea did not resolve, she was treated with amoxicillin for 7 days. Now, after 2 weeks of treatment, she reports persistent loose stool and decreased appetite. She lost 7 pounds in the first few days but has since stabilized. She has no fever and is not vomiting. Stool cultures show *Salmonella* non-*typhi*. Which is the best option for this patient?
   a. Intravenous fluoroquinolones
   b. Oral amoxicillin for 3 weeks
   c. Combination of ciprofloxacin orally and loperamide
   d. No antimicrobial treatment
   e. Oral trimethoprim-sulfamethoxazole for 7 to 10 days.

4. Which of the following statements about genital herpes infection is true?
   a. HSV-2 is the only cause of genital herpes
   b. Risk of transmission to baby is <1% for pregnant woman with recurrent HSV
   c. Cultures are more sensitive than polymerase chain reaction (PCR) assays

   d. Most women who have genital lesions at the time of delivery will transmit genital herpes to the neonate
   e. Early treatment of the primary infection will decrease future infectiousness

5. Which of these statements about the prevention of malaria is *false*?
   a. Once weekly mefloquine is effective prophylaxis against malaria, except along the Thai-Cambodia and Thai-Myanmar borders
   b. Atovaquone-proguanil effectively prevents malaria but is poorly tolerated
   c. Mefloquine can be used prophylactically in pregnant women planning travel to a malarial endemic area
   d. DEET 100% lotion appears no more effective and is more irritating than 40% DEET spray
   e. Chloroquine is an effective antimalarial medication in Haiti

6. A 36-year-old man is scheduled to travel to Mexico City for a meeting and is concerned about developing traveler's diarrhea. In addition to advising the patient about food safety, you should recommend which of the following?
   a. Ciprofloxacin (500 mg) daily, throughout the trip
   b. Doxycycline (100 mg) daily, throughout the trip
   c. Amoxicillin (250 mg) 3 times daily for 5 days if diarrhea develops
   d. Ciprofloxacin (500 mg) twice daily for 3 days if diarrhea develops
   e. Metronidazole (250 mg), 3 times daily for 3 days if diarrhea develops

7. A 23-year-old woman in the eighth month of pregnancy is evaluated because of a urinary tract infection. Which of these agents is the most appropriate for empiric treatment?
   a. Amoxicillin
   b. Norfloxacin
   c. Tetracycline
   d. Trimethoprim-sulfamethoxazole

8. A 32-year-old woman who had been vacationing in Wisconsin comes to your office because of concern for Lyme disease. The area where she vacationed is known to be highly endemic for Lyme disease and she has found and removed a tick from her body the day before. She brought the tick to show you. She has no symptoms. The patient has no medical problems or allergies and takes no medications. Physical examination findings are normal. The tick does appear to be an adult *Ixodes scapularis*. Which of the following should you prescribe?
   a. Ceftriaxone for 7 days
   b. Hydrocortisone ointment at the site of the tick bite
   c. Amoxicillin for 10 days
   d. Single-dose doxycycline

Answers

1. **Answer d.**

   According to recent American Heart Association guidelines, no prophylaxis is needed for routine upper and lower gastrointestinal tract endoscopy for patients with native valve stenosis or regurgitation without a history of infective endocarditis.

2. **Answer e.**

   In an immunocompromised host, tuberculosis can manifest as infiltrates anywhere in the lung field, including the lower lobes. In the context of AIDS, tuberculosis is often multidrug resistant.

3. **Answer d.**

   Gastroenteritis with a *Salmonella* non-*typhi* species is generally a self-limited illness in a healthy adult. Immunocompromised patients and the very old and young are at increased risk of complications, and treatment should be considered. However, the patient's symptoms are fairly mild and improving. Stool culture is not recommended for follow-up of an immunocompetent patient with *Salmonella* gastroenteritis because *Salmonella* can be excreted in the stool for more than a month after resolution of symptoms.

4. **Answer b.**

   HSV-2 is the most common cause of genital herpes, but HSV-1 can also cause genital disease (HSV-1 tends to cause milder disease with less frequent recurrence). Cultures for HSV are much less sensitive than PCR assays. Most women who transmit HSV to their babies are asymptomatic at the time of delivery. A woman with a primary infection during her third trimester or active disease at the time of delivery has a very high risk of transmitting disease to the baby; cesarean delivery should be considered. Unfortunately, although early treatment of a primary infection will result in earlier resolution of the outbreak and decreased viral shedding during treatment, it does not eradicate the virus and has no effect on future infectiousness.

5. **Answer b.**

   The atovaquone-proguanil formulation available in the United States is very effective and well tolerated. The most common adverse effects are in the gastrointestinal tract, and these are generally mild and rarely require cessation of appropriate prophylaxis. Mefloquine offers effective prophylaxis (see main text for dosing schedule). Mefloquine can be used in pregnant women when they are traveling to a malarial endemic area because the risk of severe illness to mother and fetus from a malarial infection is greater than the increased risk of stillbirth from mefloquine. Doxycycline is contraindicated in pregnancy and atovaquone-proguanil has not been approved and has not been well studied. DEET spray is preferred over lotion because clothing as well as skin can be easily treated. Increasing the concentration of DEET above 35% has little additional benefit, although a more concentrated spray will not have to be applied as frequently.

6. **Answer d.**

   Continuous use of antibiotics during travel is not recommended because of the potential for antibiotic resistance. Ciprofloxacin is the most effective of the options, and 2 to 3 days of treatment usually is adequate.

7. **Answer b.**

   Uncomplicated urinary tract infections in pregnancy are usually due to *E coli*, which is susceptible to norfloxacin or other fluoroquinolones. Amoxicillin is safer and the first choice in pregnancy. Early treatment is indicated. Screening for asymptomatic bacteriuria is indicated in pregnancy.

8. **Answer d.**

   The circumstances of a recently removed *Ixodes scapularis* tick, together with the fact that the patient vacationed in a highly endemic area, justify prompt treatment with single-dose doxycycline as a preventive measure.

IMMUNIZATION

Claudia L. Swanton, MS, CNP; Barbara J. Timm, MS, CNP; and
Heidi K. Roeber Rice, MD, MPH

The use of vaccines can be traced back to China and India before 200 BC. In 1796, Edward Jenner inoculated humans with cowpox as a vaccine against smallpox. Some 80 years later, Louis Pasteur successfully vaccinated people against smallpox. Vaccination, now considered one of the most effective public health interventions, became common practice in the 1940s with the introduction of vaccines for diphtheria and tetanus. Since that time, many infectious diseases have been well controlled through vaccination. In this chapter, we describe live and attenuated bacterial and viral vaccines and those that are composed of toxoids.

Vaccination Schedules

The Centers for Disease Control and Prevention (CDC) **Advisory Committee on Immunization Practices** (ACIP) annually reviews immunization schedules for adults and children in an effort to reduce the incidence of vaccine-preventable disease (VPD) in the United States. Despite considerable improvement in the rate of pediatric immunization, data from 2002 indicate that 50,000 to 70,000 deaths due to VPD occur annually; furthermore, 99% of these deaths occur in adults. Although it is generally assumed that childhood vaccination confers lifelong immunity, many adults are not properly vaccinated as children. Because immunity may diminish with time, adults, particularly the elderly, are increasingly susceptible to infections and serious disease. Hepatitis B, pneumococcal disease, and influenza are the most common VPDs in adults.

Recommendations for vaccination may be affected by the immune status of an individual patient. Patients may have increased risk of infection or severe disease (eg, asplenia) or reduced antibody response, thereby requiring higher or booster doses. The vaccine itself may pose potential risk of infection. Pregnancy and immunosuppression due to malignancy, human immunodeficiency virus (HIV) infection (with certain exceptions), or treatment with medications such as high-dose corticosteroids are generally considered contraindications to live-virus vaccines. With this exception, patients with other conditions (eg, inflammatory bowel disease) generally follow the ACIP-recommended vaccination schedule. Table 1 includes vaccine recommendations and contraindications to consider when caring for special populations.

- Hepatitis B, pneumococcal disease, and influenza are the most common vaccine-preventable diseases (VPDs) in adults.
- Pregnancy, immunosuppression due to malignancy, human immunodeficiency virus infection (with certain exceptions), and treatment with high-dose corticosteroids are contraindications to live-virus vaccines.

Active vs Passive Immunity

Immunity is defined as the state of being protected from a disease. Passive immunity, usually limited to several months'

Table 1 Vaccination for Special Populations

Condition	Indicated Vaccines	Possible Vaccines	Contraindicated Vaccines	Comment
HIV positive	Pneumococcal, Td/Tdap, hepatitis B, annual influenza	Hepatitis A (for MSM traveling to or living in an area with increased prevalence of hepatitis A) MMR and varicella (for patients with CD4$^+$ counts >200 cells/mm^3)	Zoster vaccine	. . .
Asplenia (functional or surgical)	Meningococcal, pneumococcal, *Haemophilus influenzae* type b	. . .	. . .	Generally administered at least 2 wk before or after splenectomy Risk of infection with encapsulated bacteria is 10–50 times higher than for the general population
Awaiting solid-organ transplantation	Td, pneumococcal (initial plus booster after 5 y), influenza (annual)	Hepatitis B booster (if titer <10 mIU/mL), hepatitis A (for at-risk patients), meningococcal (for at-risk patients, 2 doses)	Live-virus or bacterial vaccines (after transplantation)	. . .
Pregnancy	Td, influenza (injectable)	Hepatitis A and hepatitis B (for at-risk patients), meningococcal, Tdap	MMR, influenza (live, attenuated), varicella	Live vaccines should be administered at least 1 mo before pregnancy

Abbreviations: HIV, human immunodeficiency virus; HPV, human papillomavirus; MMR, measles, mumps, rubella; MSM, men who have sex with men; Td, tetanus-diphtheria; Tdap, tetanus, diphtheria, acellular pertussis.

Adapted from the Centers for Disease Control and Prevention (2009).

duration, is conferred when preformed antibodies are administered directly to a recipient. In active immunity, the immune system is stimulated by exposure to a disease-causing organism to make antigen-specific antibodies and establish **cellular immunity**. Most vaccinations induce active immunity; these vaccines usually are created from naturally occurring organisms and use either a live, attenuated form or an inactivated form. Although **attenuated vaccines** contain live virus particles, they have a very low virulence.

An **inactivated vaccine** consists of virus particles that are grown in culture and then killed. Although the destroyed virus particles are incapable of replication, the viral capsid proteins are intact. These are recognized by the immune system and evoke a response. Booster shots with inactivated vaccines are required periodically to reinforce the immune response. Newer, component vaccines use only portions of an organism; they also provoke an immune response but are unable to cause disease.

Childhood Vaccination

Rates of childhood vaccination remain suboptimal. For example, in 2005, only 85.7% of children between the ages of 19 to 35 months had received 4 doses of the diphtheria, tetanus, and acellular pertussis vaccine. Infants and children can and should receive multiple vaccinations during a single well-child visit; there is no evidence that simultaneous vaccinations decrease antibody response or increase the rate of adverse reactions. Rather, the vaccination schedule ensures that children will be immunized at the appropriate age. Most vaccines for children are given in 2 or more doses to develop adequate antibody response. Ideally, vaccination begins before an otherwise healthy neonate is dismissed home after birth. Annually updated childhood vaccination schedules, endorsed by the US Department of Health and Human Services, are available online (http://cdc.gov/vaccines/recs/schedule/).

- Active immunity is based on creation of antigen-specific antibodies by the organism. Short-duration, passive immunity is based on administration of preformed antibodies.
- Rates of childhood vaccination remain suboptimal. Ideally, vaccination begins before infants are dismissed home after birth.

Toxoid Vaccines

Tetanus

Tetanus is an acute infection attributable to an exotoxin produced by the bacterium *Clostridium tetani*. The infection presents as an acute illness with generalized rigidity and convulsive spasms of the musculoskeletal system. It most often attacks the jaw, causing lockjaw, and the muscle rigidity that spreads to rest of the body often is fatal. Treatment and prophylaxis initially was through passive immunization, but a tetanus toxoid vaccine was developed and widely used during World War II. Table 2 summarizes the composition, primary prevention or indications, adverse effects, and contraindications to tetanus vaccination.

Postexposure Treatment and Prophylaxis

A tetanus vaccine should be administered after an injury occurs. Immunoglobulin may be indicated, depending on the number of years since the last booster shot, the total number of tetanus vaccinations the patient has received, and the nature of the wound (Table 3). Persons with a diagnosis of tetanus need to start treatment with tetanus immunoglobulin because this may help remove the unbound tetanus toxins. Because of the high potency of the tetanus toxin, illness does not result in tetanus immunity. Active immunization with tetanus toxoid must be started as soon as the individual has recovered from an active infection.

- A tetanus booster, along with tetanus immunoglobulin, is recommended if a patient sustains a high-risk wound and had his last vaccination greater than 10 years before the injury.

Diphtheria

Diphtheria is an acute bacterial disease caused by the aerobic, gram-positive bacillus *Corynebacterium diphtheriae*. The incubation period for diphtheria is usually 2 to 5 days and can involve any mucous membrane. The disease is usually classified according to the site involved, and the most commonly affected sites are the pharynx and tonsils. Those infected will have malaise, sore throat, and a low-grade fever. Within 2 to 3 days, a bluish-white membrane forms and covers the tonsils and soft palate. If the membrane formation is extensive, it can cause respiratory obstruction. At this point, the patient's condition can improve or worsen, depending on the amount of toxin absorbed. With a sufficiently high level of toxin, the patient can become comatose and die within 6 to 10 days. Diphtheria is very rare in the United States because of the effectiveness of preschool vaccinations. Table 2 summarizes the composition, primary prevention or indications, adverse effects, and contraindications to diphtheria vaccination.

Postexposure Treatment and Prophylaxis

Suspected cases of diphtheria should be treated immediately. Presumptive treatment should be administered (eg, oral erythromycin or intramuscular penicillin). The disease usually is not contagious 48 hours after beginning antibiotic therapy. Close household contacts should be tested (with blood cultures) and should receive appropriate antibiotic prophylaxis and immunization boosters. Infections can be treated with diphtheria antitoxin to neutralize the unbound toxin in the blood; antitoxin is available through the CDC.

- Diphtheria, a rare bacterial disease in the United States, can cause respiratory obstruction. High levels of diphtheria toxin can be fatal.
- Suspected cases of diphtheria should receive immediate, presumptive treatment.

Pertussis

Pertussis (**whooping cough**) is an infection of the respiratory system caused by the bacterium *Bordetella pertussis*. The first symptoms of whooping cough are similar to those of a common cold (eg, runny nose, sneezing, mild cough, and low-grade fever). After about 1 to 2 weeks, the dry, irritating cough transforms into a paroxysmal cough. These severe coughing spells end in a "whooping" sound when the person inhales. Pertussis cases have increased dramatically in the United States, from approximately 1,000 cases in 1976 to nearly 26,000 cases in 2004. Most of these cases have been adults, and inadequate immunization and waning immunity have been proposed as causative factors. Table 2 summarizes the composition, primary prevention or indications, adverse effects, and contraindications to pertussis vaccination.

Postexposure Treatment and Prophylaxis

Medical treatment of pertussis is usually supportive, but antibiotic therapy is helpful. Erythromycin is preferred because it kills the bacteria in secretions, which may limit the spread of disease. Other recommended medications include azithromycin and clarithromycin. Revised CDC guidelines (published December 2005) recommend that all close contacts of persons with pertussis receive prophylactic treatment, regardless of age or vaccination status. This treatment should be initiated within 3 weeks after exposure. Close contacts who are younger than 7 years should complete the recommended vaccination schedule with minimal intervals. Close contacts aged 4 through 6 years who have not had the second booster dose should be vaccinated.

- Pertussis characteristically begins with cold-like symptoms but progresses to paroxysmal

Table 2 Tetanus, Diphtheria, and Pertussis Vaccination

Composition	Primary Prevention or Indication	Booster	Adverse Effects and Contraindications	Other Recommendations
Tetanus Vaccine				
Formaldehyde-treated toxin, administered with the diphtheria toxoid as DTaP, DT, Td, or Tdap[a]	Primary series starts at age 2 mo, with subsequent doses at 4, 6, and 15–18 mo. Children older than 7 y require 3 doses at least 1 mo apart	Every 10 y. Individuals with a contaminated wound should receive a booster shot if the previous dose was >5 y earlier	Adverse effects include localized, self-limited, type III hypersensitivity (Arthus reaction). Contraindications include severe allergies to a vaccine component. Tdap is not licensed for use in adults ≥65 y	Adults with an uncertain history of completing the primary vaccination series should begin or complete the series. Tdap should replace a single dose of Td for adults younger than 65 y who have not previously received a dose of Tdap. Health care workers should keep their Tdap vaccination status current. Caution should be taken for patients with a moderate or severe acute illness at the time of vaccination. Pregnancy is not a contraindication for Tdap; when used, administration during the second or third trimester is preferred
Diphtheria Vaccine				
Given in combination with tetanus and pertussis. Diphtheria toxoid is produced by growing toxigenic *Corynebacterium diphtheriae* in liquid media. The filtrate is incubated with formaldehyde to convert the toxin to a toxoid, which is then adsorbed onto an aluminum salt.	See notes for tetanus	See notes for tetanus	See notes for tetanus	See notes for tetanus
Pertussis Vaccine				
Purified, inactivated components of *Bordetella pertussis* cells. Acellular pertussis vaccine is available only in combination with tetanus and diphtheria. Three acellular pertussis vaccines are available as pediatric formulations (ages 6 wk through 6 y). Two acellular formulations are available for adolescents (ages 10–18 y) and adults (ages 11–64 y). None of these vaccines contain the preservative thimerosal	Children aged 11–12 y should receive 1 dose of Tdap instead of Td	Children aged 13–18 y who did not get Tdap should receive 1 dose of Tdap as a catch-up booster instead of Td	See notes for tetanus	See notes for tetanus

Abbreviations: DT, diphtheria-tetanus; DTaP, diphtheria, tetanus, acellular pertussis; Td, tetanus-diphtheria; Tdap, tetanus, diphtheria, acellular pertussis.

[a] For vaccine abbreviations, upper-case letters denote full-strength doses of diphtheria (D) and tetanus (T) toxoids and pertussis (P) vaccine. Lower-case letters denote reduced doses of diphtheria (d) and pertussis (p).

Adapted from the Centers for Disease Control and Prevention (2009).

Table 3 Tetanus Vaccination in Patients With Wounds

Vaccination History	Therapy for Clean, Minor Wounds		Therapy for High-Risk Wounds[a]	
	Td/Tdap	TIG	TD/Tdap	TIG
Unknown or <3 doses	Yes	No	Yes	Yes
≥3 doses	Yes (if last booster was >10 y earlier)	No	Yes (if last booster was >5 y earlier)	No

Abbreviations: Td, tetanus-diphtheria; Tdap, tetanus, diphtheria, acellular pertussis; TIG, tetanus immunoglobulin.
[a] Examples of high-risk wounds: 1) wounds in contact with soil, manure, or compost; 2) puncture-type wounds; 3) infected wounds; 4) compound fractures; 5) wounds with a large amount of devitalized tissue; or 6) animal or human bite.

- coughing spells that end with a "whooping" sound.
- Most recent pertussis cases have been adults; increasing prevalence of disease may be attributable to inadequate immunization and waning immunity. Treatment is mostly supportive.

Bacterial Vaccines

Anthrax

Anthrax is a zoonotic infection caused by *Bacillus anthracis*. According to the CDC, anthrax infection can occur in 3 forms: cutaneous, pulmonary, and gastrointestinal. Most **cutaneous** infections occur when the bacteria enter a cut or abrasion on the skin (eg, when handling contaminated animals or their meat, hides, or wool). A skin infection begins as a small papule that resembles an insect bite, but within 1 to 2 days, a vesicle develops, followed by a painless ulcer with a black, necrotic center. About 20% of untreated cases are fatal.

The initial symptoms of **inhalation** anthrax resemble a common cold (eg, sore throat, mild fever, muscle aches, nonproductive cough, malaise). After several days, the symptoms may progress to high fever, dyspnea, and shock. Inhalation anthrax has a case-fatality rate of 85% to 97%; this decreases to 75% with antibiotic use. The **gastrointestinal** form of anthrax may occur after consumption of contaminated meat. It is characterized by acute inflammation of the gastrointestinal tract. Initial signs of nausea, anorexia, vomiting, and fever are followed by abdominal pain, hematemesis, and severe diarrhea. Intestinal anthrax results in death for 25% to 60% of cases.

The anthrax vaccine was licensed in 1970 and used in select populations such as laboratory personnel who handle *B anthracis*, people who work with imported animal hides or furs, and veterinarians and military personnel with high risk of exposure. A controlled study of mill workers in 1962 showed that the anthrax vaccine was 92.5% effective. The current vaccine consists of aluminum hydroxide–adsorbed cell-free anthrax, which is administered prophylactically before exposure. The vaccine is administered in 6 doses; the first 3 doses are given at 2-week intervals, and the final 3 are administered 6, 12, and 18 months after the first dose. Annual boosters are recommended if there is ongoing exposure to anthrax. Most commonly noted adverse effects are mild erythema and pruritus at the injection site.

Postexposure Treatment and Prophylaxis

Treatment is different for a person who is exposed to anthrax but not yet sick. Health care providers may use antibiotics (such as ciprofloxacin, levofloxacin, doxycycline, or penicillin) for 60 or 100 days in combination with the anthrax vaccine to prevent infection. Treatment of a confirmed infection usually involves a parenteral course of ciprofloxacin or doxycycline, with 1 or 2 additional antibiotics. The success of this treatment depends on the form of anthrax and how soon the individual begins treatment.

- Anthrax may occur in 3 forms: cutaneous, pulmonary, and gastrointestinal.
- The anthrax vaccine can be administered prophylactically to prevent disease.

Haemophilus influenzae Type B Infection

Haemophilus influenzae is a gram-negative coccobacillus. Although the organism colonizes in the nasopharynx, invasive disease caused by *H influenzae* type b (Hib) can affect many organ systems. The most common types of invasive disease are epiglottitis, arthritis, meningitis, pneumonia, otitis media, and cellulitis. Hib disease is age-dependent and is uncommon in persons older than 5 years. Hib disease occurs worldwide.

The Hib polysaccharide-protein conjugate vaccine was licensed in 1987 and approved for use in children as young as 6 weeks. Repeat doses may elicit a booster response. More than 95% of vaccinated infants will develop protective antibody levels after 2 or 3 doses. Table 4 summarizes the composition, primary prevention or indications, boosters, adverse effects, and contraindications to Hib vaccination.

Table 4 *Haemophilus influenzae* Type B, Meningococcal, and Pneumococcal Vaccination

Composition	Primary Prevention or Indication	Booster	Adverse Effects and Contraindications	Other Recommendations
Haemophilus influenzae Type B Vaccine				
Polysaccharide-protein conjugate vaccine	Vaccination series begins as young as age 6 wk; dosing interval to be at least 4 wk (recommended interval of 2 mo) PRP-OMP requires 2 doses in the series and a booster PRP-T requires a 3-dose primary series and a booster	At age 12–15 mo	Adverse effects include redness, swelling, and discomfort at the site, but systemic reactions such as fever and irritability are rare Contraindicated for those with severe allergies to a vaccine component; moderate or severe illness (delay vaccination until health improves); and age younger than 6 wk or older than 59 mo	High-risk individuals older than 59 mo may be vaccinated with at least 1 pediatric dose of any *Haemophilus influenzae* type b conjugate vaccine (high-risk populations are recipients of hematopoietic stem cell transplantation and patients with functional or anatomic asplenia, immunodeficiency, or HIV infection)
Meningococcal Vaccine				
MPSV4 contains the capsular polysaccharide antigens for serogroups A and C MCV4 contains capsular polysaccharide from *Neisseria meningitidis* serogroups A, C, Y, and W-135, conjugated to the diphtheria toxoid	Indicated for college freshmen in dormitories, occupationally exposed microbiologists, US military personnel, patients with asplenia or terminal complement deficiency, and travelers to a country with an outbreak of meningococcal disease	Uncertain whether additional booster doses are needed; however, they are not recommended currently	Adverse effects include pain and redness at the injection site, fever up to 7 d after vaccination, and fatigue; severe systemic reactions are rare (less than 3%) Contraindicated for patients with moderate or severe acute illness and for those with severe allergies to the vaccine, or vaccine components	For patients with Guillain-Barré syndrome, use MPSV4 instead of MCV (CDC recommendation) Revaccinate certain populations in 3 y with MCV4, including children aged 2–10 y with high risk (eg, travelers), patients with terminal complement deficiency or asplenia (anatomic or functional), and children with HIV (administered electively) Vaccine can be used to control outbreaks of meningitis

Pneumococcal Vaccine

PCV7 consists of inactivated bacterial vaccine (conjugate)	For all infants: 4 doses total, at ages 2, 4, 6, and 12–15 mo	Revaccinate in 5 y for persons with highest risk of pneumococcal infections (patients with asplenia, chronic renal failure, nephrotic syndrome, other immunosuppressed conditions)	Adverse effects include erythema and tenderness at the injection site	PCV7 is not recommended in children older than 59 mo
PPV23 consists of inactivated bacterial vaccine (polysaccharide)	Also indicated for children 2 y and older if they are immunocompromised or have chronic illness such as HIV infection or anatomic or functional asplenia	Booster is indicated if primary vaccination was received before age 65 y	Contraindicated for patients with allergies to the vaccine or vaccine components	Healthy children between 24-59 mo should not receive PPV23
	Recommended for those in an environment or setting with increased risk: patients with cochlear implants, some American Indian populations, residents of long-term care facilities, adults aged 65 y and older			PPV23 is not effective in children younger than 24 mo
	Recommended (by ACIP) for adults 19 y and older who are asthmatic or cigarette smokers			If elective splenectomy or cochlear implant is being considered, the vaccine should be administered at least 2 wk before the procedure; if this is not possible, vaccinate as soon after surgery as possible

Abbreviations: ACIP, Advisory Committee on Immunization Practices; CDC, Centers for Disease Control and Prevention; HIV, human immunodeficiency virus; MCV4, meningococcal conjugate vaccine; MPSV4, meningococcal polysaccharide vaccine; PCV7, 7-valent pneumococcal conjugate vaccine; PPV23, 23-valent pneumococcal polysaccharide vaccine; PRP-OMP, meningococcal group B outer membrane protein polysaccharide-protein conjugate vaccine; PRP-T, polysaccharide-protein conjugate vaccine using tetanus toxoid as a protein carrier.

Postexposure Treatment and Prophylaxis

Household contacts of individuals infected with invasive Hib disease should receive **rifampin** if children younger than 12 months are in the home and the children have not received the primary vaccination series. Households with at least one contact younger than 4 years who is not completely immunized should also receive rifampin. Households with immunocompromised children should receive prophylaxis, regardless of immunization status. Prophylaxis should be started as soon as possible. Rifampin is not recommended for pregnant women or persons with liver disease.

- Invasive disease caused by *H influenzae* type b (Hib) can cause epiglottitis, arthritis, meningitis, pneumonia, otitis media, and cellulitis.
- Rifampin may be used for postexposure prophylaxis.

Meningococcal Meningitis

Meningitis, a severe, acute infection caused by the bacterium *Neisseria meningitidis*, has a case-fatality rate of 10% to 14%. Survivors have risk of developing long-term sequelae, including deafness, limb loss, and neurologic deficits. Meningeal infection is similar to other forms of acute, purulent meningitis. Symptoms include a sudden-onset fever, headache, and stiff neck; nausea, vomiting, photophobia, and altered mental status also may occur. Meningococcal disease can also present with arthritis, otitis media, pneumonia, and epiglottitis. All health care providers should report any case of invasive meningococcal disease to local or state health departments. Table 4 summarizes the composition, primary prevention or indications, boosters, adverse effects, and contraindications to meningococcal vaccination.

Postexposure Treatment and Prophylaxis

Antimicrobial chemoprophylaxis is recommended for close contacts of infected persons, including household members, caregivers of children, and anyone directly exposed to the patient's oral secretions. The preferred antibiotics are rifampin, ciprofloxacin, and ceftriaxone, which are 90% to 95% effective. Rifampin (600 mg, every 12 hours, for 2 days) should be administered as soon as possible, preferably less than 24 hours after identification of the source patient. If the period between identification and treatment is longer than 14 days, treatment has limited or no value. Because systemic antimicrobial therapy does not eradicate nasopharyngeal carriage of *N meningitidis*, the source patient should also receive chemoprophylaxis before hospital dismissal.

- Patients with meningococcal meningitis can present with a sudden-onset fever, headache, and stiff neck; nausea, vomiting, photophobia, and altered mental status also may occur.

- Antimicrobial chemoprophylaxis with rifampin, ciprofloxacin, or ceftriaxone is recommended for close contacts of infected persons.

Pneumococcal Disease

In the United States, *Streptococcus pneumoniae* causes 500,000 cases of pneumonia, 3,000 cases of meningitis, and nearly 40,000 deaths per year. Rates of complication and death are highest among the elderly and among younger adults with chronic illness. The 7-valent pneumococcal conjugate vaccine is effective in children younger than 59 months. The 23-valent pneumococcal polysaccharide vaccine contains a purified capsular polysaccharide of 23 serotypes responsible for 90% of the bacteremic pneumococcal infections in the United States. This vaccine has 60% to 70% efficacy against invasive disease and is preferred for patients older than 2 years. Table 4 summarizes the composition, primary prevention or indications, boosters, adverse effects, and contraindications to pneumococcal vaccination.

- Rates of complication and death from pneumococcal infections are highest among the elderly and among younger adults with chronic illness.
- The vaccine against *Streptococcus pneumoniae* is 60% to 70% effective against invasive disease.

Viral Vaccines

Hepatitis A

Hepatitis A virus is the most common cause of acute viral hepatitis. It is spread via fecal-oral transmission, often in household, food preparation, or child care settings. Bloodborne and sexual transmission of the disease is less commonly reported. When infected, 70% of adults will have clinical symptoms of the disease, which usually last 6 to 8 weeks. The illness most often presents with an abrupt-onset fever, malaise, anorexia, nausea, abdominal discomfort, dark urine, and jaundice. Table 5 summarizes the composition, primary prevention or indications, boosters, adverse effects, and contraindications to hepatitis A vaccination.

Postexposure Treatment and Prophylaxis

Individuals exposed to hepatitis A virus should receive hepatitis A immunoglobulin or the hepatitis A vaccine. The vaccine is indicated for healthy persons aged 12 months to 40 years. The immunoglobulin is indicated for persons younger than 1 year and those who are immunocompromised or have chronic liver disease.

- Hepatitis A virus is the most common cause of acute viral hepatitis. It often presents with an abrupt-onset

Table 5 Hepatitis A, Hepatitis B, and Human Papillomavirus Vaccination

Composition	Primary Prevention or Indication	Booster	Adverse Effects and Contraindications	Other Recommendations
Hepatitis A Vaccine				
Inactivated whole virus	All children aged 12-23 mo Children who are not vaccinated by age 2 y can still be vaccinated Also indicated for men who have sex with men, recipients of clotting factor concentrates, users of illegal drugs, persons with chronic liver disease, persons working with HAV (eg, research setting), individuals traveling to or working in countries where HAV is endemic, any person seeking protection from HAV infection	No booster recommended	Adverse effects include pain and tenderness at the injection site, headache, and diarrhea Contraindicated for patients with severe allergies (eg, anaphylaxis) after a previous vaccine dose or to a vaccine component	Safety of vaccination during pregnancy has not been determined
Hepatitis B Vaccine				
Recombinant vaccine, produced by inserting a plasmid with the HBsAg gene into baker's yeast; 2 formulations are available	All infants should be vaccinated at birth, 1 mo, and 6 mo Also indicated for persons with end-stage renal disease, persons seeking evaluation or treatment for a sexually transmitted infection, persons with HIV or chronic liver disease, health care and public safety workers exposed to blood or body fluids, sexually active individuals not in a long-term, mutually monogamous relationship, intravenous drug users, men who have sex with men, clients and staff members of institutions for persons with developmental disabilities, international travelers, household contacts of infected individuals, and any adult seeking protection from hepatitis B infection	Routine booster doses are not recommended but can be administered when antibody levels decline to less than 10 mIU/mL	Adverse effects include mild, self-limited soreness at the injection site Contraindicated for patients with severe allergies (eg, anaphylaxis) after a previous vaccine dose, hypersensitivity to yeast	Safety of vaccination during pregnancy has not been determined More than 90% of healthy adults will develop immunity upon completion of the vaccine series, but actual seroconversion rates decrease substantially with age In immunocompromised adults or children and those receiving hemodialysis, 2-4 times the normal dose may be needed to induce immunity.
Human Papillomavirus Vaccine				
Purified proteins from HPV strains 6, 11, 16, and 18	Indicated for females aged 9-26 y	Routine boosters are not recommended	Adverse effects include pain at the injection site, local swelling, and fever Contraindicated for patients with allergies to a vaccine component or to a prior dose, allergy to yeast, severe or moderate acute illness Not recommended for use during pregnancy	HPV vaccine can be administered in women with equivocal or abnormal Papanicolaou test results, positive HPV test results, or genital warts Vaccination can proceed for women who are immunosuppressed or breastfeeding Prior infection with a different HPV strain does not decrease the efficacy of the vaccine against HPV strains 6, 11, 16, and 18

Abbreviations: HAV, hepatitis A virus; HBsAg, hepatitis B surface antigen; HIV, human immunodeficiency virus; HPV, human papillomavirus.

fever, malaise, anorexia, nausea, abdominal discomfort, dark urine, and jaundice.

- Individuals aged 1 to 40 years should receive hepatitis A immunoglobulin or the hepatitis A vaccine after exposure to the virus.

Hepatitis B

The hepatitis B virus is a blood-borne pathogen. In the United States, the lifetime risk of infection is 5%, and more than 90% of those affected are 20 years or older. Of those infected, 5% to 10% become carriers of the disease. On an annual basis, hepatitis B infection causes 4,000 deaths from cirrhosis and 1,500 from hepatocellular carcinoma in the United States. Liver cancer is one of the most common and most deadly cancers worldwide because of the huge burden of viral hepatitis transmission and disease. Table 5 summarizes the composition, primary prevention or indications, boosters, adverse effects, and contraindications to hepatitis B vaccination.

A combined vaccine against hepatitis A and hepatitis B is available, and it is administered in 3 doses (0, 1, and 6 months). For travelers to endemic areas who need a faster series, an alternative 4-dose schedule can be used (administration on days 0, 7, and 21, with a final dose at 12 months).

Postexposure Treatment and Prophylaxis

The hepatitis B vaccine is recommended as part of postexposure management for unvaccinated individuals (eg, occupational exposure, sexual contact, or neonate with an HBsAg-positive mother). Exposure can also occur in infants younger than 1 year if a primary caregiver has an acute hepatitis B infection. For exposed individuals, vaccination and hepatitis B immunoglobulin are administered if indicated. For infants born to HBsAg-positive mothers, this combination is 85% to 95% effective in preventing active disease when given in the first 24 hours after birth.

- The hepatitis B virus is a blood-borne pathogen; in the United States, the lifetime risk of infection is 5%.
- For exposed individuals, vaccination and hepatitis B immunoglobulin are administered if indicated.

Human Papillomavirus Infection

Human papillomavirus (HPV) infection is a sexually transmitted infection that has been linked to **cervical cancer**. HPVs are small, double-stranded DNA viruses. Most HPVs attack the cutaneous epithelium and cause common skin warts. HPV strains 16 and 18 cause 70% of cervical cancer in women and 70% of anal cancer in men. In contrast, HPV strains 6 and 11 cause up to 90% of genital warts in women. Table 5 summarizes the composition, primary prevention or indications, boosters, adverse effects, and contraindications to HPV vaccination.

Postexposure Treatment and Prophylaxis

HPV transmission can be reduced with the use of physical barriers such as condoms, but this does not eliminate the risk. Abstaining from sexual activity is the most certain way to prevent genital HPV infection. After women become sexually active, it is important to undergo routine cervical cancer screening. If an individual is positive for 1 or more of the high-risk HPV types (other than HPV 16 and 19), postexposure vaccination is recommended.

- Human papillomavirus (HPV) strains cause 70% of cervical cancer in women, 70% of anal cancer in men, and 90% of genital warts in women.
- HPV vaccination is recommended for females 9 to 26 years of age.

Live-Virus Vaccines

Influenza

Influenza is caused by RNA viruses of the Orthomyxoviridae family (subtypes A, B, and C). Type A can affect all age groups and cause moderate-to-severe illnesses. Type B usually affects children and is milder than type A. Type C is rarely reported. Influenza activity peaks from December to March in temperate climate areas, but it can occur throughout the year in tropical areas.

The influenza virus has an incubation period of 1 to 4 days; about 50% of those infected have classic flu symptoms (ie, sudden-onset fever, chills, body aches, sore throat, headache, and nonproductive cough). These symptoms typically last from 3 to 5 days. The virus is spread by direct or indirect contact with respiratory secretions of infected persons. Complications associated with influenza include pneumonia, Reye syndrome in children, and myocarditis.

The first recorded influenza pandemic occurred in 1580, and at least 3 pandemics have occurred during the 20th century. Annually, deaths from influenza are estimated to exceed 36,000. Influenza-related deaths are the highest among the VPDs, with approximately 90% occurring among adults aged 65 years and older. Young children can also have complications that often result in hospitalization. Among the elderly in nursing homes, vaccination against influenza may reduce the incidence of illness by 30% to 40% and may be 80% effective in the prevention of influenza-related death. Table 6 summarizes the composition, primary prevention or indications, adverse effects, and contraindications to influenza vaccination.

Postexposure Treatment and Prophylaxis

The **neuraminidase inhibitors** oseltamivir and zanamivir can effectively prevent influenza A and B. Oseltamivir

Table 6 Influenza, MMR, and Varicella Vaccination

Composition	Primary Prevention or Indication	Booster	Adverse Effects and Contraindications	Other Recommendations
Influenza Vaccine				
Vaccine contains 1 type B strain and 2 type A strains considered likely to circulate in the upcoming influenza season Two types of vaccines are used: the TIV is administered intramuscularly, and the LAIV is administered intranasally (single-dose unit; half of the dose is sprayed in each nostril)	Indicated for all children aged 5-18 y, patients with chronic disorders (eg, cardiovascular or pulmonary disease, including asthma), metabolic disease (eg, diabetes mellitus), liver or renal dysfunction, immunosuppression due to medications or HIV infection, women who will be pregnant during the influenza season, health care workers, employees and residents of long-term care facilities, caregivers and household contacts of persons at high risk, and anyone who would like to be vaccinated Intranasal vaccine is approved for use only in healthy, nonpregnant patients aged 2-49 y	Yearly boosters	Adverse effects most often observed with TIV include localized skin reaction Adverse effects most often observed with LAIV include rhinorrhea, sore throat, and headache Contraindicated for patients with severe allergies to the vaccine or any vaccine component, moderate or severe acute illness, or allergies to eggs or egg products LAIV is contraindicated for children younger than 2 y, immunosuppressed patients, patients with chronic medical conditions, patients who are pregnant, and children receiving long-term aspirin therapy	Children first vaccinated between age 6 mo and 8 y should have 1 dose in the early autumn and a second dose 4 wk after the initial dose
Measles Vaccine				
Two types of live-virus vaccines are used: single-antigen vaccine combined with vaccines for mumps and rubella; and single-antigen vaccine combined with vaccines for mumps, rubella, and varicella	All children 12 mo and older should receive 2 doses of the vaccine, at least 4 wk apart (the second dose preferably is administered at age 4-6 y) Adults born in 1957 or later with no medical contraindications should receive at least 1 dose of MMR vaccine if they have no proof of prior vaccination ACIP recommends that MMR be used when any component is indicated	Indicated for individuals vaccinated before the first birthday, vaccinated with killed measles vaccine, vaccinated before 1968 with an unknown type of vaccine, and vaccinated with immunoglobulin plus a further attenuated strain or vaccine of unknown type	Adverse effects of MMR include fever (mostly due to the measles component), rash, arthralgias (25%; mostly due to the rubella component, mostly occurs in women) Rare effects include thrombocytopenia, parotitis (due to the mumps component), deafness, and encephalopathy Contraindicated for patients with severe allergies to the vaccine or any component of the vaccine (including neomycin and gelatin), moderate or severe illness, pregnant patients, recent recipients of blood products or immunoglobulin (past 3-12 mo), immunosuppressed patients (except HIV-positive patients with >200 CD4$^+$ cells/mm^3)	A tuberculin skin test can be applied on the same day or 1 mo after the MMR vaccine because the MMR vaccine can cause mild suppression of the immune system, diminishing the reactivity of the test Avoid pregnancy for at least 4 wk after the MMR vaccine

Table 6 (continued) Influenza, MMR, and Varicella Vaccination

Composition	Primary Prevention or Indication	Booster	Adverse Effects and Contraindications	Other Recommendations
Mumps Vaccine				
Live, attenuated virus	See notes for measles	See notes for measles	See notes for measles	See notes for measles
Rubella Vaccine				
Live, attenuated virus	See notes for measles	See notes for measles	See notes for measles	See notes for measles
Varicella Vaccine				
In the United States, 2 preservative-free vaccines are used: one is derived from the Oka strain of varicella-zoster virus, the other is a live, attenuated virus vaccine In 2005, a combined, live, attenuated MMR and varicella vaccine was licensed	Children should receive the first dose at age 12-15 mo and the second dose at 4-6 y Also indicated for all adolescents 13 y or older and adults who do not have evidence of varicella immunity The varicella vaccine is for children 12 mo and older The combined MMR-varicella vaccine is for children aged 12 mo through 12 y	Yearly boosters	Adverse effects include erythema and pain at the injection site, maculopapular generalized rash (5%-6%), and occasional zoster infection (mostly in children) Contraindicated for patients with severe allergies to the vaccine or vaccine components, immunosuppressed children, and persons with severe allergies to neomycin	Adults with both laboratory evidence of immunity and birth in the United States before 1980 are considered immune to varicella; exceptions are health care workers and pregnant women It is important that children do not receive other live viral vaccines within 30 d of receiving the varicella vaccine, which can reduce the efficacy of the vaccine

Abbreviations: ACIP, Advisory Committee on Immunization Practices; HIV, human immunodeficiency virus; LAIV, live, attenuated influenza vaccine; MMR, measles, mumps, and rubella; TIV, trivalent, inactivated vaccine.

(75 mg daily, for up to 6 weeks) has a protective efficacy of up to 74%. Zanamivir (10 mg daily, for 10 days) has a protective efficacy of 78% for influenza A and about 85% for influenza B. An orally inhaled powder, zanamivir can cause rare bronchospasm and oropharyngeal edema and is not recommended for individuals with underlying airway problems; otherwise, it is recommended for children 7 years and older and for adults. Amantadine and rimantadine, previously used for prevention of influenza A, are no longer effective as prophylaxis because resistance has developed against these medications.

- The influenza virus has an incubation period of 1 to 4 days. Classic flu symptoms last 3 to 5 days and include sudden-onset fever, chills, body aches, sore throat, headache, and nonproductive cough.
- Neuraminidase inhibitors such as oseltamivir and zanamivir can effectively prevent influenza.
- Egg allergy is a contraindication to influenza vaccination.

Measles, Mumps, and Rubella

Measles or **rubeola** is an acute, systemic, febrile disease that is highly contagious. Common symptoms are cough, conjunctivitis, rhinitis, erythematous maculopapular rash, and Koplik spots. Measles is still common and can be fatal in developing countries. In 1963, the first vaccine was licensed in the United States, and the incidence of measles decreased by more than 98%. However, between 1989 and 1991, a marked increase in measles was observed in the United States, which likely was attributable to high numbers of unvaccinated preschool children. Intensive efforts to vaccinate preschoolers resulted in an increase in the rate of vaccinated 2-year-olds from 70% in 1990 to 91% in 1997.

Mumps is an acute viral illness that can cause swelling of the salivary glands. Periodic outbreaks have been documented and likely are associated with decreased vaccination levels and waning immunity. Rubella is a mild infectious disease that is generally characterized by a rash, lymphadenopathy, and mild fever. Table 6 summarizes the composition, primary prevention or indications, adverse effects, and contraindications to measles, mumps, and rubella vaccination.

Postexposure Treatment and Prophylaxis

Individuals exposed to measles may receive the live measles vaccine within 72 hours after exposure; this should provide lifelong immunity and prevent the development of active disease. Passive immunity can be achieved through immunoglobulin administration within 6 days after exposure. Immunoglobulin should be considered for susceptible household members who are exposed, especially children younger than 1 year. If exposed children are older than 1 year, they should receive the live measles vaccine 5 months after administration of immunoglobulin. Immunoglobulin is not to be used to control measles outbreaks.

- Common measles symptoms include cough, conjunctivitis, rhinitis, erythematous maculopapular rash, and Koplik spots. Mumps can cause swelling of the salivary glands. Rubella is a mild infectious disease that is generally characterized by a rash, lymphadenopathy, and mild fever.
- The measles-mumps-rubella (MMR) vaccine is contraindicated in pregnant women. Women who have received the MMR vaccination are recommended to wait at least 4 weeks before attempting conception.

Poliomyelitis

Poliomyelitis was first described in 1789, and the first outbreak in the United States occurred in 1843. More than 21,000 cases were noted in the United States in 1952. Symptoms can range from flu-like illness to flaccid paralysis.

The disease is caused by poliovirus, an enterovirus that enters through the mouth and multiplies in the pharynx, gastrointestinal tract, and lymph system. The incubation period is 7 to 14 days. Infected persons are contagious for about 1 week, starting a few days before symptoms occur. Poliovirus is highly infectious. Polio at one time occurred throughout the world, but the global polio eradication program has markedly reduced its worldwide incidence. Successful vaccination since the mid-1950s has resulted in the eradication of polio from the Western hemisphere.

Inactivated poliovirus vaccine (IPV) was licensed in 1955 and used until 1961, when the monovalent oral poliovirus vaccine became licensed. In 1963, a trivalent oral vaccine was introduced and used until 1987, when an enhanced-potency version was developed. Oral poliovirus vaccine is also very effective and is believed to produce lifelong immunity after 3 doses. The oral vaccine was used almost exclusively until 2000. However, IPV now is used exclusively in the United States because rare cases of paralytic polio have been reported with the oral vaccine. The IPV is well tolerated and is associated only with minor, local skin reactions. The formulation contains very small amounts of streptomycin, polymyxin B, and neomycin, and individuals who are sensitive to these products may have an allergic reaction (the vaccine is contraindicated for individuals with anaphylaxis after exposure to those antibiotics). Caution should be used if the person has a moderate or severe acute illness.

For individuals needing vaccination, a 3-dose primary series of injectable IPV at 0, 1, and 6 to 12 months is recommended. For patients with an incomplete primary series, completion of the series should commence without restarting, regardless of the interval. The IPV is more than 95% effective when properly administered and results in 99% immunity to poliovirus after 3 doses. The duration of immunity is uncertain. Polio vaccination is not recommended for persons older than 18 years unless they plan to travel to an endemic area and have not completed the primary series.

Postexposure Treatment and Prophylaxis

If a single case of paralytic poliomyelitis is identified in a community and is shown to be caused by an infection of wild poliovirus, all unvaccinated persons in the epidemic area who are at least 6 weeks old and have uncertain vaccination histories should be vaccinated.

- Poliovirus is highly infectious. Symptoms can range from flu-like illness to flaccid paralysis.
- In the United States, inactivated poliovirus vaccine (IPV) is used exclusively because rare cases of paralytic polio have been reported with the oral vaccine.
- Vaccination for persons older than 18 years usually is not recommended unless patients plan to travel to endemic areas and have not completed the primary series.
- If a case of wild poliovirus is identified, unvaccinated persons in the epidemic area who are at least 6 weeks old and have uncertain vaccination histories should be vaccinated.

Rabies

Rabies is a viral disease in mammals that most often is transmitted through the bite of an infected animal. Most rabies cases occur in wild animals such as raccoons, skunks, bats, and foxes. Although cats, cattle, and dogs are the domestic animals most often reported rabid, domestic animal cases account for less than 10% of reported rabies cases overall. The rabies virus infects the central nervous system and causes encephalopathy and ultimately death. Approximately 16,000 to 39,000 persons come in contact with potentially rabid animals and receive rabies postexposure prophylaxis each year. Preexposure prophylactic vaccination is recommended for animal handlers, laboratory workers, persons traveling to hyperendemic areas for more than 1 month, and those with vocations involving exposure to skunks, raccoons, bats, or other animals. Rabies preexposure vaccination should include 3 doses of the vaccine administered intramuscularly, with 1 injection daily on days 0, 7, and 21 or 28.

Postexposure Treatment and Prophylaxis

Administration of rabies postexposure prophylaxis is considered a medical urgency, not a medical emergency.

Prophylaxis is occasionally complicated by adverse reactions, but these are rarely severe. For humans exposed to rabies virus, the main preventive measures are prompt and thorough wound cleansing, passive rabies immunization with human rabies immunoglobulin, and vaccination with a cell culture rabies vaccine. For persons who have never been vaccinated against rabies, postexposure vaccination should always include administration of human rabies immunoglobulin and rabies vaccine (human diploid cell vaccine or purified chick embryo cell vaccine).

Persons who have previously completed a vaccination regimen and have a documented rabies virus–neutralizing antibody titer should receive only 2 doses of vaccine, the first on day 0 and the second on day 3. Human rabies immunoglobulin is administered only once to previously unvaccinated persons to provide immediate, passive, rabies virus–neutralizing antibody coverage until the patient is actively producing antibodies. As of June 2009, the CDC recommends administering a regimen of 4 vaccine doses to previously unvaccinated persons, with the first dose administered as soon as possible after exposure (day 0). Subsequent doses should be administered on days 3, 7, 14, and 28 after the first vaccination.

- Rabies virus most often is transmitted through the bite of an infected animal. The virus infects the central nervous system and ultimately causes death.
- After exposure to rabies, the key preventive measures are prompt and thorough wound cleansing, passive rabies immunization with human rabies immunoglobulin, and vaccination with a cell culture rabies vaccine.

Rotavirus Infection

Rotavirus illness is the most common cause of severe diarrhea in children, and it is responsible for up to 500,000 deaths worldwide per year. Infection with rotavirus is considered nearly universal—almost all children have been infected within the first 5 years of life. The highest incidence is among children aged 3 to 35 months. The first infection after age 3 months is usually the most severe.

The first vaccine for this virus was licensed in 1998, but cases of intussusception were noted and the vaccine was withdrawn in 1999. A second-generation vaccine was licensed in 2006; it is a live oral vaccine containing no preservatives or thimerosal. Three doses are required, and the completed vaccine series has an efficacy of 74% in preventing all rotavirus gastroenteritis and 98% in preventing severe disease (defined as fever, vomiting, diarrhea, and changes in behavior). The duration of immunity is not definitely known, but protection lasting at least 2 seasons has been shown in a clinical trial. The newest vaccine, approved in 2008, is administered in 2 doses at ages 2 and 4 months. ACIP recommends routine, 3-dose vaccination of all infants, administered at age 2, 4, and 6 months.

The series should not be started after the infant is 12 weeks old because of limited data on the vaccine's safety in older infants. Rotavirus vaccine may be given with other vaccines. Breastfeeding infants, preterm infants, and infants who have already had rotavirus illness should be immunized (the last group may not be immune to all 5 serotypes present in the vaccine).

Potential adverse effects of the vaccine include vomiting, diarrhea, nasopharyngitis, otitis media, and bronchospasm. The rotavirus vaccine is contraindicated for infants who had an anaphylactic reaction to a prior dose. Caution should be taken when treating infants with an altered immune system, with chronic (preexisting) gastrointestinal tract disease, or with a history of intussusception. The decision to vaccinate infants with an altered immune system or a preexisting gastrointestinal tract disease should be made on a case-by-case basis. Recent recipients of blood products should delay vaccination for 6 weeks. Infants with acute, moderate-to-severe gastroenteritis or other illness should delay the vaccination until the illness improves, although vaccination can proceed for infants with mild gastrointestinal tract illness. If a household member is immunocompromised, the infant should be vaccinated and family members should use strict handwashing techniques after infant diapering.

Postexposure Treatment and Prophylaxis

Individuals exposed to rotavirus can develop the illness, but if they have been infected previously, the illness may not be as severe. Hydration is important during illness. Good hygiene practices can help prevent the spread of illness. No clinical data are available regarding the usefulness of the vaccine when it is administered after exposure to rotavirus.

- Rotavirus illness is the most common cause of severe diarrhea in children, and almost all children have been infected within the first 5 years of life.
- The live, oral vaccine currently used has an efficacy of 74% in preventing all rotavirus gastroenteritis and 98% in preventing severe disease.
- Infants should be vaccinated at ages 2, 4, and 6 months. However, decisions about vaccination of infants with an altered immune system or a preexisting gastrointestinal tract disease should be made on a case-by-case basis.

Smallpox

Smallpox is caused by the variola virus, which is transmitted through oropharyngeal or respiratory secretions. The first symptoms of the illness occur within 2 to 4 days after exposure and include fever, malaise, headache, and body aches. A rash of small, red spots develops on the tongue and mouth. These become sores that break open, and the rash spreads to the rest of the body. The rash is characterized by papules, which have a central depression and are filled with an opaque fluid. These papules subsequently become pustules and then scabs.

In May of 1980, the World Health Organization declared the world free of smallpox after a successful worldwide vaccination program. The vaccine is made from the **vaccinia virus**, a poxvirus similar to smallpox. Smallpox vaccination provides high-level immunity for 3 to 5 years and decreasing immunity thereafter. A subsequent vaccination results in even longer immunity. The vaccine is 95% effective in preventing smallpox infection.

Potential adverse effects of vaccination include rash, fever, head and body aches, eczema vaccinatum, generalized vaccinia, postvaccinal encephalitis, and myopericarditis. Inadvertent inoculation at other sites can also occur. This vaccination is contraindicated in pregnancy, in those with eczema (history or presence) or HIV infection, immunocompromised individuals, and those with a known allergy to a vaccine component.

Postexposure Treatment and Prophylaxis

Vaccination within 3 days of exposure will prevent or considerably lessen the severity of smallpox symptoms for most people. Vaccination 4 to 7 days after exposure likely offers some protection from disease or may diminish the severity of disease.

- The smallpox vaccine is made from the vaccinia virus.
- After a successful worldwide vaccination program, the World Health Organization declared the world free of smallpox in 1980.
- Vaccination is contraindicated in pregnancy, in those with eczema or human immunodeficiency virus infection, immunocompromised individuals, and those with a known allergy to a vaccine component.

Varicella Infection

Varicella or **chickenpox** is an infection caused by the varicella-zoster virus (VZV). A low-grade fever may precede the rash, but with children, the rash is often the first sign. The rash is generalized and pruritic in nature. It progresses from macules to papules to vesicles before crusting. The fever may last a few days. Varicella susceptibility results in 3 million cases of VPD in adults annually in the United States. Although these infections comprise less than 10% of the total cases of chickenpox or primary VZV infection, 20% of deaths due to VZV infection occur in adults, and the greatest morbidity and mortality occur in the elderly and immunosuppressed.

For adults, the vaccine is 95% effective in the prevention of severe disease, although breakthrough infections have been reported. Generally, breakthrough disease is mild and occurs only after intense exposure to wild virus. A person who recovers from a primary varicella infection usually has lifelong immunity; adults with a reliable history of infection with chickenpox during childhood have 97% to 99% seropositivity. Table 6 summarizes the composition, primary prevention or indications, adverse effects, and contraindications for varicella vaccination.

Postexposure Treatment and Prophylaxis

Individuals need to be vaccinated if they are exposed to varicella infection and have no evidence of immunity. The varicella vaccine is 70% to 100% effective in preventing the development of varicella infection or decreasing the severity of the infection if used within 3 days (and possibly up to 5 days) after exposure. During outbreaks of varicella infection in child care facilities or schools, ACIP recommends that children receive a second dose of varicella vaccine. Doses should be spaced by 3 months for children aged 12 months to 12 years. For children 13 years and older, 4 weeks are recommended between doses.

- Symptoms of varicella (chickenpox) include a low-grade fever and a generalized, pruritic rash that progresses from macules to papules to vesicles before crusting.
- The vaccine is 95% effective in the prevention of severe disease, although mild breakthrough infections have occurred with exposure to wild virus.
- During outbreaks of varicella infection in child care facilities or schools, children should receive a second dose of varicella vaccine.

Zoster

VZV causes chickenpox as a primary infection, but it can remain latent in the dorsal root ganglion and reactivate, resulting in herpes zoster or **shingles**. This presents as a unilateral rash that usually affects 1 to 3 dermatomes, most frequently in the thoracic region. Approximately 1 million cases of shingles occur annually in the United States, with the highest risk of severe disease in immunocompromised and elderly populations. Complications of shingles include postherpetic neuralgia, which is associated with increased age and estimated to occur in approximately 10% to 33% of cases.

A live, attenuated zoster vaccine can reduce the risks of zoster and postherpetic neuralgia. Currently, the zoster vaccine is recommended in a single dose for adults 60 years and older, and booster doses are not recommended. Although the vaccine is safe for persons who have had a previous episode of zoster, the efficacy remains uncertain. Common adverse reactions include erythema, pain, and swelling at the injection site. The vaccine is contraindicated

for persons with a history of severe reactions to gelatin or neomycin and for immunosuppressed patients.

- Complications of shingles include postherpetic neuralgia, which is associated with increased age and estimated to occur in approximately 10% to 33% of cases.
- The zoster vaccine is recommended in a single dose for adults 60 years and older.

Strategies for Increasing Immunization Rates in the Outpatient Practice Setting

Despite broad support of vaccination from professional medical organizations, vaccination rates of susceptible adults remain suboptimal. According to the CDC, the costs associated with VPD are approximately $10 billion yearly. Strategies to enhance the rate of immunization include **targeted awareness campaigns** to educate providers and the public about the importance of immunization. Funding and infrastructure development are required at local, regional, and national levels to increase the capacity of the health system and to treat the underinsured and uninsured adults who do not receive recommended vaccinations. Legislative efforts to expand and standardize adult immunization coverage by public and private insurance programs and efforts to ensure adequate support for research of vaccines and VPDs, including surveillance, have also been endorsed by the CDC.

Practice-based systematic models to maintain increased adult immunization rates include vaccination algorithms, electronic medical record reminders, community partnerships, and the creation of a culture of excellence. An **immunization registry**, a computerized information system that records immunization status of individual patients, has been proposed to increase rates of immunization. An individual's immunization record may be linked to a public health database, enhancing opportunities for a registry to create reminders. **Reminder** or **recall systems** ideally contact patients and health care providers and may incorporate phone contact, e-mail, or postal mail. An additional benefit of an immunization registry is the potential to rapidly identify susceptible individuals in the event of a disease outbreak. Issues of privacy remain one of the major obstacles to the development of such a registry.

Indicators of health care quality are becoming more prominent in health care organizations. The promotion of patient immunization as a potential quality metric may increase provider and organizational awareness of the importance of vaccination in preventing disease.

- Targeted awareness campaigns can be used to educate providers and the public about the importance of immunization.

- An immunization registry can be used to develop reminder or recall systems to facilitate timely vaccination

SUGGESTED READING

Advisory Committee on Immunization Practices. Recommended adult immunization schedule: United States, October 2007-September 2008. Ann Intern Med. 2007 Nov 20;147(10):725-9. Epub 2007 Oct 18.

Centers for Disease Control and Prevention. Epidemiology and Prevention of Vaccine-Preventable Diseases. Atkinson W, Wolfe S, Hamborsky J, McIntyre L, eds. 11th ed. Washington (DC): Public Health Foundation, 2009. Available from: http://www.cdc.gov/vaccines/pubs/pinkbook/default.htm.

Centers for Disease Control and Prevention, Vaccines & Immunizations [Internet]. Atlanta: Centers for Disease Control and Prevention [cited 2008 Oct 20]. Available from: http://www.cdc.gov/vaccines/.

Ghosh AK, editor. Mayo Clinic Internal Medicine Review. 8th ed. Rochester (MN): Mayo Clinic Scientific Press and Florence (KY): Informa Healthcare Kentucky Distribution Center; c2008. Chapter 21, Preventive Medicine; p. 839-60.

Questions and Answers

Questions

1. A 67-year-old Hmong woman sustained a deep and dirty laceration (a tetanus-prone injury) on her leg while gardening. She immigrated to the United States 5 years ago to live with her son and his family. She is not aware of having any vaccinations in the past. She takes no medications and has no known allergies. Which treatment do you recommend for tetanus prophylaxis?
   a. Tetanus immunoglobulin
   b. Primary series of tetanus toxoid
   c. Primary series of tetanus-diphtheria toxoids
   d. Primary series of diphtheria, tetanus, and pertussis vaccine
   e. Tetanus immunoglobulin and primary series of tetanus-diphtheria toxoids

2. A 5-year-old, healthy boy presents for a pre-kindergarten evaluation. His parents report that he has no known medical conditions or allergies. They provide records of his immunization history that show he has received the inactivated polio vaccine ([IPV] 2 doses at 2 and 4 months), diphtheria, tetanus, and acellular pertussis vaccine ([DTaP] 3 doses at 2, 4, and 12 months), hepatitis B vaccine ([HepB] 2 doses at 2 and 12 months), measles, mumps, rubella vaccine ([MMR] 1 dose at 12 months), and *Haemophilus influenzae* type b vaccine (1 dose at 2 months).

Which of the following would you *not* recommend to his parents in this setting?
   a. DTaP
   b. Begin the varicella series, return in 3 months for the second dose
   c. IPV
   d. Restart the HepB series, return in 4 weeks for the second dose
   e. All of the above are recommended at this time

3. A type III hypersensitivity (Arthus) reaction is most frequently associated with which vaccination?
   a. Inactive poliovirus
   b. Meningococcus
   c. Hepatitis B
   d. Diphtheria, tetanus, acellular pertussis
   e. Measles, mumps, rubella

4. A 65-year-old, recently retired man comes for travel counseling. He is planning to volunteer to do construction work in Guatemala for 3 to 6 months each year. He will be staying in an isolated rural village where malaria transmission is documented. He takes atenolol and triamterene-hydrochlorothiazide for treatment of mild hypertension but otherwise is in very good health. He received the primary series of tetanus and diphtheria toxoids while in military service and has had several boosters since then, most recently 4 to 5 years ago. He also had a primary series of polio vaccine during his military service. He recently received pneumococcal and influenza vaccinations from his primary care physician. All of the following recommendations would be appropriate *except*:
   a. Enhanced injectable polio booster
   b. Counseling with malaria chemoprophylaxis
   c. Hepatitis A vaccine
   d. Hepatitis B vaccine

5. Which of the following groups should *not* receive the live, attenuated influenza vaccine?
   a. Adults with mild-to-moderate illness
   b. Healthy children aged 2 through 5 years
   c. Healthy, pregnant women
   d. Healthy, penicillin-allergic adults
   e. Health care workers

6. Which of the following is a recombinant vaccine?
   a. *Haemophilus influenzae* type b
   b. Hepatitis B
   c. Varicella
   d. Pneumococcus
   e. Rotavirus

7. Which statement about the tetanus, diphtheria, and acellular pertussis (Tdap) vaccine is *false*?
   a. Tdap is contraindicated in pregnancy
   b. Tdap should replace a single dose of tetanus-diphtheria (Td) vaccine for adults who have not previously received a dose of Tdap and require a booster of Td
   c. Tdap vaccine is not licensed for use among adults aged 65 years and older
   d. Tdap is contraindicated in adults allergic to formaldehyde

Answers

1. Answer e.

Appropriate tetanus prophylaxis for an adult who has never received tetanus vaccinations includes both tetanus immunoglobulin and initiating the 3-dose primary series of tetanus-diphtheria toxoids (Td). The tetanus, diphtheria, acellular pertussis vaccine (Tdap) should replace a single dose of Td for adults younger than 65 years who have not previously received a dose of Tdap.

2. Answer d.

It is not necessary to restart the hepatitis B series, provided that the first 2 doses were appropriately spaced. One additional dose is required to complete the series of 3, and this should be recommended at this time. To complete the primary series of DTaP, a fourth dose is indicated. To complete the primary series of polio vaccination, a third dose of IPV is indicated. The child has not previously received the varicella vaccination. The first vaccination is recommended at this time, with a booster after at least 3 months.

3. Answer d.

Type III hypersensitivity (Arthus) reactions are rarely reported after vaccination but can occur after administering vaccines containing tetanus or diphtheria toxoids. An Arthus reaction is a local vasculitis. Arthus reactions are characterized by severe pain, swelling, induration, edema, hemorrhage, and occasionally by necrosis. These symptoms and signs usually occur 4 to 12 hours after vaccination. The Advisory Committee on Immunization Practices recommends that persons who experienced an Arthus reaction after a dose of tetanus toxoid–containing vaccine should not receive tetanus-diphtheria vaccination more frequently than every 10 years, even for tetanus prophylaxis as part of wound management.

4. Answer a.

Polio has been eradicated from the Western hemisphere and the patient therefore does not need a polio booster. For adults traveling to areas where polio is still endemic (eg, South Asia and Africa), a single booster dose of injectable polio vaccine is recommended if the primary polio vaccine series was administered previously. Unimmunized adults should have a 3-dose primary series or as many doses of the series as time permits before travel to an endemic area. Hepatitis A vaccination is recommended for nonimmune travelers to countries with an intermediate or high endemicity of infection, which includes all developing countries. Hepatitis B vaccination is recommended for nonimmune travelers to areas of high endemicity. Those with high risk of exposure include longer-term travelers and persons having direct contact with blood or secretions (including sexual contact) of potentially infected persons.

5. Answer c.

The intranasally administered preparation of live, attenuated influenza virus may be used to vaccinate only healthy, nonpregnant patients aged 2 to 49 years who have no high-risk medical conditions. Other individuals should receive the inactivated, injectable influenza vaccine.

6. Answer b.

The only recombinant vaccine currently in use is the hepatitis B vaccine. This is produced by inserting a plasmid containing the gene for HBsAg into common baker's yeast. The *Haemophilus influenzae* type b and *Streptococcus pneumoniae* vaccines are conjugate vaccines. The varicella vaccine is a live, attenuated virus. The rotavirus vaccine is a live-virus vaccine that is administered orally.

7. Answer a.

Tdap is not contraindicated in pregnancy. Tdap should replace a single dose of Td for adults younger than 65 years who have not received a dose of Tdap previously (ie, in a primary series, booster, or wound management). Tdap vaccine is not licensed for use among adults aged 65 years and older. Tdap is contraindicated for individuals with an allergy to aluminum or formaldehyde and those with a history of neurologic or immediate hypersensitivity reactions.

8

MATERNAL AND CHILD HEALTH

Heidi K. Roeber Rice, MD, MPH; Brian C. Brost, MD

The habits and health of mothers and children have life-long significance to the well-being of a nation and the world. Healthy People 2010, a statement of national health objectives, aims to increase the quality and years of healthy life and to eliminate health disparities. It includes maternal, infant, and child health as focus areas. Early recognition and detection of problems, followed by treatment and ongoing assessment, can lead to considerable reductions in preventable morbidity and mortality for women and children. This chapter provides an overview of issues necessary for adequate maternal and child health (MCH).

Epidemiology: Health Indicators

The terms commonly used in epidemiologic reports comparing populations are presented in the Table. Public health officials often consider infant and maternal mortality as indicators of the health and social well-being of a region or country.

Maternal Death

Since the 1980s, the overall maternal mortality rate in the United States has fluctuated between 7 and 8 per 100,000 live births. Although maternal death is rare in the United States, a high proportion of these deaths potentially are preventable. The leading cause of maternal death in the first trimester is **ectopic pregnancy**. Risk factors for ectopic pregnancy include prior pelvic inflammatory disease, prior ectopic pregnancy, prior tubal surgery, and advancing maternal age. Other major causes of maternal death include preeclampsia or eclampsia, embolism, hemorrhage, infection, and complications of obstetric anesthesia.

Infant Death

The infant mortality rate (death before the first birthday) in the United States declined steadily during the period from 1975 to 1995, with an overall rate of 7.2 deaths per 1,000 live births. Two-thirds of these infant deaths occurred during the neonatal period, particularly among infants **born prematurely**. According to figures released in 2008 by the US Centers for Disease Control and Prevention (CDC), the US infant mortality rate ranked 29th in the world, among the highest of industrialized nations. Nevertheless, the approval of synthetic pulmonary surfactants, the recommendation that infants be placed on their backs when sleeping, and other major advances may have contributed to the continued decrease in the infant mortality rate during the 1990s.

Although the overall rates of infant mortality have declined in the United States, increases have been noted among critical measures of risk, including **low birth weight** (LBW) and **very low birth weight** (VLBW) infants. Of significant concern are the persistent disparities in infant mortality rates between whites and other racial groups. The rate of infant mortality of blacks remains twice that of whites.

The infant mortality rate has 2 components, neonatal and postneonatal. **Neonatal death** is most frequently a result of congenital malformations, deformations, and chromosomal

Table Maternal and Child Health Epidemiologic Terms

Term	Definition
Fetal death	Fetal death in utero after gestation of ≥20 wk
Fetal death rate	$\dfrac{\text{No. of fetal deaths}}{\text{No. of live births } + \text{ No. of fetal deaths}}$
Infant death	Death of infants aged <1 y
Infant mortality rate (in a population)	$\dfrac{\text{No. of deaths of infants aged } <1 \text{ y}}{1,000 \text{ live births}}$
Low birth weight	Birth weight <2,500 g
Maternal death	Death (from any cause) while pregnant or within 42 d after the end of pregnancy
Maternal mortality rate (or ratio)	$\dfrac{\text{No. of maternal deaths}}{100,000 \text{ live births}}$
Neonatal death	Death of an infant ≤28 d after birth
Neonatal period	First 28 d of life
Perinatal death	$\dfrac{\text{No. of stillbirths } + \text{ No. of neonatal deaths}}{1,000 \text{ total births}}$
Postneonatal period	Infant age from 29 d through 1 y
Postpartum period	Six-week period immediately after birth
Preterm birth	Birth before 37 wk of pregnancy
Very-low birth weight	Birth weight <1,500 g

abnormalities. Other causes include disorders related to premature delivery, LBW, and complications of pregnancy. Common causes of **postneonatal death** include sudden infant death syndrome (SIDS), birth defects, injuries, and homicide.

Perinatal Death

Because only live births are included in the calculation of infant mortality rates, perinatal and fetal mortality rates provide a more complete picture of perinatal health. The perinatal mortality rate includes stillbirths and the deaths of live-born infants through the first 28 days of life. This rate has declined steadily since 1980; however, as with many disparate health indicators, the gap between whites and nonwhites has continued to increase.

- The US maternal mortality rate is between 7 and 8 per 100,000 live births. The leading cause of maternal death in the first trimester is ectopic pregnancy.
- The US infant mortality rate is 7.2 deaths per 1,000 live births. More than half of infant deaths may be attributed to congenital birth defects, preterm delivery

and low birth weight (LBW), sudden infant death syndrome (SIDS), and respiratory distress syndrome.
- The US perinatal mortality rate has declined steadily since 1980.

MCH Programs and Services Management

Health Resources and Services Administration

The Health Resources and Services Administration (HRSA) is part of the US Department of Health and Human Services. HRSA administers many programs that increase and promote access to health care among vulnerable populations.

The **MCH Bureau** administers the MCH block grant; this grant is a federal-state partnership (established by Title V of the Social Security Act) to improve the health of low-income women and their families through the development of family-centered, community-based systems of care, to support research and training of MCH professionals, and to develop and support systems and programs that address health and safety issues of women and children.

The **Bureau of Primary Health Care** manages the Health Center Program, which funds a national network of health centers, including those for the community, for migrants, for the homeless, and for public housing residents. These health centers deliver preventive and primary care services to patients, regardless of their ability to pay; charges for health care services are set according to income.

Medicaid and State Children's Health Insurance Program

Public programs such as the State Children's Health Insurance Program (SCHIP) and Medicaid insure almost 30% of children in the United States. Eligibility for public programs is decided on the basis of the family's income compared with federal poverty guidelines. The SCHIP exists in every state. This federal-state partnership, administered by the Centers for Medicare and Medicaid Services, is designed to **cover uninsured children** in families with incomes that are modest but too high to qualify for Medicaid.

US Department of Agriculture

The **Supplemental Nutrition Assistance Program** (formerly the Food Stamp Program) is a federal assistance program that helps low-income individuals purchase food. The program is administered through the US Department of Agriculture (USDA), but benefits are distributed by individual states. Nearly one-third of households that rely on this program are single-parent households with children; furthermore, nearly 60 percent of the program's households with children are single-parent households.

The **Special Supplemental Nutrition Program for Women, Infants, and Children** (WIC), also administered by the USDA, provides federal grants to states for supplemental foods, health care referrals, and nutrition education. The program is geared toward low-income women who are pregnant or in the postpartum period (breastfeeding or not) and for infants and children up to 5 years old. During 1992–2005, the number of women participating in WIC increased by 60%, and this figure continues to rise.

- The US Department of Health and Human Services administers programs that aim to increase and promote access to health care among vulnerable populations, improve the health of low-income women and their families, and deliver preventive and primary care services.
- The Children's Health Insurance Program (SCHIP) and Medicaid insure almost 30% of children in the United States.

- The US Department of Agriculture (USDA) administers assistance programs that provide low-income persons with aid to purchase food and receive health care referrals and nutrition education.

Obstetrics

Preconception Counseling and Prenatal Care

Because many women are unaware of their pregnancy during a critical period of development, unknowing exposure to **teratogens** may result in major morphologic abnormalities or embryonic death (Figure). When taken early in pregnancy, medications may cause fetal death or have no effect at all. Before implantation, the embryo is highly resistant to teratogens; however, between the third and eighth weeks of gestation, organs are rapidly developing and are particularly vulnerable.

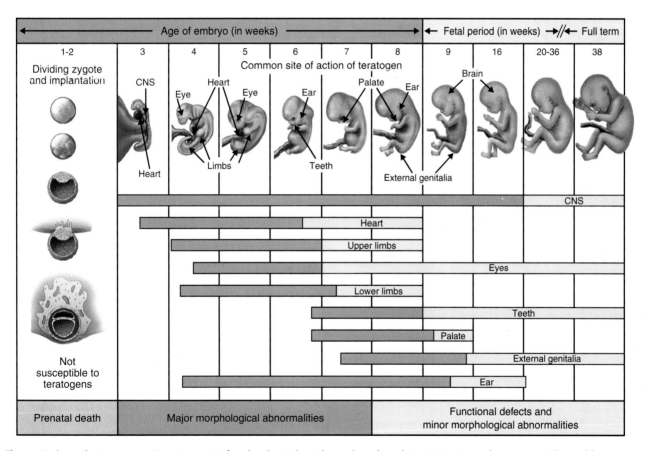

Figure Embryonic Exposure to Teratogens. Before implantation, the embryo is resistant to teratogenic exposure. The rapid development of organs between gestational weeks 3 and 8 is associated with particular vulnerability to teratogens. Dark blue bars indicate the periods of development that are most susceptible to insult. Exposure during the periods indicated in light blue are more likely to result in minor structural anomalies. CNS denotes central nervous system. (Adapted from Hill M. University of South Wales [UNSW] Embryology: an educational resource for learning concepts in embryological development [Internet]. Sydney, Australia: Dr. Mark Hill; ©2009 [cited 23 September 2009]. Available from: http://embryology.med.unsw.edu.au/Medicine/images/hcriticaldev.gif)

Preconception counseling may improve outcomes for the mother or baby. It consists of a medical evaluation to detect maternal health conditions and provides an opportunity for interventions before conception. This may occur in the context of routine care or during treatment of other medical conditions. Preconception counseling and prenatal care includes 3 primary components: **risk assessment, risk reduction (treatment of medical conditions), and patient education**.

Prenatal care is more likely to be effective when initiated early and continued throughout pregnancy. Since 1990, the proportion of infants whose mothers received prenatal care during the first trimester increased from 76% to 83%, with higher rates of increase among black, Hispanic, and Native American women. This increase may be due partly to improved access to Medicaid programs and coverage for pregnancy-related services. Nearly three-quarters of women receive adequate prenatal care, and the likelihood of early entry into prenatal care increases with maternal age. **Risk factors for late or no prenatal care** include being younger than 20 years, being unmarried, and having a low level of education. With fewer than half of pregnant girls aged 15 years and younger receiving adequate prenatal care, **prevention of adolescent pregnancy** and **education of women** about the need for early, continuous, and regular prenatal care are important public health issues.

Preterm Birth and Risk Assessment

Approximately **11% to 12% of singleton births** in the United States are preterm and the rate continues to increase. This public health concern has an economic cost exceeding $26 billion per year. Preterm and LBW infants have elevated risk of death, neurodevelopmental disabilities, cognitive impairment, and behavior disorders, even though half of these deliveries are associated with no known risk factors.

Potential causes of preterm labor include hemorrhage (placental abruption, uterine distortion), cervical incompetence, cervical inflammation, maternal infection or fever, and hormonal changes (resulting in maternal or fetal stress). Evidence of complications associated with uteroplacental insufficiency, hypertension, insulin-dependent diabetes mellitus, drug abuse, smoking, or alcohol use may prompt a physician to recommend premature delivery. Demographic factors for preterm labor include nonwhite race, extremes of maternal age (<17 or >35 years), low socioeconomic status, and low prepregnancy weight.

Premature rupture of membranes is defined as the rupture of membranes before the onset of labor. Although most women will start having contractions within 24 hours of leaking fluid, prolonged rupture of membranes at term increases risk of complications because of **oligohydramnios** and the potential for **intrauterine infection** of the membranes or fetus. The earlier in gestation that premature rupture occurs, the longer the potential latency period before the onset of labor.

Cervical incompetence (painless, preterm dilation in the absence of contractions) occurs in approximately 1% of all pregnancies and may be responsible for as many as 20% to 25% of second-trimester losses. Risk factors for cervical incompetence include a history of cervical procedures, cervical trauma, maternal exposure to diethylstilbestrol in utero, and uterine anomalies. Painless delivery with a prolapsing amniotic sac (resembles an hourglass shape on ultrasound), generally at less than 22 weeks' gestation, is often the initial presentation of cervical incompetence. Subsequent pregnancies can be monitored with serial ultrasounds of the cervix or prophylactically treated with transvaginal cerclage. Cervical **cerclage** with a suture may reinforce the tissue and prevent miscarriage or preterm birth for most women with cervical incompetence. Rarely, abdominal cerclage may be required.

Predictors of Preterm Birth

Methods used to predict preterm birth include home monitoring of uterine activity, detection of bacterial vaginosis or fetal fibronectin in the vagina, and cervical length assessment. Fetal fibronectin is a membrane protein that binds placental membranes to the deciduas; it is associated with a negative predictive value when identifying patients who will not deliver within the subsequent 1 or 2 weeks. Bacterial vaginosis has been associated with risk of preterm delivery, but eradication of asymptomatic bacterial vaginosis has not reduced this risk. Shorter cervical lengths in the second trimester are associated with an increased risk of preterm labor and delivery.

Maternal periodontal disease is associated with an increased risk of preterm birth and LBW. Treatment of pregnant women improves periodontal disease and is safe but does not markedly alter rates of preterm birth, LBW, or fetal growth restriction.

Urinary tract infections are common in pregnant women, as is a positive urine culture in the absence of symptoms (asymptomatic bacteriuria). As bacteriuria is associated with an increased risk of preterm birth, LBW, and perinatal mortality, treatment of asymptomatic bacteriuria during pregnancy greatly reduces the incidence of upper urinary tract infections and lowers the rate of preterm delivery.

Pregnancy Monitoring

Fundal height is the distance from the top of the uterus to the pubic bone; after the midpoint of pregnancy, its measurement in centimeters usually matches closely to the number of weeks' gestation and thus is routinely monitored at prenatal visits. Discrepancies may be noted with noncephalic presentation, growth restriction or macrosomia, incorrect menstrual dating, abnormalities of amniotic fluid, or multiple gestations. An ultrasound examination may help determine the cause when fundal height is not consistent with anticipated growth.

Intrapartum Evaluation

The goal of intrapartum evaluation is to **monitor maternal wellbeing** and **prevent fetal oxygen deprivation**. Antepartum complications, suboptimal uterine perfusion, placental dysfunction, or other intrapartum events may be associated with adverse outcomes.

Auscultation of fetal heart rate is performed externally or internally. Either continuous electronic fetal heart monitoring or intermittent auscultation of fetal heart sounds at regular intervals (every 30 minutes in the active phase and every 15 minutes during the second [pushing] phase) is equally appropriate for patients not at high risk. Internal fetal heart rate monitoring is performed by attaching an electrode to the fetal scalp and connecting to a monitor. Amniotic membranes must be ruptured and the cervix at least partially dilated before the electrode can be placed. Electronic monitoring is associated with a high false-positive rate of predicted adverse outcomes, and electronic fetal monitoring also is associated with an increased rate of operative interventions (eg, vacuum, forceps, and cesarean delivery). Use of electronic fetal monitoring has not reduced the rates of cerebral palsy.

Fetal **scalp stimulation** (painful stimulus applied to the boney portion of the fetal scalp) can be used to induce accelerations, a reassuring sign of fetal well-being. Fetal **vibroacoustic mulation** uses a handheld electronic device on the gravid abdomen to wake a sleeping fetus and thus potentially shorten the time needed for fetal heart rate testing. Fetal **scalp blood sampling** may be performed during labor to assist in the determination of fetal well-being. Decreased pH or elevated levels of lactate may indicate fetal hypoxia when fetal heart tones are nonreassuring. Fetal scalp hemorrhage is a complication, and false-positive results may be a factor in unnecessary cesarean delivery.

Obstetric Procedures

Repair of obstetric laceration and **cesarean delivery** are the 2 most common obstetric procedures according to hospital discharge data. Other common procedures include artificial rupture of membranes, episiotomy, and medical induction of labor. Complications of labor and delivery can include the presence of meconium, breech presentation or malpresentation, tocolysis, and precipitous labor.

Low Birth Weight

Preterm babies often have LBW because they are born early, but full-term infants with intrauterine growth restriction also may be small. LBW is associated with **long-term disabilities** such as cerebral palsy, autism, mental retardation, vision and hearing impairments, and other developmental disabilities. In addition, although LBW babies are a low proportion of pregnancies, expenditures for the care of these infants exceed half of all newborn costs.

Preterm delivery with LBW is the leading cause of neonatal death not associated with birth defects. The smallest (VLBW) infants have the highest risk of death. Survival of LBW infants improves with increasing gestational age, even among very preterm infants. Neonatal death rates are lowest when LBW infants are delivered at level III hospitals.

Cigarette smoking is the greatest known risk factor, accounting for 20% to 30% of all LBW cases in the United States. However, alcohol and illegal substances also pose major risks for LBW and poor infant outcomes. Other maternal risk factors include a prior LBW infant, maternal age younger than 15 or older than 45 years, low prepregnancy weight, maternal poverty, low education level, multiple births, vaginal infection, and low weight gain during pregnancy. Maternal medical conditions such as chronic hypertension, diabetes mellitus, lupus, thrombophilias, organ transplant, and renal disorders also are associated with a higher incidence of LBW infants.

- Preconception counseling and early prenatal care may improve pregnancy outcomes through risk assessment, risk reduction, and patient education.
- Preterm infants have elevated risk of death, neurodevelopmental disabilities, cognitive impairment, and behavioral disorders. Premature membrane rupture and preterm labor are 2 common causes of preterm birth and neonatal morbidity.
- Predictors of preterm birth include shorter cervical lengths in the second trimester and urinary tract infections. Treatment of infections may reduce risk.
- Fundal height after the midpoint of pregnancy is a marker of fetal growth.
- The fetal heart rate is monitored during labor to try to detect fetal oxygen deprivation.
- Repair of obstetric laceration and cesarean delivery are the 2 most common obstetric procedures.
- Preterm infants and full-term infants with intrauterine growth restriction may have low birth weight (LBW). LBW is associated with infant death, numerous long-term disabilities, and tremendous cost of care. Tobacco use is the greatest known risk factor for LBW.

Special Issues and Considerations in Pregnancy

Medical Risk Factors

During pregnancy and delivery, anatomic and physiologic alterations in many organ systems accommodate the increase in metabolic demands (brought on by the fetus, placenta, and uterus) and mechanical changes necessitated by the enlarging uterus. Increases in maternal blood volume and cardiac output are paralleled by increases in renal plasma flow and glomerular filtration, but increased glomerular filtration may overwhelm the ability of the renal tubules to reabsorb solutes. Thus, slightly increased glucose and protein loss in the urine is normal during pregnancy.

The most commonly reported conditions that contribute to maternal morbidity are **diabetes mellitus** and **hypertension**. Both preexisting and gestational diabetes mellitus are associated with health risks to pregnant women and infants. Women with diabetes mellitus before pregnancy are 3 to 4 times more likely than nondiabetic mothers to have a child with 1 or even multiple birth defects. Poor glucose control from conception throughout organogenesis is associated with a significant increase in congenital birth defects. Excellent control of glucose levels before and during the course of pregnancy can markedly reduce the risks of birth defects and stillbirth.

Diabetes mellitus in pregnancy has an estimated incidence of 2% to 3%; of these cases, 90% are categorized as gestational diabetes. Universal screening for gestational diabetes is controversial, but most pregnant women are screened at 24 to 28 weeks' gestation; screening is earlier for women with high risk factors. Risks associated with gestational diabetes mellitus include macrosomia, polyhydramnios, shoulder dystocia, higher rates of cesarean delivery, and the diagnosis of diabetes mellitus later in life for the mother.

Hypertension may be either chronic or limited to the duration of pregnancy. Chronic hypertension increases the risk of preeclampsia, fetal growth restriction, premature birth, placental abruption, and stillbirth. Other conditions increasing maternal or fetal risk during pregnancy can include eclampsia, which involves seizures (and usually is preceded by preeclampsia). Women with a **seizure disorder** have 2- to 3-fold increased risk of an infant with a birth defect, even when no anticonvulsant medications are taken.

Preeclampsia

A serious complication occurring in approximately 5% of pregnancies is preeclampsia. Although hemorrhage and embolism are the leading pregnancy-related causes of maternal death in the United States, preeclampsia is the third-leading cause. The vasospasm associated with this condition results in maternal hypertension with concomitant proteinuria (>300 mg protein in a 24-hour urine sample) after 20 weeks' gestation. Screening urinalysis and regular blood pressure monitoring may identify this condition while it is mild and asymptomatic. However, as symptoms progress, patients may experience headache, upper

abdominal pain, and shortness of breath. More severe preeclampsia must be aggressively managed with blood pressure control and fluid management, as well as intravenous magnesium sulfate prophylaxis to prevent seizures or eclampsia. Delivery is the definitive treatment for this condition, with the infant's risk of preterm delivery or placental abruption balanced against maternal risk of stroke or severe hemorrhage due to coagulopathy.

Numerous interventions have been explored in an effort to prevent the development of preeclampsia. However, the risk or severity of preeclampsia does not appear to be decreased by a high-protein or low-salt diet, supplementation with calcium, magnesium, zinc, or vitamins C and E, consumption of fish oils, or daily low-dose aspirin.

Nutrition, Dietary Intake, and Anemia

All pregnant women should be screened for anemia (hemoglobin or hematocrit levels) at the first prenatal visit. Pregnancy is normally associated with erythroid hyperplasia, but a disproportionate increase in plasma volume commonly results in hemodilution during pregnancy. Anemia in pregnancy is defined as a hemoglobin level <11 g/dL; however, using this definition, up to 50% of pregnant women are anemic.

The most common causes of true anemia in pregnancy are deficiencies of iron (~75%) and folate; however, hemoglobin electrophoresis may identify an underlying hemoglobinopathy. Decreased serum iron and ferritin levels with increased transferrin levels confirm iron deficiency. Infants born to anemic mothers usually have normal hematocrit levels but decreased total iron stores, and early dietary iron supplementation is required.

The US Preventive Services Task Force (USPSTF) "recommends routine screening for iron-deficiency anemia in asymptomatic pregnant women" (grade B recommendation). The USPSTF "concludes that evidence is insufficient to recommend for or against routine iron supplementation for nonanemic pregnant women" (grade I statement).

Women should be counseled to eat a well-balanced, varied diet at all times, but this should be particularly emphasized during pregnancy. Some authorities recommend universal **prenatal iron supplementation** (27-30 mg daily) because iron-deficiency anemia is associated with adverse outcomes, the average diet and endogenous iron stores of women are often insufficient to meet the requirements of pregnancy, and supplementation appears to be safe.

Additional dietary considerations in pregnancy include avoidance of large amounts of certain large predatory fish such as tuna, mackerel, and swordfish, which may have high levels of mercury and polychlorinated biphenyls (compounds associated with adverse neurologic effects for the developing baby). Oysters, sushi, and raw shellfish may be contaminated with *Vibrio cholera*, hepatitis A virus, or parasites and therefore should be avoided in pregnancy. In addition, listeriosis outbreaks from contaminated deli meat and unpasteurized dairy products have been associated with chorioamnionitis and fetal death.

To prevent neural tube defects, all women of reproductive age should consume 400 mcg of **folic acid** (folate) daily. This may be achieved through consumption of folate-rich foods, fortified foods, or supplements. For women who have had a previous fetus or child with a neural tube defect, 4 mg daily is recommended for at least 2 to 3 months before conception and throughout the first 3 months of pregnancy.

Maternal Weight Gain and Activity Recommendations

Caloric requirements increase during the second and third trimesters of gestation. For women with a normal body mass index, gaining approximately **25 to 35 pounds** during pregnancy is recommended. Obese and morbidly obese women may need less weight gain during pregnancy to ensure adequate growth of the fetus. Excessive weight gain may result in elevated risk of macrosomia, cesarean delivery, and long-term maternal weight retention.

Teenagers and black women tend to gain less than the recommended amount of weight during pregnancy and have particularly high risk of LBW infants. Inadequate maternal weight gain is associated with increased risk of intrauterine growth restriction, preterm birth, and perinatal mortality in observational studies. Maternal weight gain is susceptible to early intervention and represents an opportunity for prevention of poor birth outcomes.

Contact sports and high-impact activities are generally not recommended during pregnancy, but many other types of exercise are safe during pregnancy. Moderate activity levels may be recommended, with suggestions to monitor heart rate and avoid overexertion, particularly for conditioned athletes. While activities may require modification, especially as pregnancy advances, no specific limitations are universally recommended.

- Seizure disorders, preexisting or gestational diabetes mellitus, and hypertension are common causes of maternal and fetal morbidity and mortality.
- Preeclampsia (hypertension and proteinuria in the second half of pregnancy) is the third-leading pregnancy-related cause of death. Definitive therapy is delivery.
- Iron supplementation in pregnancy can be recommended because the average diet and endogenous iron stores are often insufficient. Folic acid supplementation is recommended to prevent neural tube defects.
- Inadequate maternal weight gain is associated with increased risk of intrauterine growth restriction,

preterm birth, and perinatal mortality. Women with a normal body mass index should gain approximately 25 to 35 pounds; obese and morbidly obese women may need less weight gain.

Infectious Diseases and Immunization in Pregnancy

Human Immunodeficiency Virus, Syphilis, Hepatitis, and Herpes

Because targeted testing does not readily identify infected women, the USPSTF strongly recommends **universal screening** of pregnant patients for human immunodeficiency virus (HIV), syphilis, and hepatitis B (grade A recommendation). The number of HIV-positive infants born to HIV-infected mothers has declined considerably through increasing use of prophylaxis before, during, and after pregnancy to reduce perinatal transmission. Screening typically is performed at the first prenatal visit, but women with increased risk of infection should be retested in the third trimester. Testing is currently performed on a voluntary basis and requires informed patient consent.

A young patient with gonorrhea, chlamydia, or trichomoniasis has a 25% risk of reinfection in the following year. These patients and their partners have increased risk of infection and should be screened regularly and administered appropriate treatment. Testing is performed on the basis of clinical findings or risk factors for sexually transmitted infection (STI). The USPSTF "recommends against routinely providing screening for chlamydial infection for women aged 25 and older, whether or not they are pregnant, if they are not at increased risk" (grade C recommendation.)

Patients should be asked about symptoms of herpes simplex virus infection. **Vertical (perinatal) transmission** rates during delivery are approximately 50% for primary infections and about 0% to 3% for recurrent infections. Women with recurrent outbreaks should be counseled about decreasing the risk of vertical transmission with cesarean delivery and using acyclovir from about 36 weeks' gestation until delivery. Neonatal herpes infection may result in localized facial lesions, or it may affect the central nervous system and cause disseminated disease. Neonatal herpes is associated with considerable mortality.

Group B Streptococcus

Group B streptococcus (GBS) bacteria are commonly found in the gastrointestinal and genital tracts, with **colonization** rates of up to 40% in women. GBS infection increases risk of developing chorioamnionitis and premature labor or premature rupture of membranes. Infection is diagnosed by culturing swab samples from the maternal perineum and perianal region, ideally at a prenatal visit between

35 and 37 weeks' gestation. If GBS is noted in the urine during prenatal screening, women should be treated for a urinary tract infection, and **intrapartum antibiotic prophylaxis** for a presumed heavy colonization should be administered.

Treatment of GBS colonization occurs at presentation for delivery. Most newborns delivered from a colonized mother will have no signs of infection. Nevertheless, without antibiotic treatment during labor, up to 1% to 2% will have early onset GBS infection with pneumonia, sepsis, or meningitis. Intrapartum prophylaxis antibiotics can reduce the risk of early onset neonatal infection by 30-fold.

Immunizations

Women exposed to live-attenuated vaccines during pregnancy should be referred to a maternal-fetal medicine specialist. Box 1 lists the absolutely contraindicated vaccines during pregnancy. When possible, it is preferable to immunize women 3 to 4 months before conception. **Live-virus vaccines generally are contraindicated** in pregnancy.

Influenza vaccination (with inactivated virus) is indicated for all women who will be pregnant during the flu season (October-March). **Maternal influenza immunization** also confers some protection to infants during the first 6 months of life, when administration of infant influenza vaccine is contraindicated. The postpartum period is an ideal opportunity to vaccinate women, particularly those who are nonimmune to rubella and varicella (as determined during prenatal tests).

- Universal, voluntary screening for human immunodeficiency virus (HIV), syphilis, and hepatitis B typically is performed at the first prenatal visit. Women with increased risk of infection should be retested in the third trimester.
- Colonization with group B streptococcus (GBS) bacteria is common. Antibiotic prophylaxis should be administered when the patient presents for delivery.
- Live-attenuated vaccines are contraindicated during pregnancy. Influenza vaccination (with inactivated virus) is indicated for all women who will be pregnant during the flu season (October-March).

Box 1 Vaccines Contraindicated in Pregnancy

Measles, mumps, rubella

Yellow fever (except if exposure is unavoidable)

Varicella

Live, attenuated influenza virus (intranasal)

Zoster

Substance Abuse and Personal Safety

Tobacco

Smoking during pregnancy increases the risk of ectopic pregnancy, spontaneous abortion, preterm delivery, placental abruption, placenta previa, LBW, and stillbirth. Fetal mortality rates are 35% greater than average for women who smoke.

The USPSTF "strongly recommends that clinicians ask all pregnant women about tobacco use and provide augmented pregnancy-tailored counseling to those who smoke" (grade A recommendation). Smoking is the **most modifiable risk factor** for adverse obstetric outcomes. Furthermore, pregnancy is a unique opportunity for smoking cessation because women are more likely to quit smoking when pregnant than at any other period in life (approximately 46% of smokers quit during pregnancy). Brief counseling can improve cessation rates (use the 5 A's [Ask, Advise, Assess, Assist, and Arrange], as detailed in Chapter 5).

Some studies estimate that a 5% reduction in perinatal deaths and 10% decrease in LBW infants would occur if women stopped smoking during pregnancy. Stopping smoking in the first trimester is the ultimate goal, but even a reduction in tobacco use results in improved infant birth weight. Newborn birth weight is directly associated with the number of cigarettes smoked during pregnancy. Smoking cessation by the third trimester usually results in delivery of infants of normal birth weight.

Intense efforts are needed postpartum because **60% to 80% of women resume smoking** within the first postpartum year. Mothers should be reminded that exposure to tobacco smoke during and after pregnancy is one of the major factors known to increase the rate of SIDS, childhood asthma, and infantile colic.

Alcohol

The USPSTF "recommends screening and behavioral counseling interventions to reduce alcohol misuse by adults, including pregnant women, in primary care settings" (grade B recommendation). Among pregnant women, 12% admit to alcohol use in the past month. Drinking at any time during pregnancy can cause miscarriage or preterm delivery; the rate of fetal death is 77% higher for women who use alcohol.

Maternal alcohol use is the leading cause of mental retardation in infants, and it is one of the leading preventable causes of neurodevelopmental disorders. Fetal alcohol spectrum disorders, caused by exposure to alcohol during pregnancy, encompass a pattern of growth deficiencies, facial deformities, central nervous system impairment, behavior disorders, and impaired intellectual development. **No level of alcohol use is known to be safe.** Smoking, drug use, and poor diet are common in women using alcohol in pregnancy, and these also may contribute to how severely a child is affected.

Illicit Drug Exposure

Use of illegal drugs during early pregnancy may cause **birth defects** and **spontaneous abortion**. During the final 12 weeks of pregnancy, illicit drug use is more likely to stunt fetal growth and cause preterm birth and fetal death. Nevertheless, the USPSTF "concludes that the current evidence is insufficient to assess the balance of benefits and harms of screening adolescents, adults, and pregnant women for illicit drug use" (grade I statement).

Illicit drugs have numerous adverse effects on the fetus. Marijuana may impair fetal growth, mainly in women who are regular users. Cocaine may increase risk of miscarriage, preterm labor or delivery, and LBW. Infants exposed to cocaine tend to have smaller heads, increased risk of urinary tract defects, neurologic disorders, and behavior disturbances; placental abruption is an uncommon but potentially deadly consequence of cocaine use in pregnancy. Use of heroin may result in impaired fetal growth, premature rupture of membranes, increased risk of birth defects, and stillbirth. Most babies of heroin users suffer from withdrawal symptoms after birth. Methamphetamine causes an increase in maternal blood pressure and heart rate, placing the fetus at increased risk of stroke, brain damage, and fetal death.

Violence, Personal Safety, and Abuse Issues

Women and children are the most frequent victims of domestic violence. For abuse that started before or during pregnancy, studies suggest that it may escalate during the postpartum period. The estimated incidence of abuse during pregnancy is from 1% to 20%.

Numerous **risk factors for family violence** have been identified. They include low income status, low maternal education, nonwhite race, large family size, young maternal age, single-parent household, parental psychiatric disturbances, and presence of a stepfather. Factors associated with intimate partner violence include young age, low income status, pregnancy, mental health problems, alcohol or substance use by victims or perpetrators, separated or divorced status, and history of childhood sexual or physical abuse.

Currently, little evidence supports improved maternal or fetal outcomes after screening and early intervention. However, some recommend **routine screening for domestic violence** because of patient acceptance of screening, minimal cost, low risks, and considerable potential benefit. The American College of Obstetricians and Gynecologists recommends screening for intimate partner violence at the first prenatal visit, at least once per trimester, and during the postpartum visit.

- Tobacco use is the most modifiable risk factor for adverse obstetric outcomes. Nearly half of smokers quit during pregnancy, but the majority of those who quit will resume smoking within the first postpartum year.
- Alcohol consumption is one of the leading preventable causes of neurodevelopmental disorders. No level of alcohol use is known to be safe in pregnancy.
- Exposure to illicit drugs can cause birth defects, impair growth, and result in preterm birth or fetal death.
- Domestic violence or abuse that started before or during pregnancy may escalate during the postpartum period. Routine screening for domestic violence is recommended, at least once per trimester and during the postpartum visit.

Postpartum Health

Breastfeeding

Breast milk is widely acknowledged to be the **most complete form of nutrition for infants**. In addition to supporting growth, immunity, and development, benefits include decreased incidence of neonatal diarrheal illness, fewer respiratory and ear infections, and reduced family cost. In addition, breastfeeding improves long-term maternal health—breastfeeding mothers have less postpartum bleeding, earlier return to prepregnancy weight, and have reduced risk of osteoporosis and premenopausal breast cancer.

Breastfeeding rates for all women decrease substantially between birth and 6 months. The highest rates of nursing are reported among older (>35 years) and college-educated women, whereas infants less likely to breastfeed are born to younger mothers, those with lower education levels or low income, or those receiving benefits from the WIC program. Infants with highest risk of poor health and development are less likely to be breastfed. Non-Hispanic black infants are the least likely to be breastfed (55%), whereas Asians and Pacific Islanders are most likely (81%), followed by Hispanics (79%). Education of new mothers, health care providers, and hospital maternity ward employees, improved employer support, and greater societal acceptance are needed to increase breastfeeding rates.

Although breastfeeding is widely encouraged, **universal breastfeeding is not always recommended** in the United States. Mothers who use illicit drugs, have active tuberculosis, are HIV positive, or take certain prescription medications should not breastfeed. Although nearly all medicines are present in breast milk to some degree, few are absolutely contraindicated while nursing.

Without intervention, 15% to 30% of infants born to HIV-positive mothers will be infected before or during delivery. If all HIV-positive mothers breastfeed, another 10% to 20% will be infected. Nutritional support for newborns in developing countries is particularly important, especially for those born to HIV-positive mothers. The risk of HIV transmission through breastfeeding may be reduced by preventing any oral or breast lesions, using antiviral medications, and exclusively nursing during the first 6 months (with subsequent transition to other nutritional sources). In the developed world, breastfeeding is generally not recommended in HIV-positive mothers. However, in areas of the world where the rate of infant mortality is high because of infectious diseases or limited access to clean water or affordable substitutes, breastfeeding may be the safest option, even when the mother is HIV positive.

Depression

The precipitous decrease in estrogen and progesterone levels at delivery in conjunction with the postpartum disruption of maternal routines and sleep cycles may contribute to maternal **postpartum blues**; sadness that continues longer than 2 weeks after delivery is considered **postpartum depression**. Risk factors for postpartum depression include a history of mood disorders, increased life stressors (eg, illness or complications of pregnancy), marital discord, or unwanted or unplanned pregnancy. Postpartum depression can be disabling for a new mother and can compromise her ability to care for her infant. Early identification and treatment of this condition may prevent the development of **postpartum psychosis**. Although rare, it presents usually within the first 2 weeks after delivery. The risk of postpartum psychosis is higher for women who have bipolar disorder.

Contraception

Addressing contraception is an essential component of routine gynecologic and postnatal care. Roughly half of all pregnancies in the United States are unplanned, which has important health, economic, and social consequences. **Unplanned pregnancy** is a risk factor for late entry into prenatal care and is associated with LBW, prematurity, and higher rates of infant illness and death. Women with certain medical conditions and those receiving medications that increase the risk of birth defects should be routinely asked and counseled about family planning. Effective contraception will facilitate planning and optimization of conditions before attempting pregnancy. When counseling about contraceptive methods, the discussion should include convenience, efficacy, affordability, and noncontraceptive effects of hormonal methods (Box 2).

Postpartum contraceptive selection must also consider sexual activity, breastfeeding pattern, menstruation, and medical and social factors. Within the first 6 months postpartum, **lactational amenorrhea** in women who are exclusively breastfeeding is 98% effective in preventing pregnancy. As breastfeeding decreases and menstruation resumes, risk of pregnancy increases. Although hormonal

Box 2 Currently Available Contraceptive Methods

Reversible methods

Intrauterine devices, contraceptive implants, and injectable contraceptives

Very low pregnancy rate

Minimally influenced by compliance

Oral contraceptives

Very low pregnancy rate if taken consistently and correctly

Actual pregnancy rates are increased because of incorrect use

Other methods, including diaphragms, cervical caps, condoms, spermicides, withdrawal, and periodic abstinence

Actual pregnancy rates are much higher than perfect-use rates

Permanent methods

Tubal ligation

Vasectomy

Adapted from Ghosh AK (ed). Mayo Clinic: internal medicine review. 8th ed. Rochester (MN): Mayo Clinic Scientific Press; Informa Healthcare; c2008. Used with permission of Mayo Foundation for Medical Education and Research.

contraception is not known to have adverse effects on infant growth, use of a combined (estrogen and progestin) oral contraceptive is generally not advised during the first 6 months postpartum because of potentially decreased milk volume. Progestin-only products may be started anytime postpartum, and intrauterine devices may be considered 4 weeks after delivery.

- Breast milk is the most complete form of nutrition for infants and reduces incidence of illness and disease. Breastfeeding also improves long-term maternal health. Few medications are absolutely contraindicated while nursing.
- Postpartum sadness or depression may be attributable to the precipitous decrease in estrogen and progesterone levels and the disruption of maternal routines and sleep cycles.
- Postpartum contraception choice must consider sexual activity, breastfeeding pattern, menstruation, and medical and social factors. When counseling about contraceptive methods, the discussion should include convenience, efficacy, affordability, and noncontraceptive effects of hormonal methods.

Pediatrics

Newborn Assessment

The transition from fetus to newborn is a normal physiologic process. Although immediate cord clamping is common, recent evidence suggests that delaying clamping until cessation of cord pulsations may decrease rates of anemia in the infant. Neonates are routinely dried and suctioned immediately after delivery. **Apgar scores** are measured to determine quickly whether a newborn requires immediate medical care. Each of 5 criteria—1) appearance, 2) pulse, 3) grimace, 4) activity, and 5) respiration—is graded as 0, 1, or 2, resulting in an Apgar score between 0 and 10. Note that this metric is not predictive of long-term health. Skin-to-skin care of the newborn is recommended in the immediate postpartum period to maintain thermoregulation.

Newborn assessment further includes evaluation of length and weight, head size, changes in skin color, signs of birth trauma, malformations, evidence of respiratory distress, level of arousal, posture, tone, presence of spontaneous movements, and symmetry of movements. A Ballard assessment is a specified set of procedures (neuromuscular and physical assessment) used to determine the gestational age of a newborn. A newborn with any anatomic malformation should be evaluated for other associated anomalies. Total and direct bilirubin levels should be measured in newborns with jaundice, and a complete blood count is recommended for newborns with a pale or ruddy complexion. Infants experiencing difficulty during transition, of abnormal size, or requiring additional observation (eg, because of gestational age, complications of pregnancy or delivery) may require admission to a neonatal intensive care unit.

Metabolic Screening

The public health programs of all states now require newborn screening for **phenylketonuria** and **congenital hypothyroidism**. Other tests in the screen may include sickle cell disease, galactosemia, congenital adrenal hyperplasia, homocystinuria, maple syrup urine disease, biotinidase deficiency, and tyrosinemia. Some states also test for cystic fibrosis, additional metabolic disorders, and congenital infections. Although screening is universally available, continued efforts are needed to ensure quality of screening tests, to provide diagnostic tests for newborns with positive screening results, and to make treatment available for children with diagnosed congenital disorders.

Eye Prophylaxis and Vitamin K Prophylaxis

Shortly after birth, infants are treated with erythromycin eye ointment to prevent **gonococcal infection**, which can result in permanent blindness. Without prophylactic treatment immediately after delivery, infants born of women with untreated gonococcal infections have a 30% to 40% rate of congenital infection and blindness. The USPSTF "strongly recommends prophylactic ocular topical medication for all newborns [to protect] against gonococcal ophthalmia neonatorum" (grade A recommendation).

Vitamin K is an essential component of blood clotting; normally, low levels are present at birth. To prevent **hemorrhagic disease** of the newborn, most babies receive an injection of vitamin K in the upper thigh soon after delivery.

Sudden Infant Death Syndrome

SIDS is the acute and unexplained death of a seemingly healthy infant. SIDS is the **leading cause of postneonatal death** among all racial and ethnic groups and accounts for nearly one-third of all cases of postneonatal death. The rate of SIDS among blacks is 1.4 per 1,000 live births—a rate that is twice that of whites.

Most SIDS-related deaths occur in children who are from **2 to 4 months old**; it rarely occurs in children younger than 1 month or older than 6 months. Although the exact cause is unknown, it is likely multifactorial, including some element of **biological vulnerability** (eg, heart or brain defect) combined with an **environmental stressor** (eg, sleeping on the stomach). Brain abnormalities that affect breathing and arousal likely have a role in SIDS, and SIDS also may be linked to long QT syndrome.

Male babies are more likely to die of SIDS than females, particularly if they are also premature or LBW infants. Babies who sleep on their stomachs are at much greater risk than those who sleep on their backs. Tobacco exposure during or after pregnancy is associated with a considerably higher risk of SIDS. More SIDS cases occur when the weather is cooler, when infants are placed in loose bedding, and during bedsharing with an older child or adult. Other infants at risk are born of mothers who had inadequate prenatal care, placental abnormalities, or low weight gain or are younger than 20 years. Childhood immunizations do not appear to have a role in SIDS.

- Newborn assessment begins immediately after birth (Apgar score, physical examination). Screening for metabolic diseases is a part of public health programs throughout the United States.
- Neonates are promptly treated prophylactically with ocular topical medication to protect against gonococcal ophthalmia neonatorum. Vitamin K is administered to prevent hemorrhagic disease.
- Sudden infant death syndrome (SIDS) is the leading cause of postneonatal death. The cause likely is multifactorial and involves biological vulnerability and environmental stressors.

Child Health Supervision

Immunization

The number of reported cases of vaccine-preventable diseases has decreased steadily in the past decade. Data from the 2004 CDC National Immunization Survey showed that 80.9% of children aged 19 to 35 months received the recommended series of vaccines (4 doses of diphtheria, tetanus, and pertussis vaccine; 3 doses of poliovirus vaccine; 1 dose of measles, mumps, rubella vaccine; and 3 doses of *Haemophilus influenzae* type b vaccine). Overall, 76.0% received the preceding series plus the varicella vaccine. Still, **racial and ethnic disparities in vaccination rates** persist. Non-Hispanic black children and American Indian/Alaska Native children had the lowest rates for each of the major vaccines, and non-Hispanic white children had the highest vaccination rates. Further details of childhood vaccination are presented in Chapter 7.

Weight and Height

Weight, height, and head circumference are all an integral part of each well-child visit. These data are recorded on pediatric growth charts to monitor consistency in growth patterns.

Obesity

Obesity is defined as a body mass index of at least 30 kg/m^2. During the past 2 decades, the prevalence of childhood obesity has risen greatly worldwide, more than doubling for preschoolers (aged 2-5 years) and adolescents (aged 13-19 years), and it has more than tripled for children aged 6 to 11 years. Obesity in childhood causes various health complications and increases the risk of many diseases and poor health conditions later in life, including coronary heart disease, type 2 diabetes mellitus, cancer (endometrial, breast, and colon cancer), hypertension, dyslipidemia, stroke, and osteoarthritis. Young people also have risk of serious psychosocial burdens due to societal stigmatization associated with obesity.

The obesity **epidemic** is a serious public health problem. Immediate action is required to reduce the prevalence and health and social consequences. Obesity prevention should focus on specific **eating and physical activity behaviors** that are likely to promote maintenance of a healthy weight. Currently, evidence regarding the best ways to prevent childhood obesity is limited. Primary care physicians should assess children for obesity risk to improve early identification of elevated body mass index, medical risks, and unhealthy eating and physical activity habits.

Developmental Milestones

Identification and treatment of developmental disabilities are important for child health. Assessment of normal developmental milestones occurs on a regular basis through well-child care. Gross motor skills (eg, control of the head, sitting, walking), fine motor skills (eg, holding a spoon, grasping small items between thumb and finger), sensory (eg, seeing, hearing, touching), language development (eg, speech, comprehension), and social abilities are assessed routinely to detect developmental delays. Failure to achieve milestones in one domain may require additional evaluation and assessment for **early intervention services** that may prevent progressive delays in other developmental areas.

Special Needs

Historically, services for children with special health care needs have been difficult for families to access and for providers to coordinate. Care for children with special care needs should be coordinated through an accessible **medical home** in the child's community that accepts all insurance, is family centered, and provides care that is continuous, comprehensive, coordinated, compassionate, and culturally appropriate to the family's background. Early intervention is best, with educational, vocational, mental health, and support services for children and families.

Child Care

Nearly three-quarters of women with children younger than 18 years are in the labor force (employed or looking for work). Employed mothers with children aged 6 to 17 years are more likely than women with younger children to be employed full-time. The ability to find high-quality, affordable child care remains a challenge for many working families, and strategies to promote policies that support and protect child health and safety in this setting remain a public health opportunity.

Injury Prevention

Childhood death rates generally have declined during the past decades. **Unintentional injury** continues to be the primary cause of death for children of all ages; this public health concern is also an opportunity for prevention. Injuries account for 13.1 deaths per 100,000 preschool children (age, 1-4 years) and 8.7 deaths per 100,000 school-aged children (age, 5-14 years). **Motor vehicle crashes** are the most common causes of unintentional injury or death among children aged 1 to 14 years, followed by deaths due to drowning, fires, and burns. Many of these deaths are potentially preventable. Other leading causes of childhood death that are less likely to be preventable include birth defects, malignant neoplasm, and cardiac disease.

State government–based **child protective services** receive approximately 3 million reports yearly alleging the maltreatment of children. Over half of these reports are received from community professionals, with the remaining received from family, friends, relatives, or neighbors. Victimization occurs most frequently among the youngest children. Among the estimated 1,300 children who die annually in the United States of abuse and neglect, children younger than 1 year accounted for 41% of fatalities and children younger than 6 years accounted for 85%. Most fatalities involved a parent.

- Approximately 80% of US children aged 19 to 35 months have received the recommended series of vaccines, although racial and ethnic disparities in vaccination rates persist.
- The prevalence of childhood obesity has risen greatly worldwide during the past 2 decades. Prevention should focus on specific eating and physical activity behaviors that are likely to promote maintenance of a healthy weight.
- Assessment of normal developmental milestones should occur routinely to detect developmental delays. Care for children with special needs should be coordinated through a medical home.
- Unintentional injury is the primary cause of death for children of all ages. Of the children who died of abuse and neglect, children younger than 1 year accounted for 41% of fatalities and children younger than 6 years accounted for 85%.

Adolescent Health Care

Adolescents (age, 13-19 years) account for approximately 10% of the US population. Generally, adolescents are a healthy group, but they are also in a time of physical and emotional growth and exploration. During this period, many **lifelong health habits** are formed, including diet, exercise, and the use of health care services. This opportunity to introduce preventive health care issues begins with addressing risk-taking behaviors such as experimentation with cigarettes and drugs, sex, or inattentive driving habits.

The National Center for Health Statistics reports that the leading cause of adolescent death is unintentional injury, with motor vehicle crashes being the leading cause in this age group. The second- and third-leading causes of adolescent death are homicide and suicide. Adolescents and young adults between the ages of 20 and 24 years are at much higher risk of contracting STIs than are older adults. About 3 million new STIs, not including HIV, occur among teenagers each year. In addition, an estimated one million teenagers become pregnant yearly.

Results of the Substance Abuse and Mental Health Services Administration's 2001 National Household Survey on Drug Abuse show that the percentage of adolescents (defined by the survey as age 12-17 years) who reported using alcohol in the previous month increased to 17.3%,

with similar rates between boys and girls. Rates of binge drinking and heavy alcohol use were higher among boys. Use of marijuana, the most common illicit drug, continues to increase. Researchers speculate that the decline in adolescent cigarette smoking is a result of an increased perception of risk and disapproval of smoking, increased price, and declining accessibility.

Contraception and Prevention of STIs

Adolescents commonly choose not to use contraception because of fear of adult discovery, fear and misconception about hormonal methods or pelvic examinations, a sense of invincibility, or reluctance to acknowledge sexual activity. However, states are required (by Titles XIX and XX of the Social Security Act) to provide family planning assistance to minors who desire assistance and meet financial eligibility requirements; assistance is provided without regard to marital status, age, or parenthood status. Further, the US Supreme Court has ruled that states may not prohibit the availability of contraceptives to minors.

Abstinence is the most efficacious method of preventing pregnancy and STIs. Oral contraceptive pills may be considered, but adolescents may be less compliant than adults. A skin patch, vaginal ring, or progesterone injection may improve compliance. Barrier methods such as a diaphragm, cervical cap, or female condom tend not to be popular with this age group because of discomfort during insertion. Few adolescents are candidates for an intrauterine device, which generally is not recommended for nulliparous women or those not in mutually monogamous relationships. All adolescents should be encouraged to use male latex condoms because they also provide some protection against STIs.

Although genital human papillomavirus is considered the most common STI in the United States, for adolescents, chlamydia and gonorrhea are the first and second most common STIs, respectively. Syphilis is less common among young people. Active STIs can increase the likelihood of contracting HIV, and untreated infections can lead to **pelvic inflammatory disease**. All sex partners of an infected patient should be evaluated, tested, and treated. Pelvic inflammatory disease caused by chlamydia or gonorrhea is the leading preventable cause of scarring, which can result in tubal pregnancy or infertility.

Several guidelines exist for screening adolescents for chlamydia or gonorrhea. The USPSTF "recommends screening for chlamydial infection for all sexually active, nonpregnant young women aged 24 and younger and for older nonpregnant women who are at increased risk" (grade A recommendation). The USPSTF "recommends screening for chlamydial infection for all pregnant women aged 24 and younger and for older pregnant women who are at increased risk" (grade B recommendation).

The USPSTF "recommends that clinicians screen all sexually active women, including those who are pregnant, for gonorrhea infection if they are at increased risk for infection" (grade B recommendation).

- Adolescence is when lifelong health habits are established. It is an opportunity to introduce preventive health care issues by addressing risk-taking behaviors.
- For adolescents, contraception commonly is unused or is associated with poor compliance. All adolescents should be encouraged to use male latex condoms because they also provide some protection against sexually transmitted infections (STIs).
- Chlamydia and gonorrhea are the first and second most common STIs among young people, respectively. Untreated infections increase the likelihood of contracting HIV or developing pelvic inflammatory disease.

SUGGESTED READING

Cox SM, Werner CL, Hoffman BL, Cunningham FG. Williams obstetrics. 22nd ed. New York: McGraw-Hill Medical Publishing Division; c2005.

Preventive Services Task Force (USPSTF) Recommendations [Internet]. Rockville (MD): Department of Health and Human Services (US), Agency for Healthcare Research and Quality (AHRQ); [cited 23 September 2009]. Available from: http://www.ahrq.gov/clinic/USpstfix.htm

U.S. Department of Health and Human Services. Healthy people 2010: understanding and improving health. Boston (MA): Jones and Bartlett Publishers; c2000.

U.S. Department of Health and Human Services, Health Resources and Services Administration. Women's Health USA 2007. Rockville (MD): U.S. Department of Health and Human Services; c2007.

U.S. Department of Health and Human Services, Health Resources and Services Administration, Maternal and Child Health Bureau. Child Health USA 2006. Rockville (MD): U.S. Department of Health and Human Services; c2006.

Questions and Answers

Questions

1. Of the following statements regarding the health of pregnant women in the United States, which is true?
   a. Preeclampsia is the primary cause of pregnancy-related death
   b. Maternal risk for domestic violence decreases
   c. Influenza vaccination should be deferred until completion of pregnancy
   d. Screening for human immunodeficiency virus (HIV), syphilis, and hepatitis B is recommended at the first prenatal visit
   e. They should be counseled to eat at least 1 serving of large predatory fish daily

2. A healthy 34-year-old woman presents 10 weeks after her last menstrual period to establish care for her first pregnancy. She has no risk factors for sexually transmitted infection and takes no medications. Which of the following is strongly recommended by the United States Preventive Services Task Force (grade A recommendation)?
   a. Screening for illicit drug use
   b. Screening for tobacco use with augmented counseling if she is a smoker
   c. Booster dose of measles, mumps, and rubella (MMR) vaccine
   d. Screening for chlamydial infection
   e. Routine iron supplementation

3. As a public health provider, you are providing care for pregnant refugees with human immunodeficiency virus (HIV) in a primitive central African refugee camp. Of the following messages, which will you *not* include as you counsel your patient?
   a. Taking HIV medications as directed may reduce the risk of the baby becoming infected with HIV
   b. Breastfeeding is not recommended
   c. A balanced diet is important for the health of the mother and child
   d. Moderate, regular exercise is recommended
   e. Smoking and alcohol are to be avoided

4. Which of the following statements regarding preterm birth is *false*?
   a. Cervical incompetence has painless cervical dilation
   b. Treatment of asymptomatic bacterial vaginosis has been shown to decrease the risk of preterm labor
   c. Preterm delivery is associated with low birth weight
   d. Preterm delivery with low birth weight is a leading cause of neonatal death
   e. Preterm birth includes singletons born before 37 weeks' gestation

5. The Special Supplemental Nutrition Program for Women, Infants, and Children (WIC) program is administered by which government agency?
   a. Maternal and Child Health (MCH) Bureau
   b. Health Resources and Services Administration (HRSA)
   c. US Department of Agriculture (USDA)
   d. Supplemental Nutrition Assistance Program
   e. Centers for Medicare and Medicaid Services

6. A healthy 32-year-old woman presents for her initial prenatal visit. This is her third pregnancy, and she is at 14 weeks' gestation. Her obstetric history is remarkable for the development of preeclampsia during her first pregnancy, which resulted in the preterm delivery at 33 weeks' gestation. At the time of delivery, the child was noted to have spina bifida. Her second pregnancy was unremarkable. She takes fluoxetine for depression, has no known allergies, and is a conditioned athlete. Her most recent tetanus booster was 10 years earlier, and review of prenatal test results indicate that she is not immune to rubella. Management during her initial visit should include which of the following?
   a. Activity restrictions, with no lifting greater than 10 pounds
   b. Administration of the measles, mumps, rubella (MMR) vaccine
   c. Recommendation to consume 0.4 mg of folate daily
   d. Recommend limiting alcohol intake to 3 drinks daily
   e. Administration of the tetanus, diphtheria, acellular pertussis (Tdap) vaccine

7. Which of the following is the leading cause of childhood death (ages 1-17 years) in the United States?
   a. Homicide
   b. Unintentional injury
   c. Malignant neoplasm
   d. Heart defects
   e. Sudden infant death syndrome

8. Which term most appropriately describes the mortality rate that includes stillbirths and live-born infants who die within the first 28 days of life?
   a. Postneonatal mortality rate
   b. Maternal mortality rate
   c. Neonatal mortality rate
   d. Infant mortality rate
   e. Perinatal mortality rate

Answers

1. Answer d.

Screening for HIV, syphilis, and hepatitis B is recommended at the first prenatal visit. Preeclampsia is the third-leading, pregnancy-related cause of death, after hemorrhage and embolism. The literature suggests that the risk for domestic violence increases during the postpartum period, particularly if the abuse began during pregnancy. Influenza vaccination (with inactivated virus) is indicated for women who are or will be pregnant during the flu season (October-March). Large amounts of large predatory fish such as tuna, mackerel, and swordfish are not recommended because they may have high levels of mercury and polychlorinated biphenyls.

2. Answer b.

The USPSTF "strongly recommends that clinicians ask all pregnant women about tobacco use and provide augmented pregnancy-tailored counseling to those who smoke" (grade A recommendation). The USPSTF "concludes that the current evidence is insufficient to assess the balance of benefits and harms of screening adolescents, adults, and pregnant women for illicit drug use" (grade I statement). The MMR and other live-virus vaccines are contraindicated in pregnancy. The USPSTF "concludes that evidence is insufficient to recommend for or against routine iron supplementation for nonanemic pregnant women" (grade I statement). The USPSTF "recommends against routinely providing screening for chlamydial infection for women aged 25 and older, whether or not they are pregnant, if they are not at increased risk" (grade C recommendation).

3. Answer b.

In the developed world, breastfeeding is generally not recommended for HIV-positive mothers. However, in areas of the world where the rate of infant mortality is high due to infectious diseases or limited access to clean water or affordable substitutes, breastfeeding may be the safest option, even when the mother is HIV positive. Although prenatal care and well-balanced nutritional support are strongly recommended for pregnant and lactating women, the lack of these 2 factors is not a contraindication to breastfeeding. Regular, moderate exercise may continue during pregnancy. Counseling to avoid smoking and alcohol are appropriate messages.

4. Answer b.

Bacterial vaginosis has been associated with risk of preterm delivery, but eradication of asymptomatic disease has not

reduced this risk. Cervical incompetence is defined as painless, preterm dilation in the absence of contractions. Preterm infants (those born before 37 weeks' gestation) are often of low or very low birth weight; this is the leading cause of neonatal death not associated with congenital defects, and the smallest are at highest risk.

5. Answer c.

Both the WIC program and the Supplemental Nutrition Assistance Program (formerly the Food Stamp Program) are federal assistance programs administered through the USDA. The United States Department of Health and Human Services, through the HRSA, administers the Maternal and Child Health (MCH) Bureau.

6. Answer e.

With a 10-year period since her most recent tetanus toxoid vaccination, she is due for a booster. Use of the tetanus-diphtheria or Tdap vaccine is not contraindicated in pregnancy, and either may be given during the second or third trimesters. While MMR is recommended upon completion of pregnancy to address her lack of immunity to rubella, the vaccine is contraindicated in pregnancy because it contains live virus. Contact or high-impact activity should be avoided during pregnancy, but many other exercise activities are safe in pregnancy, particularly for the conditioned athlete, and are associated with health benefits. Therefore, activity restrictions limiting lifting to 10 pounds are not appropriate. Folate supplementation is indicated in pregnancy, but for women with a previous fetus or child with neural tube defect, 4 mg of folic acid daily in the 1 to 3 months before pregnancy is recommended. There is no known level of alcohol consumption known to be safe during pregnancy.

7. Answer b.

The leading cause of death for all children aged 1 through 17 years is unintentional injury. Motor vehicle crashes are the most frequent cause of unintentional injury or death in this group.

8. Answer e.

The definition of perinatal mortality includes stillbirths and the deaths of live-born infants through the first 28 days of life. Neonatal mortality includes the deaths of infants within the first 28 days of life, postneonatal mortality between 29 days and 1 year, and infant mortality refers to the death of live-born children up to 1 year of age.

9

OBESITY, NUTRITION, AND PHYSICAL ACTIVITY

Donald D. Hensrud, MD, MPH

Obesity

Obesity is defined as an increase in body fat. Because direct measurement of body fat is impractical, surrogate measures of body fat such as weight and body mass index (BMI) are used clinically, in epidemiologic and other research studies, and by the general public. **Body mass index** is calculated as follows: (body weight in kg)/(height in m)^2. BMI correlates with body fat and health outcomes better than weight alone or combined weight-height measures, which is why it is used as the standard for classification of obesity. Table 1 shows the current classification and disease risks of obesity. BMI performs well in predicting health risks in populations and in most people—the health risks associated with obesity begin to increase in the overweight range. However, muscular individuals may have a high proportion of lean vs fat tissue; these people have high BMI and yet have low health risks.

Health risks are associated with body fat distribution in a manner independent of BMI. Individuals with a greater **abdominal distribution** of weight have increased obesity-associated health risks (Table 1), including overall risk of death. The precise mechanisms of these relationships are not entirely clear, but visceral and subcutaneous abdominal fat appear to increase insulin resistance and release of free fatty acids into the bloodstream. Most studies have shown that the waist measurement is as good as the waist-to-hip ratio when predicting health risks associated with abdominal fat distribution. However, it should be recognized that the risks associated with abdominal fat distribution are continuous and that threshold values were established primarily to facilitate clinical classification. Increased abdominal fat distribution is associated particularly with **metabolic syndrome**, of which the main features are 1) increased waist measurement (>102 cm in men and >88 cm in women); 2) elevated blood pressure (>130/85 mm Hg) or hypertension; 3) elevated fasting blood glucose (>110 mg/dL) or type 2 diabetes mellitus; 4) dyslipidemia, with high-density lipoprotein (HDL) cholesterol <40 mg/dL for men and <50 mg/dL for women; and 5) triglycerides, >150 mg/dL for both sexes. When 3 of these 5 factors are present, a diagnosis of metabolic syndrome can be established. Metabolic syndrome is associated with an increased risk of cardiovascular disease.

Epidemiology

The prevalence of obesity has increased markedly over the past few decades in the United States (Table 2). This increase has occurred across all ethnic groups and all ages, including childhood and adolescence. Obesity prevalence similarly has increased in almost all areas of the world. The latest National Health and Nutrition Examination Survey (NHANES) showed that in 2003-2004, the prevalence of at least overweight was 66% and the prevalence of obesity was 32%. Class III or extreme obesity (BMI >40 kg/m^2) affects 1 in 20 Americans (4.8%), including 14.7% of black females. Childhood obesity prevalence increased 2- to 3-fold from 1980-2000. This is of particular concern because obese children are now being diagnosed with type 2 diabetes mellitus (formerly termed "adult onset"), and obese children have greater risk of becoming obese adults.

Table 1 Classification of Overweight and Obesity and Associated Disease Risks

Weight Classification	BMI, kg/m² [a]	Obesity Class	Disease Risks	
			Low Waist Cir	High Waist Cir[b]
Underweight	<18.5	...	...	...
Normal	18.5-24.9	...	...	...
Overweight	25.0-29.9	...	Increased	High
Obesity	30.0-34.9	I	High	Very high
	35.0-39.9	II	Very high	Very high
Extreme obesity	≥40	III	Extremely high	Extremely high

Abbreviations: BMI, body mass index; cir, circumference.
[a] BMI is calculated as (body weight in kg)/(height in m)².
[b] Defined as >102 cm for men and >88 cm for women.
Adapted from The Practical Guide (2000).

Only recently has the increasing prevalence of obesity shown signs of slowing in any subgroup. From 1999-2004, the prevalence of obesity among women did not increase. The Behavioral Risk Factor Surveillance System (a national telephone survey) has reported a similar increase in obesity during the same period. However, the reported prevalence estimates are lower, probably because this survey uses self-reported weight.

Health Risks

Overweight and obesity are associated with numerous comorbid conditions (Box 1) and are considered responsible for a large number of excess deaths each year. Some reports have estimated this to be up to 300,000 deaths per year; however, others have estimated a much lower number of deaths due to obesity and reported no relationship between overweight and increased mortality rate. Among causes of death due to obesity, cardiovascular disease ranks first.

Causes

Ultimately, obesity results from an **imbalance between energy intake and energy expenditure**. The factors that

Table 2 Prevalence of Obesity in the United States

Group	1960-1962	1971-1974	1976-1980	1988-1994	1999-2000	2003-2004
Men, %	10.7	12.1	12.7	20.6	27.5	31.1
Women, %	15.8	16.6	17.0	25.9	33.4	33.2
Total, %	13.4	14.5	15.0	23.3	30.5	32.2

Data from Flegal KM, Carroll MD, Ogden CL, Johnson CL. Prevalence in trends in obesity among US adults, 1999-2000. JAMA. 2002;288:1723-7 and data from Ogden et al (2006).

Box 1 Health Complications of Obesity

Cancer (breast, colon, endometrium, and others)

Coronary heart disease

Degenerative arthritis

Dyslipidemia (hypertriglyceridemia; low level of high-density lipoprotein cholesterol; small, dense low-density lipoprotein cholesterol)

Gastroesophageal reflux disease

Hepatobiliary problems (cholelithiasis, nonalcoholic fatty liver disease)

Hypertension

Increased overall mortality rate

Infertility

Menstrual irregularities

Respiratory problems (obesity hypoventilation syndrome, obstructive sleep apnea, restrictive lung disease)

Skin infections and slow wound healing

Stroke

Type 2 diabetes mellitus

Urinary stress incontinence

influence this simple energy balance equation are complex, pervasive, and powerful, as evidenced by the rapid increase in the prevalence of obesity in the relatively recent past. These factors involve genetic, neurologic, psychologic, behavioral, nutritional, and environmental relationships. The recent increase in obesity prevalence implicates predominantly environmental influences, perhaps in conjunction with genetic susceptibility.

Increased energy intake may occur because people underestimate calorie intake by an average of 20%, although studies report a wide range. Obese individuals may underestimate their energy intake by more than twice this amount. This is not necessarily a conscious act—the volume of food does not correlate tightly with its calorie content. Dietary factors associated with increased energy intake or obesity are listed in Box 2.

Total energy expenditure (TEE) consists of resting energy expenditure or basal metabolic rate (60%-75% of TEE), the thermic effect of food (10% of TEE), and activity energy expenditure (15%-30% of TEE). The main determinant of basal metabolic rate is lean body mass. A low metabolic rate is a commonly perceived reason for weight gain among the public. However, because 20% to 35% of excess weight is composed of lean tissue, basal metabolic rate increases with increased weight. The thermic effect of food is the energy required to digest, assimilate, and store nutrients in the body. Activity energy expenditure is the most variable component of TEE; it can be further divided into **exercise and nonexercise activity** (activities throughout the day). Both components of activity energy expenditure

Box 2 Dietary Factors Associated With Increased Energy Intake or Obesity

Eating away from home

Energy-dense food

Increased intake of snacks, soft drinks, and pizza

Increased portion size

Increased refined carbohydrates, particularly simple sugars

Increased variety of available foods (other than vegetables and fruits)

Data from Hensrud DD. Diet and obesity. Curr Opin Gastroenterol. 2004 Mar;20(2):119-24.

can be intentionally increased to help prevent weight gain, promote weight loss, and maintain weight loss. Increased physical activity may be more important to prevent primary weight gain and maintain weight loss (ie, prevent weight regain), whereas decreased energy intake through diet may be more important to facilitate weight loss.

Other factors that promote weight gain include smoking cessation, medications such as corticosteroids and some antidepressants, depression and other psychological conditions, and pregnancy. A common belief among patients is that low thyroid function is contributing to increased weight, but hypothyroidism and other endocrine disorders are uncommon contributors to obesity (account for <1% of obese individuals).

Prevention and Treatment

After obesity has developed, long-term results from the treatment of obesity are generally poor. Because of this reason and the fact that obesity has been increasing in all segments of the population, interest in the prevention of obesity has increased. Environmental strategies have attempted to **change the built environment** through community and grassroots efforts (eg, community programs, creation of bicycle paths, modification of building design with more accessible stairs). However, little evidence to date shows widespread and sustained effectiveness from these initiatives.

The treatment of obesity should involve **dietary restriction** of calories, **increased energy expenditure** from physical activity, and **behavioral modification**. Many methods can be used to decrease overall calorie intake and none has been shown to be clearly superior. Increased physical activity can be implemented through exercise, an increase in nonexercise activity, or both. The specific types of behavioral changes should be tailored to the individual. Both individual and group weight loss programs can be effective. Lifestyle changes in these areas are more effective than temporary restrictive programs. Strategies associated with long-term successful weight maintenance among people

who have lost weight include various dietary changes to decrease calorie intake, a marked increase in daily physical activity (approximately 1 hour of daily exercise, commonly walking), and approaching behavioral modification as a lifestyle change.

- Body mass index (BMI) correlates well with body fat and health outcomes. Waist measurement is a strong predictor of health risks associated with abdominal fat distribution.
- The prevalence of obesity has increased during the past several decades. As of the early 2000s, prevalence of at least overweight was 66% and the prevalence of obesity was 32%.
- Overweight and obesity are associated with numerous comorbid conditions. The largest cause of death due to obesity is cardiovascular disease.
- Increased physical activity may be more important to prevent primary weight gain and maintain weight loss, whereas decreased energy intake through diet may be more important to facilitate weight loss.
- After obesity has developed, long-term results of treatment are generally poor. However, lifestyle changes are more effective than temporary restrictive measures.

Nutrition and Disease Prevention

The importance of diet and nutrition in the prevention of disease is summarized in this statement from the Surgeon General's Report on Nutrition and Health in 1988: "For the two of three adult Americans who do not smoke and do not drink excessively, one personal choice seems to influence long-term health prospects more than any other: what we eat."

An estimated 365,000 deaths occur each year because of suboptimal diet and activity habits. Dietary factors play a prominent role in 5 of the 10 leading causes of death for Americans: heart disease, cancer, stroke, diabetes mellitus, and cerebrovascular disease. In the period since the release of the report, a great deal has been learned about the relationships between nutrition and disease prevention.

Hyperlipidemia and Coronary Heart Disease

Hyperlipidemia is a major risk factor for heart disease. Total serum cholesterol consists of low-density lipoprotein (LDL) cholesterol, HDL cholesterol, and very-low-density lipoprotein cholesterol (estimated as one-fifth of serum triglycerides). **HDL cholesterol and triglycerides have an inverse relationship** (eg, as body weight increases, triglycerides increase and HDL cholesterol decreases). Box 3 lists the lifestyle habits that raise HDL cholesterol and lower triglycerides.

Box 3 Lifestyle Changes That Affect Serum Lipid Levels

Raise high-density lipoprotein cholesterol

Weight loss

Exercise

Smoking cessation

Increased alcohol consumption

Decreased trans fat consumption

Lower triglycerides

Weight loss

Exercise

Decreased alcohol consumption

Decreased sweet consumption

Improved blood glucose control for people who have diabetes mellitus or impaired fasting blood glucose

Saturated Fat, Trans Fat, and Unsaturated Fat

The main determinants of LDL cholesterol, in decreasing order of impact, are dietary saturated fat, trans fat, and cholesterol. In most cases, saturated fat and cholesterol are found together (eg, in meat, full-fat dairy products), and processed foods (eg, pastries, fast foods) also contain these ingredients. Trans fats naturally occur in very small amounts in food. Usually, they are created through hydrogenation of liquid vegetable fats and are added to food to prolong shelf life and improve texture. Although trans fats constitute only 2% to 3% of calories in our diet (whereas 11% is from saturated fat), they raise LDL cholesterol and also lower HDL cholesterol. Because trans fats have health risks and no known benefits, efforts have been made to decrease their presence in the food supply. New York City has banned trans fats from restaurants. Addressing this issue from a public health perspective has generated controversy and practical challenges in implementation, but overall, it appears to have been successful.

Increased intake of monounsaturated and polyunsaturated fats (as substitutes for saturated and trans fats) will lower LDL cholesterol. Carbohydrate appears to slightly lower LDL and HDL cholesterol. Monounsaturated fats are found in olive oil, canola oil, nuts, and avocados. Polyunsaturated fats are found primarily in vegetable oils. The Therapeutic Lifestyle Change diet (created by the National Cholesterol Education Program) has established dietary guidelines for fat consumption, with the goal of decreasing serum cholesterol levels (Table 3). Other dietary components that affect either serum lipids or the risk of coronary heart disease (CHD) are listed in Box 4.

Fiber

Soluble fiber such as that found in beans, oat bran, apples, and psyllium lowers serum LDL cholesterol by up to 10%.

Table 3 Therapeutic Lifestyle Change Diet Recommendations from the National Cholesterol Education Program

Diet Component	Recommended Daily Consumption[a]
Total fat	25%-35% of calories
Saturated fat	<7% of calories
Monounsaturated fat	Up to 20% of calories
Polyunsaturated fat	Up to 10% of calories
Cholesterol	<200 mg
Fiber	20-30 g
Protein	Approximately 15% of calories

[a] Total calories to maintain desirable weight.
Adapted from Grundy SM, Becker D, Clark LT, Cooper RS, Denke MA, Howard WJ, et al; National Cholesterol Education Program (NCEPP) Expert Panel on Detection, Evaluation, and Treatment of High Blood Cholesterol in Adults (Adult Treatment Panel III). Executive Summary of the Third Report of the National Cholesterol Education Program (NCEPP) Expert Panel on Detection, Evaluation, and Treatment of High Blood Cholesterol in Adults (Adult Treatment Panel III) JAMA 2001;285:2486-97. Used with permission.

The magnitude of this effect decreases as dietary saturated fat decreases. Insoluble fiber from wheat bran and other whole grains and vegetables lowers the risk of CHD through mechanisms that are not completely understood. The effect of fiber is most apparent when it is present in foods (as opposed to isolated in a supplement). This may be partly because fiber is a marker for other beneficial nutrients in plant foods that also have positive effects on health.

Nuts

The association between nuts and reduced risk of CHD has been shown in a number of epidemiologic studies. Although nuts are relatively high in fat, most contain a large proportion of monounsaturated fat. Walnuts have a relatively high content of omega-3 fatty acids. Of note, studies have shown that people tend to compensate for the calories in

Box 4 Dietary Factors That May Lower Serum Low-Density Lipoprotein Cholesterol or Decrease the Risk of Coronary Heart Disease

Fiber (whole grains, vegetables, fruits)

Nuts

Fish (omega-3 fatty acids)

Dark chocolate

Alcohol

Olive oil, canola oil

Soybeans

Stanol- and sterol-containing food products

nuts by not consuming as many calories from other sources, perhaps because of the effect of nuts on satiety.

Sterols and Stanols

Sterols and stanols are cholesterol-like substances found in plant foods; when consumed, they lower serum LDL cholesterol by up to 10% or 15%. Vegetables, fruits, nuts, and whole grains contain sterols and stanols, as well as soluble and insoluble fiber, vitamins, and other phytochemicals. All of these plant foods are associated with a reduced risk of CHD. In recent years, a number of food products containing sterols or stanols have appeared on the market.

Fish

Fish, particularly fatty fish such as salmon, mackerel, herring, and lake trout, are a good source of **omega-3 fatty acids**, which can decrease the risk of sudden cardiac death. For this reason, the American Heart Association (AHA) recommends at least 2 servings of fish per week. Children and women of childbearing age should limit their consumption of fish, particularly larger fish higher on the food chain, because of mercury and polychlorinated biphenyl contamination.

Soy

Soy-containing foods lower serum LDL cholesterol when substituted for animal foods such as meat and full-fat dairy products. It is unclear whether soy protein, isoflavones, or other components have additional lipid-lowering effects.

Alcohol

Alcohol has mixed effects on health. From a heart disease standpoint, alcohol reduces risk by raising HDL cholesterol and thinning blood by increasing fibrinolytic activity and interfering with platelet aggregation. However, it also increases blood pressure and triglyceride levels. Moderate alcohol consumption is defined as no more than 1 drink per day for women and 2 per day for men. Overall, people who consume moderate amounts of alcohol have lower risk of CHD than people who consume no alcohol. Moderate consumption also decreases the risk of ischemic stroke.

Wine, particularly red wine, is commonly believed to be associated with a stronger effect on heart disease than other types of alcohol. Red wine is made with grape skins that contain phenolic antioxidant compounds such as resveratrol. However, the evidence overall suggests that alcohol itself is responsible for the vast majority of health effects of wine, and the additional benefit from antioxidants and other substances is relatively small. In addition, studies have shown people who consume wine have better overall health habits compared with people who consume hard liquor or beer. Wine is more often consumed with meals. People who consume wine often have better overall health habits than people who don't, which may also explain some of its perceived health benefits.

There are no formal recommendations to consume alcohol for health benefits. Excess alcohol consumption is responsible for an estimated 85,000 deaths yearly from cancer, accidents, homicide, suicide, and other causes. The societal toll from alcohol abuse is also quite large. Thus, individual risk factors, family history, and intrapersonal characteristics may influence the decision to drink. For people who choose to consume alcohol, moderate consumption may have some beneficial health effects, but more than moderate consumption elevates risk of noncardiac death and increases the risk of hemorrhagic stroke, although this type of stroke is less common.

AHA Diet and Lifestyle Guidelines

The AHA incorporates many of these food-related findings in the 2006 edition of their Diet and Lifestyle Guidelines (Box 5). These guidelines are less quantitative than previous guidelines and attempt to encourage qualitative, practical changes in diet.

Potential Effect of Diet on Serum Lipids

The effect of diet on serum lipids sometimes is perceived to be modest. However, results appear to be dependent on the degree of dietary changes. An intensive, randomized, controlled trial showed that a low-fat diet reduced LDL

Box 5 American Heart Association 2006 Diet and Lifestyle Recommendations for Cardiovascular Disease Risk Reduction

---

Balance calorie intake and physical activity to achieve or maintain a healthy body weight

Consume a diet rich in vegetables and fruits

Choose whole-grain, high-fiber foods

Consume fish, especially oily fish, at least twice a week

Limit intake of saturated fat to <7% of calories, trans fat to <1% of energy, and cholesterol to <300 mg/d

  Choose lean meats and vegetable alternatives

  Select fat-free (skim), 1% fat, and low-fat dairy products

  Minimize intake of partially hydrogenated fat

Minimize intake of beverages and foods with added sugars

Choose and prepare foods with little or no salt

If alcohol is consumed, do so in moderation

When eating food prepared outside the home, follow the AHA Diet and Lifestyle Recommendations

---

Adapted from Lichtenstein et al (2006). Used with permission.

cholesterol by about 10%, whereas comprehensive dietary changes (increasing consumption of soluble fiber, plant sterols, soy protein, and almonds) reduced LDL cholesterol by over 30%; the latter results were comparable to those from treatment with a statin.

The potential effect of diet in the treatment and prevention of CHD is illustrated by select randomized, controlled trials. The Lyon Diet Heart Study randomized 800 people who had sustained a myocardial infarction to either follow a Mediterranean diet or receive usual care. The **Mediterranean diet** contained less meat and butter and more vegetables, fruits, beans, and canola oil margarine. When the data were analyzed after 2 years and again after 4 years, those subjects following the Mediterranean diet had a marked, statistically significant reduction in risk of a major cardiac event, including recurrent myocardial infarction or sudden cardiac death.

The Lifestyle Heart Trial randomized 40 people with angiographically documented CHD either to a 10%-fat vegetarian diet along with exercise and stress management or to usual care. After 5 years, the diameter stenosis decreased by 3% in the experimental group, whereas it increased by 11% in the usual care group. The usual care group also had more symptoms and events, despite a greater proportion of statin use.

In the studies described above, one trial used a low-fat diet and the other a higher-fat diet (mostly monounsaturated fat along with smaller amounts of omega-3 fatty acids). Both diets incorporated generous amounts of vegetables, fruits, whole grains, and legumes. Either a low-fat diet or a higher-fat diet can be cardioprotective if the type of fat is heart-healthy and overall food choices emphasize a variety of other health-supporting foods. Both studies were tertiary prevention trials, which overlapped preventive measures with treatment of established disease. However, these dietary patterns are also likely to be beneficial for the primary prevention of CHD.

- Hyperlipidemia is a major risk factor for heart disease. Changes in lifestyle habits can raise high-density lipoprotein (HDL) cholesterol and lower triglycerides.
- The main determinants of low-density lipoprotein (LDL) cholesterol are dietary saturated fat, trans fat, and cholesterol. Increased intake of monounsaturated and polyunsaturated fats (as substitutes for saturated fat), soluble fiber, plant sterols and stanols, and soy lowers LDL cholesterol.
- Risk of coronary heart disease (CHD) can be decreased by consuming insoluble fiber, nuts, fatty fish, and moderate amounts of alcohol.
- Either a low-fat diet or a higher-fat diet can be cardioprotective if the type of fat is heart-healthy and overall food choices emphasize various health-supporting foods.

- A Mediterranean diet, which emphasizes vegetables, fruits, beans, whole-grain carbohydrates, and olive oil or canola oil margarine (while limiting intake of meat and butter) considerably reduces risk of a major cardiac event.

Hypertension and Type 2 Diabetes Mellitus

Hypertension

Primary lifestyle choices that affect blood pressure are weight, salt intake, exercise, and alcohol. Although many other nutrients are associated with decreased hypertension, their clinical effects often are minor. Two randomized, controlled trials evaluated the effect of comprehensive dietary changes on blood pressure. In both of the **Dietary Approaches to Stop Hypertension** (DASH) trials, subjects were randomized to a diet of 8 to 10 servings of vegetables and fruits daily, low-fat dairy products, decreased meat, increased beans and nuts, and whole grains or to a typical American diet of 37% fat and 3 to 5 servings of vegetables and fruits daily. The studies controlled for 4 lifestyle factors known at that time to affect blood pressure. Among people with hypertension, blood pressure decreased by 11.4/5.5 mm Hg in those randomized to the DASH diet. Notably, blood pressure decreased among all subjects (mean decrease, 5.5/3.0 mm Hg) and in all subgroups following the DASH diet, suggesting that this diet also could be used for prevention of hypertension.

Consistent with these study data, increased consumption of vegetables and fruits has been associated with reduced risk of ischemic stroke, for which hypertension is a risk factor. Table 4 lists the magnitude of the effects of

Table 4 Effect of Lifestyle Changes on Systolic Blood Pressure

Intervention	Estimated Effect, mm Hg
Weight loss (per 10 kg lost)	5-20
Dietary Approaches to Stop Hypertension trial diet	8-14
Sodium restriction	2-8
Physical activity	4-9
Alcohol restriction	2-4

Data from Chobanian AV, Bakris GL, Black HR, Cushman WC, Green LA, Izzo JL Jr, et al; National Heart, Lung, and Blood Institute Joint National Committee on Prevention, Detection, Evaluation, and Treatment of High Blood Pressure; National High Blood Pressure Education Program Coordinating Committee. The Seventh Report of the Joint National Committee on Prevention, Detection, Evaluation, and Treatment of High Blood Pressure: the JNC 7 report. JAMA. 2003 May 21;289(19):2560-72. Epub 2003 May 14. Erratum in: JAMA. 2003 Jul 9;290(2):197.

diet and other lifestyle factors on systolic blood pressure. Implementing lifestyle changes in these areas will likely have some effect on preventing hypertension as well.

Type 2 Diabetes Mellitus

Up to 70% of individuals with type 2 diabetes mellitus are overweight or obese. Physical activity, particularly exercise, will help decrease body weight and the risk of diabetes mellitus, independent of the effect on weight loss. Eating a low-glycemic diet (one that minimizes the increase in blood glucose after eating) also has a small effect on decreasing risk. Decreasing the prevalence of obesity has the strongest potential effect on reducing the incidence of type 2 diabetes mellitus.

- The primary lifestyle choices that affect blood pressure are weight, salt intake, exercise, alcohol, and the Dietary Approaches to Stop Hypertension (DASH) diet.
- The DASH diet emphasizes intake of vegetables and fruits, low-fat dairy products, beans, nuts, and whole grains, while reducing the consumption of meat.
- Decreasing the prevalence of obesity may greatly reduce the incidence of type 2 diabetes mellitus.

Cancer

The term "cancer" encompasses many different diseases, each with its own risk factors. An estimated one-third of all cancers are related to diet. The American Institute for Cancer Research comprehensively reviewed the relationship between diet, physical activity, and cancer in 2007. Compared with their previous report in 1997, this report increased emphasis on the relationship between obesity and cancers of the breast, uterus, colon, kidney, pancreas, and others. Obesity is responsible for an estimated 14% of cancers in men and 20% in women. Box 6 lists nutrition and physical activity guidelines for the prevention of cancer from the American Cancer Society.

Breast Cancer

Risk factors for breast cancer include obesity, particularly abdominal obesity, and weight gain as an adult. Alcohol use also increases the risk of breast cancer, and the risk begins to increase even with low levels of consumption. Contrary to previous beliefs, total dietary fat does not seem to have a clinically significant effect on the risk of breast cancer, although some studies suggest monounsaturated fat may be protective. Physical activity is protective against breast cancer and probably is effective for tertiary prevention. Breastfeeding is also protective.

Box 6 American Cancer Society Nutrition and Physical Activity Guidelines

Maintain a healthy weight throughout life
  Balance calorie intake with physical activity
  Avoid excessive weight gain throughout life
  Achieve and maintain a healthy weight if currently overweight or obese
Adopt a physically active lifestyle
  Adults—engage in ≥30 min of moderate-to-vigorous physical activity, above usual activities, on ≥5 d/wk; 45-60 min of intentional physical activity is preferable
  Children and adolescents—engage in ≥60 min of moderate-to-vigorous physical activity, ≥5 d/wk
Eat a healthy diet, with an emphasis on plant foods
  Choose foods and drinks in amounts that help achieve and maintain a healthy weight
  Eat ≥5 servings of various vegetables and fruits daily
  Choose whole grains instead of processed (refined) grains
  Limit intake of processed and red meats
If alcoholic beverages are consumed, limit intake (no more than 1 drink/d for women or 2 drinks/d for men)

Adapted from Kushi et al (2006). Used with permission.

Colorectal Cancer

The risk of colorectal cancer is increased by red meat consumption, and processed meat is associated with even greater risk. Obesity, abdominal obesity, and alcohol use also increase risk. Physical activity and eating vegetables and fruits are protective, and folic acid appears to mitigate the increased risk from alcohol. Previously, dietary fiber was thought to protect against colorectal cancer. However, it now appears that fiber-containing foods are protective and this effect is not directly attributable to fiber itself.

Prostate Cancer

Prostate cancer risk is probably increased by diets high in calcium and dairy products. Risk may be decreased by foods containing lycopene, found in high concentration in tomatoes, and selenium.

Other Cancers

Endometrial cancer risk is increased by obesity, particularly abdominal obesity. Stomach cancer risk is increased by consuming salt and smoked foods. Cancers of the pancreas, mouth, upper gastrointestinal tract, and lung may be decreased by vegetable and fruit intake.

- About one-third of cancers are related to diet. Obesity is responsible for 14% of cancers in men and 20% in women.

- Physical activity is protective against breast and colon cancer.
- Vegetables and fruits appear to decrease the risk of cancers of the mouth, lung, pancreas, upper gastrointestinal tract, and colorectum.
- Consumption of red and processed meats increases the risk of colorectal cancer. Alcohol use increases the risk of breast and colorectal cancer.

Micronutrients, Whole Foods, and Patterns of Eating

It is possible to study the relationships between diet and health at various levels. At the micronutrient level, insufficient consumption of some nutrients affects the risk of developing specific diseases. For example, vitamin D deficiency and inadequate calcium intake may lead to osteoporosis. When strong evidence supports the role of an individual micronutrient, supplementation may be recommended. However, when the evidence is incomplete, there may be risks of unintended or adverse effects.

At the whole-food level, epidemiologic studies have consistently shown that nuts are associated with a reduced risk of CHD. However, excessive emphasis sometimes is placed on individual foods. Although nuts have a place in a healthy diet, they are energy dense, and excessive consumption could lead to a relatively large calorie intake.

At the level of eating patterns, several are associated with beneficial effects. For example, traditional **Mediterranean or Asian patterns of eating** have been associated with reduced risk of many chronic diseases. Although the specific types of food differ, these patterns share features that are collectively responsible for the beneficial effects, including generous consumption of **plant products**. The main difference between the Mediterranean and Asian eating patterns is the higher total fat intake in the Mediterranean diet, although the fats typically are heart-healthy monounsaturated fats. The common features of these and other patterns of eating that improve health and reduce disease risk are summarized in Table 5.

Dietary Guidelines

The Dietary Guidelines for Americans are the primary dietary recommendations for all healthy Americans to follow to achieve good health. They are reviewed and updated every 5 years. The 2005 Dietary Guidelines were intended, for the first time, primarily to be used by policy makers, health care providers, nutritionists, and nutrition educators; it was not for use by the general public. Twenty-three key recommendations in 9 focus areas were outlined, with additional key recommendations for specific populations.

The MyPyramid.gov Web site was created in 2006 to replace the 1992 Food Guide Pyramid as a tool to help the public implement the Dietary Guidelines for Americans. The site offers personalized eating plans and interactive tools (eg, menu planner, food tracker). The effectiveness of this tool and whether it represents the best scientific evidence are subjects of controversy.

Table 5 Summary of Dietary Patterns Associated With Improved Health and Reduced Risk of Disease

Consumption Level	Food
High	Fresh or frozen vegetables
	Fresh or frozen fruits
Moderate	Whole-grain carbohydrates (eg, whole-grain breads, pastas, cereals, and cooked grains)
	Beans, including soybeans
	Olive oil, canola oil, and nuts as added sources of fat
	Fish
Low	Meat
	Full-fat dairy products
	Refined carbohydrates, including sugar-containing foods
	High-calorie "fast foods"
	Processed food
	Alcohol

- Insufficient levels of some micronutrients affect the risk of developing specific diseases.
- Eating patterns associated with a reduced risk of chronic disease share features that are collectively responsible for the beneficial effects, including generous amounts of vegetables, fruits, whole-grain carbohydrates, nuts, beans, and other plant products.
- Low-fat traditional Asian diets and Mediterranean diets with higher total fat, primarily from monounsaturated fat, are associated with reduced risk of disease.
- The Dietary Guidelines for Americans are the primary dietary recommendations for all healthy Americans. MyPyramid.gov is a tool to help the public implement these guidelines.

Vitamins and Supplements

Vitamin deficiencies generally are uncommon in the United States, but they have been observed for individual nutrients and within specific patient populations. Table 6 lists common vitamins and signs and symptoms of their deficiency states. Increasing evidence supports the benefits of vitamin D for bone health and other conditions. Vitamin D

Table 6 Signs and Symptoms of Vitamin Deficiencies

Vitamin	Signs and Symptoms of Deficiency
Vitamin A	Night blindness, xerosis, Bitot spots, keratomalacia
Vitamin B_1 (thiamine)	Dry beriberi—neuropathy
	Wet beriberi—congestive heart failure
	Wernicke-Korsakoff syndrome—ophthalmoplegia, ataxia, psychosis
Vitamin B_2 (riboflavin)	Angular stomatitis (cracks at the corners of the mouth), glossitis (smooth, red tongue), cheilosis (vertical cracks in the lips), seborrheic dermatitis, burning eyes
Vitamin B_3 (niacin)	Pellagra—diarrhea, dementia, dermatitis, glossitis
Vitamin B_6 (pyridoxine)	Glossitis, cheilosis, seborrheic dermatitis, microcytic anemia, peripheral neuritis
Vitamin B_9 (folic acid)	Megaloblastic anemia, smooth sore tongue, thrombocytopenia, diarrhea, fatigue
Vitamin B_{12} (cobalamin)	Weakness, megaloblastic anemia, smooth sore tongue, neurologic dysfunction (impaired position and vibratory sense)
Vitamin C	Scurvy—hyperkeratosis, corkscrew hairs, perifollicular petechiae, bleeding gums, arthritis
Vitamin D	Rickets (in children, bone deformities), osteomalacia (in adults, bone pain), osteoporosis
Vitamin E	Hemolytic anemia, ataxia, neuropathy
Vitamin K	Bleeding, bruising

deficiency is common, affecting 20% to 50% of the population. Therefore, in recent years, the recommended intake and serum levels of vitamin D has increased. Occult Vitamin B_{12} deficiency increases with age and affects approximately 10% to 15% of individuals aged 65 years and older.

Dietary supplements include vitamins, minerals, herbs, and other substances. More than half of American adults take dietary supplements, at a cost exceeding $23 billion per year. The Dietary Supplement Health and Education Act of 1994 requires the US Food and Drug Administration (FDA) to regulate dietary supplements. Under this act, the FDA does not have to approve a dietary supplement before it is sold to consumers; only the manufacturer is responsible for ensuring safety before marketing. Since 2007, supplement makers have been required to follow Current Good Manufacturing Practices, but supplements are not subject to the same quality control measures that are applied to the manufacture of pharmaceutical agents. There have been examples of supplements that either do not contain the correct amount of an ingredient or contain ingredients that are not supposed to be present.

In situations not related to deficiency, few dietary supplements are associated with evidence of benefit; others

are harmful, and many have little evidence of either benefit or harm. Manufacturers do not have to disclose information on the benefits of dietary supplements (ie, they do not have to prove efficacy before marketing). Structure-function health claims are permitted, except for those that claim to cure or prevent a disease. For example, a manufacturer may claim that a dietary supplement aids digestion, but it cannot state that it prevents colon cancer. The FDA must prove a dietary supplement is unsafe before restricting its sale; this has happened with ephedra.

Few dietary supplements are formally recommended. The 2005 Dietary Guidelines for Americans recommend only the following: 1) adults aged 50 years and older should consume extra vitamin B_{12}; 2) women who may become pregnant or are in the first trimester of pregnancy should consume folic acid; and 3) older adults, adults with dark skin, and people with insufficient sun exposure should consume extra vitamin D. Extra vitamins can be consumed through fortified foods or dietary supplements. Some evidence supports use of certain supplements in specific populations. In one randomized, controlled trial, omega-3 fatty acids were associated with a reduced risk of recurrent major cardiac events among subjects who previously had a myocardial infarction. Omega-3 fatty acids will also lower serum triglycerides when taken in gram doses. Studies have shown that glucosamine reduces joint symptoms in some patients with osteoarthritis. A combination of antioxidants, including vitamin C, vitamin E, β-carotene, zinc, and copper delayed the progression of age-related macular degeneration in people with early disease. In another study of women who had or were at high risk for cardiovascular disease, folic acid, vitamin B_6, and vitamin B_{12} reduced the risk of age-related macular degeneration.

Preliminary data for some dietary supplements have not been supported in clinical trials. Vitamin E showed promise of reducing the risk of CHD in laboratory, animal, and epidemiologic studies, but clinical trials have shown little benefit; in fact, meta-analyses have suggested a slight increase in mortality rates. Folic acid, vitamin B_6 (pyridoxine), and vitamin B_{12} concentrations are inversely associated with blood homocysteine concentration, but randomized clinical trials have reported little improvement in homocysteine values after supplementation with these vitamins.

Some dietary supplements may cause harm or interact with other medications. For example, 2 large, randomized, controlled trials showed β-carotene supplementation increased the risk of lung cancer and overall mortality rate among smokers and former smokers. St John's wort was popular as a treatment for mild depression. However, it induces cytochrome P450 enzyme activity and interacts with numerous medications, including protease inhibitors (used to treat human immunodeficiency virus infection), oral contraceptives, and others. People who take dietary supplements should follow the recommendations listed in Box 7.

Box 7 General Recommendations for People Who Take Dietary Supplements

Find accurate information about the benefits and risks of supplements before taking them

Tell your health care provider about any supplements you are taking, and discuss the benefits and risks

If any unusual reactions occur, stop taking the supplement

Stop taking dietary supplements 2 weeks before surgery

- Vitamin deficiencies generally are uncommon in the United States. For most nutrients, a beneficial effect of dietary supplements has not been demonstrated.
- The US Food and Drug Administration (FDA) does not approve dietary supplements before they are marketed, and they must prove a dietary supplement is unsafe before restricting its sale.
- Precautions should be taken for some dietary supplements that may cause harm or interact with other medications.

Physical Activity and Exercise

Physical activity is defined as any bodily movement produced by skeletal muscles that results in energy expenditure. Exercise is physical activity that is planned, structured, and repetitive. Physical fitness involves personal (genetic and training-induced) attributes such as cardiorespiratory endurance, muscular strength, and endurance that affect the ability to perform physical activities.

Benefits

The health benefits of physical activity and exercise are broad, strong, and well documented (Box 8). Health benefits appear to increase linearly with the total amount of physical activity, up to approximately 2,000 calories per week of energy expended. Health benefits also increase with increasing intensity of physical activity; this increase is nonlinear, ie, a substantial benefit occurs with initiation of even mild-intensity physical activity, with increasing but diminishing returns as the level of intensity increases. Despite the known benefits, more than half of American adults are not regularly physically active, and almost one-fourth are not active at all. The main risk of physical activity and exercise is musculoskeletal injury. This risk can be decreased by gradually building up to the desired level of physical activity and by avoiding excessive amounts of activity and exercise. The risk of sudden death and acute myocardial infarction may be transiently increased during exercise. However, physically active or fit individuals have a much lower risk of cardiovascular disease during nonexercise time, thus lowering their overall risk by 25% to 50%.

Box 8 Major Benefits of Exercise and Physical Activity

Decreased overall mortality

Improved weight control and decreased risk of obesity

Decreased blood pressure and risk of hypertension

Improved glucose control and decreased risk of type 2 diabetes mellitus

Improved serum lipids (increased high-density lipoprotein cholesterol, decreased triglycerides)

Increased fitness

Decreased risk of coronary heart disease (and death from heart disease)

Decreased risk of stroke

Decreased risk of breast, colon, and endometrial cancers

Improved mood and decreased risk of depression

Increased bone strength and reduced risk of osteoporosis

Decreased risk of Alzheimer disease

Improved balance and reduced risk of falls

Improved quality of life

Improved stress management

Improved sleep

Improved immune function

Guidelines

The AHA and the American College of Sports Medicine (ACSM) released updated guidelines for physical activity in 2007 (Table 7). Their recommendations are intended for average, healthy adults to maintain health and reduce the risk of chronic disease. These activities should be in addition to the light-intensity activities of daily life. Bouts of activity should be in increments of at least 10 minutes, and combinations of moderate- and vigorous-intensity exercise

Table 7 2007 Physical Activity Recommendations for Adults from the American Heart Association and American College of Sports Medicine

Activity	Definition
1. Moderate-intensity physical activity (at least 30 min, 5 d/wk) OR Vigorous-intensity physical activity (at least 20 min, 3 d/wk)	Moderate-intensity physical activity means working hard enough to accelerate the heart rate (eg, brisk walking) Vigorous-intensity physical activity means working hard enough to breathe rapidly and substantially increase heart rate (eg, jogging)
2. Resistance activities that increase muscular strength and endurance (at least 2 d/wk)	Perform 8-10 strength-training exercises (eg, weight lifting), with 8-12 repetitions per exercise resulting in fatigue

Data from Haskell et al (2007).

can be performed. To lose weight or maintain weight loss, 60 to 90 minutes of daily physical activity may be necessary.

In 2008, the US Department of Health and Human Services released physical activity guidelines for Americans. These guidelines are very similar to the AHA/ACSM guidelines described above. However, the government guidelines specify at least 150 minutes of moderate-intensity physical activity or 75 minutes of vigorous-intensity physical activity per week (instead of recommending the number of minutes per day and days per week). This allows people more flexibility in how they achieve the activity goals during the week.

Assessment

Physical activity can be assessed by questionnaire or by taking measurements. Fitness can be assessed by submaximal or maximal oxygen consumption on a **treadmill exercise test** using a standard (Bruce) protocol. The use of exercise testing as a routine screening tool for CHD is discouraged by the US Preventive Services Task Force and the AHA. Even for patients with stable coronary artery disease, routine screening is not recommended. The AHA acknowledges the possible value of screening certain populations (Box 9).

- Health benefits appear to increase with the total amount and intensity of physical activity, up to a point.
- The most recent guidelines for physical activity recommend 150 minutes of moderate-intensity physical activity or 75 minutes of vigorous-intensity physical activity per week.
- Fitness can be assessed by submaximal or maximal oxygen consumption on a treadmill exercise test using a standard protocol.

Box 9 Populations That May Benefit From Exercise Testing

Subjects with diabetes mellitus who are beginning a vigorous exercise program

Patients with multiple risk factors who need guided risk-reduction therapy

Men (>45 y) and women (>55 y) starting a vigorous exercise program, involved in occupations that affect public safety, or are at risk of coronary heart disease (have risk factors such as peripheral vascular disease)

Data from Gibbons RJ, Balady GJ, Bricker JT, Chaitman BR, Fletcher GF, Froelicher VF, et al. ACC/AHA 2002 guideline update for exercise testing: summary article: a report of the ACC/AHA Task Force on Practice Guidelines (Committee to Update the 1997 Exercise Testing Guidelines). Circulation. 2002 Oct 1;106(14):1883-92.

SUGGESTED READING

Haskell WL, Lee IM, Pate RR, Powell KE, Blair SN, Franklin BA, et al. Physical activity and public health: updated recommendation for adults from the American College of Sports Medicine and the American Heart Association. Circulation. 2007 Aug 28;116(9):1081-93. Epub 2007 Aug 1.

Kushi LH, Byers T, Doyle C, Bandera EV, McCullough M, McTiernan A, et al; American Cancer Society 2006 Nutrition and Physical Activity Guidelines Advisory Committee. American Cancer Society Guidelines on Nutrition and Physical Activity for cancer prevention: reducing the risk of cancer with healthy food choices and physical activity. CA Cancer J Clin. 2006 Sep-Oct;56(5):254-81 Erratum in: CA Cancer J Clin. 2007 Jan-Feb;57(1):66.

Lichtenstein AH, Appel LJ, Brands M, Carnethon M, Daniels S, Franch HA, et al. Diet and lifestyle recommendations revision 2006: a scientific statement from the American Heart Association Nutrition Committee. Circulation. 2006 Jul 4;114(1):82-96. Epub 2006 Jun 19. Erratum in: Circulation. 2006 Dec 5;114(23):e629. Circulation. 2006 Jul 4;114(1):e27.

Ogden CL, Carroll MD, Curtin LR, McDowell MA, Tabak CJ, Flegal KM. Prevalence of overweight and obesity in the United States, 1999-2004. JAMA. 2006 Apr 5;295(13): 1549-55.

The Practical Guide: Identification, Evaluation, and Treatment of Overweight and Obesity in Adults [Internet]. Bethesda (MD): National Institutes of Health, October 2000, Publication No. 00-4084 [cited 17 Mar 2009]. Available online at: http://www.nhlbi.nih.gov/guidelines/obesity/practgde.htm

U.S. Department of Health and Human Services and U.S. Department of Agriculture. Executive Summary: Dietary Guidelines for Americans, 2005 [Internet]; [cited 2009 Mar 17]. Washington, DC: U.S. Government Printing Office, January 2005. Available from: http://www.health.gov/dietaryguidelines/dga2005/document/html/executivesummary.htm

U.S. Food and Drug Administration, Dietary Supplements [Internet]. Silver Spring (MD): U.S. Food and Drug Administration; [cited 17 Mar 2009]. Available from: http://www.cfsan.fda.gov/~dms/supplmnt.html

Questions and Answers

Questions

1. You are working for a national insurance company and are tasked with determining the effect of obesity on health risks for the US population. You examined recent data to estimate future changes in the prevalence estimates of obesity and found that the prevalence of obesity has been increasing in recent years in all groups *except*:
   a. Men
   b. Women
   c. Children
   d. Blacks
   e. Hispanics

2. A 52-year-old man has a body mass index of 28 kg/m², waist measurement of 96.5 cm, and blood pressure of 135/88 mm Hg. His fasting lipid profile is as follows: total cholesterol, 216 mg/dL; high-density lipoprotein (HDL) cholesterol, 43 mg/dL; low-density lipoprotein (LDL) cholesterol, 147 mg/dL; and triglycerides, 130 mg/dL. His fasting blood glucose

level is 98 mg/dL. He is wondering about health risks associated with his weight and body fat distribution and has heard about metabolic syndrome. Which of his health parameters qualifies as part of metabolic syndrome?

a. Waist measurement
b. Blood pressure
c. HDL cholesterol
d. Triglycerides
e. Fasting blood glucose

3. A 33-year-old woman is interested in improving her health by increasing her physical activity. You tell her the latest recommendations from the Department of Health and Human Services include:

a. 20 minutes of exercise at the target heart rate, 3 times per week
b. 30 minutes of light physical activity, 7 days per week
c. 30 minutes of vigorous exercise, 5 days per week
d. 150 minutes of moderate-intensity physical activity each week
e. 210 minutes of vigorous-intensity physical activity each week

4. According to guidelines from the American Heart Association, which of the following people should undergo a treadmill exercise stress test?

a. An 18-year-old male who is trying out for the football team in his high school
b. A 35-year-old woman who is going to start training for a marathon
c. A 50-year-old, sedentary woman with type 2 diabetes mellitus
d. A 52-year-old, sedentary, male policeman
e. A 63-year-old woman with stable coronary heart disease

5. A 50-year-old woman has a blood pressure of 140/90 mm Hg. Which of the following will best help lower her blood pressure?

a. Increasing her consumption of vegetables and fruits
b. Decreasing her intake of sugar
c. Increasing her intake of fish
d. Decreasing her intake of coffee
e. Increasing her intake of foods containing plant sterols

6. A 62-year-old man with a history of alcohol abuse is brought to the emergency department by friends. He is talking about going to Russia to start a rock-and-roll band. He tries to walk to the bathroom but has trouble with his balance. Upon further examination, he has difficulty looking to either side with his eyes. What is the most likely nutrient deficiency?

a. Thiamine
b. Riboflavin
c. Niacin
d. Vitamin B_6 (pyridoxine)
e. Vitamin B_{12} (cobalamin)

7. To sell a dietary supplement, a manufacturer must do which of the following?

a. Prove efficacy
b. Prove safety
c. Provide quality control data on composition of the supplement
d. Submit an application to the Food and Drug Administration (FDA)
e. Follow Current Good Manufacturing Practices

Answers

1. Answer b.

According to National Health and Nutrition Examination Survey data, which is derived from representative samples of the US population, the prevalence of obesity has been increasing in all age, sex, and ethnic groups for the past few decades. However, since 1999, the prevalence of obesity has stabilized in women while continuing to increase in all other groups. This is the first sign of slowing of the obesity epidemic. Nevertheless, some ethnic groups and body mass index categories among women show a slight increase; it is difficult to determine whether this is a marked increase or continuation of the trend.

2. Answer b.

The criteria for metabolic syndrome in men are waist measurement >102 cm, blood pressure >130/85 mm Hg, HDL cholesterol <40 mg/dL, triglycerides >150 mg/dL, and fasting blood glucose >110 mg/dL. The patient's blood pressure (135/88 mm Hg) is the only parameter that qualifies as part of metabolic syndrome. Total and LDL cholesterol are not part of metabolic syndrome. For women, a waist measurement >88 cm and HDL cholesterol <50 mg/dL are part of metabolic syndrome.

3. Answer d.

More recent recommendations have included moderate-intensity physical activity and allowed people to break up the activity in multiple sessions during the day. The latest recommendations (2008) from the Department of Health and Human Services allows greater flexibility in exercise scheduling by recommending a total amount of moderate-intensity (150 minutes) or vigorous-intensity (75 minutes) physical activity per week. How people obtain this activity is up to them.

4. Answer d.

The policeman is involved in an occupation that involves public safety (and could be in a situation of increased physical exertion); therefore, a treadmill exercise test is recommended. The 18-year-old and 35-year-old have very low risk of heart disease, and testing is not recommended before starting an exercise program. If the 50-year-old was planning to start an exercise program, a treadmill exercise test is reasonable, but she is sedentary, and it therefore is not recommended. A routine exercise stress test is not recommended for anyone with stable coronary heart disease.

5. Answer a.

Vegetables and fruits are primary components of the Dietary Approaches to Stop Hypertension diet, which can lower blood pressure in people with and without hypertension. Sugar, fish, and plant sterols have no direct effect on blood pressure. Coffee and caffeine may increase blood pressure after consumption in people who do not regularly consume coffee, but tolerance develops (with regular consumption, it has little effect on blood pressure).

6. Answer a.

Thiamine deficiency can lead to wet beriberi (congestive heart failure), dry beriberi (various neurologic symptoms), or Wernicke-Korsakoff syndrome (psychosis, ophthalmoplegia, and ataxia). The patient's findings are consistent with Wernicke-Korsakoff syndrome. Riboflavin deficiency is associated with glossitis, angular stomatitis, cheilosis, seborrheic dermatitis, and burning eyes. Niacin deficiency results in pellagra (diarrhea, dementia, dermatitis, and glossitis). Vitamin B_6 deficiency is associated with glossitis, cheilosis, seborrheic dermatitis, microcytic anemia, and peripheral neuritis. Vitamin B_{12} deficiency can lead to weakness, megaloblastic anemia, smooth sore tongue, and neurologic dysfunction.

7. Answer e.

Since 2007, manufacturers have been required to follow Current Good Manufacturing Practices. According to the Dietary Supplement Health and Education Act of 1994, proof of efficacy is not required before selling a dietary supplement. Manufacturers are supposed to have data on the safety of dietary supplements but do not have to show proof (as is required for pharmaceutical drugs), nor do manufacturers have to prove composition of supplements. There have been many examples of dietary supplements that do not contain the amount of supplement that is listed. Manufacturers do not have to apply for approval from the FDA before selling a supplement.

10

SECONDARY PREVENTION 1: CANCERS AND PRINCIPLES OF SCREENING

Martha P. Millman, MD, MPH; Paul J. Limburg, MD

Principles of Screening

Evaluating Performance Characteristics and Effectiveness of Screening Tests

Screening tests are used to differentiate between persons with and without the condition of interest in a defined population. To interpret the results of a screening test or program, several key performance characteristics should be considered, including sensitivity, specificity, positive predictive value, negative predictive value, and number needed to screen (Table 1).

Terminology

Sensitivity refers to the proportion of people in the tested population with the condition of interest who were correctly identified by the test.

$$\text{Sensitivity} = \frac{\text{true positives}}{\text{true positives} + \text{false negatives}}$$

Specificity refers to the proportion of people in the tested population without the condition of interest who were correctly identified by the test.

$$\text{Specificity} = \frac{\text{true negatives}}{\text{true negatives} + \text{false positives}}$$

The **positive predictive value** indicates the probability of having the condition of interest, given that the screening test was positive. This number is predicated by the disease prevalence in the given population.

$$\text{Positive predictive value} = \frac{\text{true positives}}{\text{true positives} + \text{false positives}}$$

The **negative predictive value** indicates the probability of not having the condition of interest, given that the screening test was negative. This number is also predicated by the prevalence of the disease in the given population.

$$\text{Negative predictive value} = \frac{\text{true negatives}}{\text{true negatives} + \text{false negatives}}$$

Examples of the effect of disease prevalence are shown using 2×2 contingency tables in Tables 2 and 3.

The **number needed to screen** indicates the number of people that need to be evaluated to identify 1 person who has the condition of interest. This value incorporates the absolute risk reduction provided by the screening test (see Chapter 4 for details). This number is often used when assessing the utility and feasibility of a screening strategy.

$$\text{Number needed to screen} = \frac{1}{\text{absolute risk reduction}}$$

Levels of Prevention

The timing of screening or treatment (or both) during the natural progression of disease can be categorized as primary, secondary, or tertiary prevention. **Primary prevention** is defined as the prevention of disease occurrence

Table 1 2×2 Contingency Table

| | | Target Disorder | | |
		Disease Present	Disease Absent	
Diagnostic Test Results	Positive	True-positive a	False-positive b	a+b
	Negative	c False-negative	d True-negative	c+d
		a+c	b+d	a+b+c+d

$$\text{Prevalence} = \frac{a+c}{a+b+c+d}$$

Test characteristics

$$\text{Sensitivity} = \frac{a}{a+c}$$

$$\text{Specificity} = \frac{d}{b+d}$$

Frequency-dependent properties

$$\text{Positive predictive value} = \frac{a}{a+b}$$

$$\text{Negative predictive value} = \frac{d}{c+d}$$

Adapted from Litin SC, Mauck KF. General internal medicine. In: Ghosh AK, ed. Mayo Clinic internal medicine review. 8th ed. Rochester (MN): Mayo Clinic Scientific Press; c2008. p. 329. Used with permission of Mayo Foundation for Medical Education and Research.

through amelioration of risk factors. Examples include immunizations, adopting a healthy lifestyle, or removing a colon polyp during a screening colonoscopy. **Secondary prevention** is defined as the early detection and amelioration of disease at a preclinical or presymptomatic stage. Examples include statin therapy for asymptomatic coronary artery disease or cancer screening to detect early, asymptomatic disease. **Tertiary prevention** is defined as the prevention or reduction of future negative health effects through treatment of existing clinical disease. Examples include β-blocker therapy or aspirin therapy after a myocardial infarction to reduce the risk of a subsequent cardiac event.

Desirable Characteristics of Screening Strategies

A screening strategy optimally would have the disease, test, and host characteristics as described below. The **disease** should be common, cause substantial morbidity and mortality, have a long preclinical phase (during which the disease is curable or modifiable), and have an effective and acceptable treatment. The **test** should be inexpensive, safe, acceptable, easy to administer, technically easy to perform,

Table 2 2×2 Table for Test With 90% Sensitivity, 95% Specificity, and 10% Prevalence

| | | Target Disorder | | |
		Disease Present	Disease Absent	
Diagnostic Test Results	Positive	90 a	45 b	135 a+b
	Negative	c 10	d 855	c+d 865
		a+c 100	b+d 900	a+b+c+d 1,000

$$\text{Prevalence} = \frac{a+c}{a+b+c+d} = \frac{100}{1,000} = 10\%$$

Test characteristics

$$\text{Sensitivity} = \frac{a}{a+c} = \frac{90}{100} = 90\%$$

$$\text{Specificity} = \frac{d}{b+d} = \frac{855}{900} = 95\%$$

Frequency-dependent properties

$$\text{Positive predictive value} = \frac{a}{a+b} = \frac{90}{135} = 66.7\%$$

$$\text{Negative predictive value} = \frac{d}{c+d} = \frac{855}{865} = 98.8\%$$

Adapted from Litin SC, Mauck KF. General internal medicine. In: Ghosh AK, ed. Mayo Clinic internal medicine review. 8th ed. Rochester (MN): Mayo Clinic Scientific Press; c2008. p. 330. Used with permission of Mayo Foundation for Medical Education and Research.

highly sensitive, and have a highly specific confirmatory test. The **host** should be at risk for the disease, have access to the screening and treatment services, be likely to comply with confirmatory testing and treatment, and have a projected functional life expectancy to warrant screening and treatment.

Screening strategies include **mass screening**, which is applied relatively indiscriminately to a population, with the intention of improving the aggregate health of the population (not necessarily improving the health of each individual in the population). **Case finding** refers to screening that aims to detect asymptomatic disease in a given individual; screening is performed on the basis of the person's risk factors and is intended to improve the health of that person.

United States Preventive Services Task Force Guidelines for Screening

As with any screening test, the potential benefits of early detection should outweigh the possible harms that may be directly or indirectly related to the procedure and to

Table 3 2×2 Table for Test With 90% Sensitivity, 95% Specificity, and 2% Prevalence

		Target Disorder			
		Disease Present	Disease Absent		
Diagnostic Test Results	Positive	18 a	49 b	67 a+b	
	Negative	c 2	d 931	c+d 933	
		a+c 20	b+d 980	a+b+c+d 1,000	

$$\text{Prevalence} = \frac{a+c}{a+b+c+d} = \frac{20}{1,000} = 2\%$$

Test characteristics

$$\text{Sensitivity} = \frac{a}{a+c} = \frac{18}{20} = 90\%$$

$$\text{Specificity} = \frac{d}{b+d} = \frac{931}{980} = 95\%$$

Frequency-dependent properties

$$\text{Positive predictive value} = \frac{a}{a+b} = \frac{18}{67} = 26.9\%$$

$$\text{Negative predictive value} = \frac{d}{c+d} = \frac{931}{933} = 99.8\%$$

Adapted from Litin SC, Mauck KF. General internal medicine. In: Ghosh AK, ed. Mayo Clinic internal medicine review. 8th ed. Rochester (MN): Mayo Clinic Scientific Press; c2008. p. 331. Used with permission of Mayo Foundation for Medical Education and Research.

subsequent therapy (or both). Thus, the **appropriateness of screening in specific clinical settings** must be determined. It is important to remember that symptomatic patients should undergo diagnostic, rather than screening, evaluation.

The United States Preventive Services Task Force (USPSTF) is an independent panel of private-sector experts in primary care prevention that is sponsored by the Agency for Healthcare Research and Quality. The task force formulates **evidence-based guidelines** for screening, counseling, and chemoprevention as they pertain to disease prevention. The USPSTF grades their recommendations on the basis of the strength of evidence and magnitude of the benefit (benefits minus harms). USPSTF recommendation grades are described in Table 4. In addition to providing graded recommendations, the USPSTF grades the quality of the overall evidence for a service on a good-fair-poor scale (Table 5).

Biases in Screening

Lead-time bias reflects the period between early detection of occult disease by screening and the typical point during

Table 4 USPSTF Recommendation Grades

Grade	Explanation
A	The USPSTF recommends the service. There is high certainty that the net benefit is substantial.
B	The USPSTF recommends the service. There is high certainty that the net benefit is moderate or there is moderate certainty that the net benefit is moderate to substantial.
C	The USPSTF recommends against routinely providing the service. There may be considerations that support providing the service in an individual patient. There is at least moderate certainty that the net benefit is small.
D	The USPSTF recommends against the service. There is moderate or high certainty that the service has no net benefit or that the harms outweigh the benefits.
I statement	The USPSTF concludes that the current evidence is insufficient to assess the balance of benefits and harms of the service. Evidence is lacking, of poor quality, or conflicting, and the balance of benefits and harms cannot be determined.

Abbreviation: USPSTF, United States Preventive Services Task Force.
Adapted from U.S. Preventive Services Task Force Grade Definitions [Internet]; May 2008; [cited 18 Aug 2009]. Rockville (MD): Agency for Healthcare Research and Quality. Available from: http://www.ahrq.gov/clinic/uspstf/grades.htm.

the disease course at which diagnosis is made on the basis of clinical findings. The inclusion of this period may result in the apparent improved survival for patients who are screened and treated, but the offered treatment may have no benefit on disease duration or outcome.

Length-time bias results from the variable rates of disease progression. Slow progression in a subset of patients could make the disease easier to detect by screening. However, the patient group with more indolent disease may be overrepresented in screening and treatment studies.

Overdiagnosis bias implies improved survival due to the detection of disease by screening; however, the disease is not clinically significant in terms of symptoms or death. Disease detected at this early stage is considered a **pseudo-disease** because no clinical symptoms are apparent.

- Screening tests are used to differentiate between persons with and without the condition of interest within a defined population.
- Primary prevention is defined as the prevention of disease occurrence through amelioration of risk factors. Secondary prevention is defined as the early detection and amelioration of disease at a preclinical or presymptomatic stage. Tertiary prevention is defined as the prevention or reduction of future negative health effects through treatment of existing clinical disease.
- An optimal screening strategy tests for a treatable, common disease with a long preclinical phase.

Table 5 USPSTF Levels of Certainty Regarding Net Benefit

Level of Certainty	Description
High	The available evidence usually includes consistent results from well-designed, well-conducted studies in representative primary care populations. These studies assess the effects of the preventive service on health outcomes. This conclusion is therefore unlikely to be strongly affected by the results of future studies.
Moderate	The available evidence is sufficient to determine the effects of the preventive service on health outcomes, but confidence in the estimate is constrained by such factors as: • The number, size, or quality of individual studies • Inconsistency of findings across individual studies • Limited generalizability of findings to routine primary care practice • Lack of coherence in the chain of evidence As more information becomes available, the magnitude or direction of the observed effect could change, and this change may be large enough to alter the conclusion.
Low	The available evidence is insufficient to assess effects on health outcomes. Evidence is insufficient because of: • The limited number or size of studies • Important flaws in study design or methods • Inconsistency of findings across individual studies • Gaps in the chain of evidence • Findings not generalizable to routine primary care practice • Lack of information on important health outcomes More information may allow estimation of effects on health outcomes.

Abbreviation: USPSTF, United States Preventive Services Task Force.
Adapted from U.S. Preventive Services Task Force Grade Definitions [Internet]; May 2008; [cited 18 Aug 2009]. Rockville (MD): Agency for Healthcare Research and Quality. Available from: http://www.ahrq.gov/clinic/uspstf/grades.htm.

The screening test should be inexpensive, safe, easy to administer and perform, and be highly specific and sensitive. The host should be at risk for the disease, compliant with treatment, and have a sufficient life expectancy to warrant screening and treatment.
• The United States Preventive Services Task Force (USPSTF) formulates evidence-based guidelines for screening, counseling, and chemoprevention as they pertain to disease prevention.
• Biases in screening may improperly suggest prolonged survival because of screening (lead-time bias), inadvertently focus on more indolent disease (length-time bias), or increase the identification of patients with clinically nonsignificant disease (overdiagnosis bias).

Cancer

Although cancer is the second-leading overall cause of death in the United States, because of a reduction in heart disease deaths, cancer became the leading cause of death in 1998 for those younger than 85 years. Cancer death rates peaked in 1990-1991 but declined by 18.4% in men and 10.5% in women by 2004. The 5-year cancer survival rate for children increased from 58% in 1975 to 80% in 2003. The reduction in cancer deaths is attributed to a reduction in carcinogen exposure (lung cancer), early detection or prevention through treatment of premalignant lesions (cervical and colorectal cancer [CRC]), and more effective treatment (many cancers). The 10 leading types of cancer incidence and deaths in the United States are shown in Table 6. The trends in annual, age-adjusted incidence rates for the most common cancers since 1975 are shown in Figure 1. The trends in annual, age-adjusted death rates for select cancers since 1930 are shown in Figure 2.

Cancer risk is associated with **genetic and environmental risk factors**. In 2001, 37% of cancer deaths in high-income counties were attributed to lifestyle factors: 29% were associated with smoking, 3% with obesity, 3% with low intake of fruits and vegetables, and 2% with lack of physical activity. Compared with nonobese individuals, the risk of death from cancer is 52% higher in obese men and 62% higher in obese women. Obesity is associated with higher death rates for patients with endometrial, cervical, breast, kidney, or colon cancers and with multiple myeloma.

Racial disparities in cancer incidence and deaths persist in the United States. Compared with non-Hispanic whites, blacks have a higher incidence of colorectal, liver, lung, prostate, stomach, and cervical cancer. Similarly, mortality rates are higher for blacks with breast, colorectal, liver, lung, prostate, stomach, or cervical cancer. The incidence and mortality rates for liver, stomach, and cervical cancer are higher for Hispanics than for non-Hispanic whites.

Level of education also appears to affect cancer survival. In the United States, cancer-related death rates are higher for those with less than 12 years of education. In a review of lung, colorectal, prostate, and breast cancer deaths, a relative risk of 1.16 to 3.36 is noted for patients with less than 12 years' education. The disparity in deaths

Table 6 Ten Leading Cancer Types for the Estimated New Cancer Cases and Deaths, Stratified by Sex (United States, 2009).

Males			Females		
Cancer	No.	%	Cancer	No.	%
Estimated New Cases[a]					
Prostate	192,280	25	Breast	192,370	27
Lung and bronchus	116,090	15	Lung and bronchus	103,350	14
Colon and rectum	75,590	10	Colon and rectum	71,380	10
Urinary bladder	52,810	7	Uterine corpus	42,160	6
Melanoma of the skin	39,080	5	Non-Hodgkin lymphoma	29,990	4
Non-Hodgkin lymphoma	35,990	5	Melanoma of the skin	29,640	4
Kidney and renal pelvis	35,430	5	Thyroid	27,200	4
Leukemia	25,630	3	Kidney and renal pelvis	22,330	3
Oral cavity and pharynx	25,240	3	Ovary	21,550	3
Pancreas	21,050	3	Pancreas	21,420	3
All sites	766,130	100	All sites	713,220	100
Estimated Deaths					
Lung and bronchus	88,900	30	Lung and bronchus	70,490	26
Prostate	27,360	9	Breast	40,170	15
Colon and rectum	25,240	9	Colon and rectum	24,680	9
Pancreas	18,030	6	Pancreas	17,210	6
Leukemia	12,590	4	Ovary	14,600	5
Liver and intrahepatic bile duct	12,090	4	Non-Hodgkin lymphoma	9,670	4
Esophagus	11,490	4	Leukemia	9,280	3
Urinary bladder	10,180	3	Uterine corpus	7,780	3
Non-Hodgkin lymphoma	9,830	3	Liver and intrahepatic bile duct	6,070	2
Kidney and renal pelvis	8,160	3	Brain and other nervous system	5,590	2
All sites	292,540	100	All sites	269,800	100

[a] Excludes basal and squamous cell skin cancers and in situ carcinoma except urinary bladder. Estimates are rounded to the nearest 10.
Adapted from Jemal et al (2009). Used with permission.

from lung cancer and CRC (for men) between those with and without higher education is greater than the disparity between blacks and whites for the same cancers. This disparity has been attributed to risk exposure (smoking, obesity) and to limited access to or use of health care.

- Cancer risk is associated with genetic and environmental risk factors.
- Racial disparities in cancer incidence and deaths persist in the United States, with blacks and Hispanics having greater cancer incidence and death rates than whites.
- Lower levels of education are associated with decreased cancer survival.

Bladder Cancer

Bladder cancer is the fourth most common incident cancer, and it is the leading type of genitourinary tract cancer among men in the United States. Risk factors include age, tobacco exposure, and occupational exposures such as aryl amines (through work in the chemical industry, rubber manufacturing, and gas production). Fifty percent of patients with a diagnosis of bladder cancer have a history of smoking. The incidence is twice as high in whites compared with blacks and is 2.5 times more frequent in men than women.

Fortunately, more than 50% of bladder cancers are low grade and superficial at the time of diagnosis. However, bladder cancer tends to recur frequently and thus requires

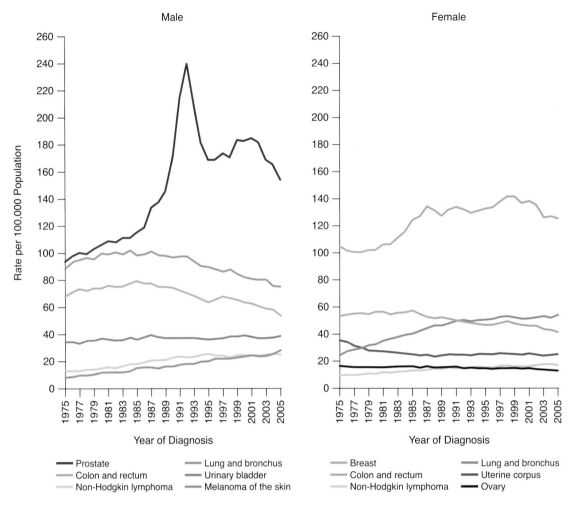

Figure 1 Annual Age-Adjusted Cancer Incidence Rates for Selected Cancers, Stratified by Sex (United States, 1975-2005).[a] Rates are age-adjusted to the 2000 US standard population and adjusted for delays in reporting. (Adapted from Jemal et al [2009]. Used with permission.)

periodic surveillance and retreatment. In contrast, high-grade bladder cancer has a poor prognosis. Although screening for **hematuria** could be considered (present for most patients with bladder cancer), the sensitivity and thus the positive predictive value of this approach at a population level is low. **Urine cytology** also has a low sensitivity (34%) for screening purposes. Limited data suggest that bladder cancer screening increases detection rates but does not appreciably change the clinical outcome. The lack of evidence that bladder cancer screening favorably affects morbidity or mortality, coupled with the low positive predictive value of existing tests, has led the USPSTF to recommend against screening of general or high-risk populations.

- Risk factors include age, tobacco exposure, and occupational exposures.
- Bladder cancer tends to recur frequently and thus requires periodic surveillance and retreatment.

Brain Cancer

Primary central nervous system malignancies are the second cause of cancer deaths in those younger than 20 years. Central nervous system malignancies are diverse and thus may be metastatic or primary tumors in adults. Currently, population screening is not recommended. However, diagnostic imaging of patients should be considered when they have a known cancer and a symptom suggestive of a central nervous system lesion.

- Central nervous system malignancies are diverse and thus may be metastatic or primary tumors in adults.

Breast Cancer

Breast cancer is the leading, nonskin cancer diagnosis among women, accounting for 27% of new cancer diagnoses annually in the United States. The incidence of breast

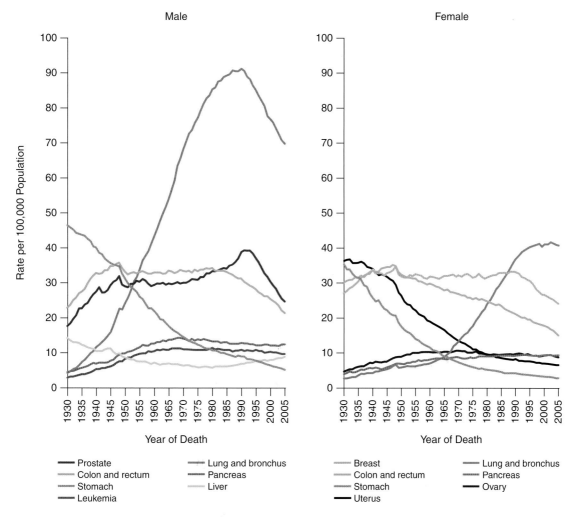

Figure 2 Annual Age-Adjusted Cancer Death Rates for Selected Cancers, Stratified by Sex (United States, 1930-2005). Rates are age-adjusted to the 2000 US standard population and adjusted for delays in reporting. Due to changes in diagnostic coding, numerator information has changed over time. Rates for cancers of the lung and bronchus (male and female), colon and rectum (male and female), liver (male), uterus (female), and ovary (female) are affected by these changes. The designation of uterus includes uterine cervix and uterine corpus. (Adapted from Jemal et al [2009]. Used with permission.)

cancer increases with age from 28 per 100,000 for women in their early 50s to 43 per 100,000 for women in their early 70s. Breast cancer is the second-leading cause of cancer death among US women, accounting for 15% of female cancer deaths annually. The cumulative lifetime risk of breast cancer is estimated to be 1 in 8 women. Breast cancer deaths declined from 32 per 100,000 in 1990 to 24 per 100,000 in 2004. The estimated 5-year breast cancer survival rate from the time of diagnosis is 89%. The decline in mortality rate is typically attributed to improved early detection and to advances in treatment.

Risk Factors

Risk factors include age, personal history of breast cancer or breast biopsy showing atypical hyperplasia (relative

risk, 3.7), personal history of ovarian or endometrial cancer, family history of breast or ovarian cancer, nulliparity or first pregnancy after age 30 (relative risk, 2.0), obesity (relative risk, up to 1.45). Although harder to quantify, radiotherapy of the chest wall during adolescence also appears to be associated with increased breast cancer risk.

A family history of breast cancer increases the relative risk; for those with only 1 first-degree relative who is affected, the relative risk is 1.8; if 2 first-degree relatives are affected, the relative risk is 2.9. This risk is lower if the affected relative was postmenopausal at the time of diagnosis and higher if the relative was premenopausal. A woman with a *BRCA1* or *BRCA2* gene mutation has a 50% to 85% lifetime risk of breast cancer.

Early menarche, late menopause, prolonged postmenopausal hormone therapy, and alcohol intake exceeding

2 drinks per day also have been associated with an increased breast cancer risk. Higher socioeconomic status has been correlated with twice the breast cancer risk. Breastfeeding, higher parity, normal weight, and physical exercise are correlated with a lower risk.

Detection

For average-risk women, early detection strategies typically include clinical breast examination and screening mammography. **Clinical breast examination** has a sensitivity of 54% and a specificity of 94%. Clinical breast examination is estimated to identify 5% of breast cancers not detected during screening mammography.

Mammography has a sensitivity of 75% to 95% for women aged 50 years or older. The sensitivity of mammography is lower for younger women and for women who take hormone replacement therapy or have denser breasts because of reduced ability to differentiate between abnormal lesions and normal surrounding tissues. The specificity of mammograms to detect breast cancer is 95% to 99% and the positive predictive value is 5% to 10%. Breast cancer is identified for 20% to 50% of women undergoing diagnostic breast biopsies; the diagnostic yield is higher for older women, who have additional risk because of age. Randomized controlled trials have shown a 20% to 30% decline in breast cancer deaths that is attributed to the use of screening mammography in women 50 years and older. Screening women in their 40s is potentially beneficial; the data show a decline in breast cancer deaths of 15% after 14 years of follow-up. Data on the impact of screening women older than age 70 are mixed in terms of all-cause mortality.

Magnetic resonance imaging (MRI) may be appropriate for populations with a lifetime breast cancer risk of 20% or higher. It has a sensitivity of 71% to 100% and specificity of 81% to 99%. However, its impact on breast cancer deaths has not yet been estimated because of a lack of long-term efficacy data.

Prophylaxis

Chemoprevention with **tamoxifen** may be acceptable for high-risk women and can reduce breast cancer risk by up to 50%. This intervention strategy must be weighed against the associated risks of tamoxifen therapy—specifically, the risks of venous thromboembolism, pulmonary emboli, stroke, endometrial cancer, and cataract progression should be considered.

Prophylactic mastectomy or bilateral oophorectomy could be considered for patients with a familial syndrome (ie, BRCA1 or BRCA2 mutation) or other extremely high-risk settings. In such situations, a mastectomy can reduce breast cancer risk by 90% and bilateral oophorectomy can reduce risk by 50%, particularly for younger women.

Cost-Effectiveness and Recommendations

According to a 1997 Markov model, the cost-effectiveness ratio for screening was estimated to be $105,000 per year of life saved for women in their 40s and $21,400 for women in their 50s and 60s. A USPSTF study showed a cost of $34,000 to $80,000 per year of life saved for women screened after age 65 years. This was considered cost-effective for women who had not been screened regularly in the past.

At present, clinical breast examination and annual screening mammography for women aged 50 to 69 years are generally recommended, even though screening and diagnostic procedures are also associated with anxiety and risks. **Radiation exposure** (4-5 mGy per 2-view bilateral mammogram) is estimated to increase the risk of breast cancer death to 80 additional cases per 1,000,000 women screened annually for 10 years, but 90,000 cases of breast cancer are expected to be diagnosed by mammography-directed screening in this population. Additional recommendations vary. The American Cancer Society (ACS) recommends screening with clinical breast examinations and mammography, starting at age 40. They also recommend annual MRI screening as an adjunct to mammography for women with known BRCA1 or BRCA2 mutations, women with 1 or more first-degree relatives with BRCA1 or BRCA2 mutations, women with a 20% or higher lifetime risk of breast cancer development, or women with a history of chest radiotherapy during adolescence. The ACS notes that evidence is insufficient to support MRI screening of women with dense breast parenchyma, a history of atypical ductal hyperplasia, lobular carcinoma in situ or atypical lobular hyperplasia on breast biopsy, or a history of breast cancer or ductal carcinoma in situ.

The USPSTF "recommends against teaching breast self-examination" (grade D recommendation). The USPSTF "recommends biennial screening mammography for women aged 50 to 74 years" (grade B recommendation). In November 2009, the USPSTF recommended that "the decision to start regular, biennial screening mammography before the age of 50 years should be an individual one and take patient context into account, including the patient's values regarding specific benefits and harms" (grade C recommendation). The USPSTF "concludes that the current evidence is insufficient to assess the additional benefits and harms of screening mammography in women 75 years or older" (grade I statement). The USPSTF "recommends that women whose family history is associated with an increased risk for deleterious mutations in BRCA1 or BRCA2 genes be referred for genetic counseling and evaluation for BRCA testing" (grade B recommendation). Furthermore, the USPSTF "recommends against routine use of tamoxifen or raloxifene for the primary prevention of breast cancer in women at low or average risk for breast cancer" (grade D recommendation). However, the USPSTF also "recommends that clinicians discuss chemoprevention with women at high risk for breast cancer and at low risk for adverse effects of chemoprevention" (grade B recommendation).

- The cumulative lifetime risk of breast cancer is estimated to be 1 in 8 women.
- A woman with a *BRCA1* or *BRCA2* gene mutation has a 50% to 85% lifetime risk of breast cancer.
- Early detection strategies typically include clinical breast examination and screening mammography.
- Prophylaxis with tamoxifen, mastectomy, or oophorectomy may be considered for women with extremely high risk.

Cervical Cancer

Cervical cancer incidence and mortality rates have declined with the 1941 introduction of routine cytologic evaluation (Papanicolaou test). Cervical cancer has a **long preclinical phase**—progression from dysplasia to invasive cancer may take up to 10 or 15 years. Cervical cancer is strongly associated with human papillomavirus (HPV) infection, particularly strains HPV 16 and HPV 18. Other risk factors include age, early onset of sexual activity, multiple sexual partners, a history of sexually transmitted disease, smoking, human immunodeficiency virus infection, or immunosuppression. The Papanicolaou test has a sensitivity of 55% to 80% and a specificity of 80% to 90%. Liquid-based cytologic assays have a sensitivity that is 12% to 17% higher than the traditional Papanicolaou test.

Although no randomized controlled trials have evaluated the effectiveness of screening with Papanicolaou tests, case-control and observational studies support its use (Table 7). The USPSTF "strongly recommends screening for cervical cancer in women who have been sexually active and have a cervix" (grade A recommendation).

Table 7 Estimated Reduction in Invasive Cervical Cancer After Papanicolaou Test Screening

Frequency of Screening	Reduction in Invasive Cancer
Every 10 y	64%
Every 5 y	84%
Every 3 y	91%
Every 2 y	92.5%
Every 1 y	93%

Adapted from IARC Working Group On Evaluation Of Cervical Cancer Screening Programmes. Screening for squamous cervical cancer: duration of low risk after negative results of cervical cytology and its implication for screening policies. Br Med J (Clin Res Ed). 1986 Sep 13;293(6548):659-64. Used with permission.

Screening should begin within 3 years of the onset of sexual activity or age 21 (whichever comes first) and should be repeated at least every 3 years until age 65. The USPSTF "concludes that the evidence is insufficient to recommend for or against routine use of new technologies to screen for cervical cancer" (grade I statement). New technologies were defined as "liquid-based cytology, computerized re-screening, or algorithm-based screening." Although HPV testing is often used to stratify risk when a Papanicolaou smear shows abnormal findings, the USPSTF "concludes that the evidence is insufficient to recommend for or against the routine use of human papillomavirus (HPV) testing as a primary screening test for cervical cancer" (grade I statement).

The ACS recommends that cervical cancer screening start 3 years after the onset of sexual activity but no later than age 21. Also, they recommend annual screening with a conventional Papanicolaou test or every 2 years if the liquid-based cytologic assay is used. Less frequent testing (every 2-3 years) is acceptable after age 30 for women with previous negative screening results and low risk factors. The recommendation suggests offering women the option to discontinue screening after age 70 years if 3 Papanicolaou tests within the previous 10 years had negative findings.

Because most cervical cancers are associated with HPV infection, a vaccine that is effective against the 4 most common HPV strains has been developed. By decreasing the risk of HPV infection, the risk of cervical, vaginal, and vulvar cancer development is thus reduced.

- Progression from dysplasia to invasive cancer may take up to 10 or 15 years.
- Screening should begin within 3 years of the onset of sexual activity or age 21 (whichever comes first) and should be repeated at least every 3 years until age 65.
- A vaccine that is effective against the 4 most common human papillomavirus (HPV) strains has been developed.

Colorectal Cancer

CRC is the second-leading cause of cancer death in the United States for men and women per aggregate statistics (it is the third-leading cause for each group when the data for men and women are evaluated separately). CRC ranks third in cancer incidence for both men and women and ranks fourth in aggregate analysis. Specifically, it accounts for 9% of cancer deaths and 10% of incident cancers. CRC mortality rates have declined from 31 to 22 per 100,000 men and from 20 to 15 per 100,000 women between 1990 and 2004. Ninety percent of CRC cases develop in persons 50 years or older. Survival is inversely associated with presentation stage, and the 5-year survival rate among patients with localized CRC is 90%.

Risk Factors

Major risk factors include age, personal history of 1 or more colorectal adenomas, inflammatory bowel disease (ulcerative colitis or Crohn disease), and heritable syndromes such as familial adenomatous polyposis (FAP) or Lynch syndrome (ie, hereditary nonpolyposis colorectal cancer [HNPCC]). Lynch syndrome is the most common heritable syndrome associated with increased CRC risk and can be diagnosed clinically on the basis of the Amsterdam II criteria: 1) at least 3 family members affected with cancer of the colorectum, endometrium, small bowel, ureter, or renal pelvis; 2) at least 1 affected family member is a first-degree relative of 2 other affected family members; 3) affected family members are from at least 2 successive generations; and 4) at least 1 affected family member was diagnosed at age younger than 50 years. Even in the absence of an identifiable syndrome, a family history of CRC with 1 or 2 first-degree relatives affected is associated with an approximately 2-to-3–fold or 3-to-4–fold increase in CRC risk, respectively. CRC among 2 or more second-degree relatives raises the personal risk by about 2-to-3–fold as well.

Most CRCs are thought to develop from **adenomatous polyps**. The risk of a polyp containing a malignant focus is associated with histologic characteristics and size. Polyps are defined as "advanced" and have higher risk of disease if they have high-grade dysplasia, villous or tubulovillous morphology, are at least 10 mm in diameter, or show some combination of these features. The presence of multiple adenomas (≥3) also increases CRC risk.

Detection

The average time from normal mucosa to invasive cancer is estimated to be 10 to 20 years. Effective screening tests can identify and remove adenomas and thereby truly prevent subsequent malignancy. Multiple test options have been endorsed for CRC screening among average-risk adults (ie, those with no known risk factors other than age). These tests include a sensitive guaiac-based or immunochemical fecal occult blood test (FOBT) every year, flexible sigmoidoscopy every 5 years, or colonoscopy every 10 years starting at age 50.

The ACS, US Multisociety Task Force on Colorectal Cancer, and the American College of Radiology have also endorsed double-contrast barium enema every 5 years, computed tomography (CT) colonography every 5 years, or stool DNA testing, the latter at an uncertain time interval. However, only the FOBT has been shown to reduce CRC mortality rates (by 15%-33%) in randomized, controlled trials. Appropriate FOBT performance requires serial sampling from up to 3 consecutive stool samples (testing a single sample obtained after in-office digital rectal examination is inadequate). Flexible sigmoidoscopy is up to 90% sensitive for the area of colon visualized, which is approximately 60 cm of the most distal portion of the colon and rectum. Double-contrast barium enema is 48% to 75% sensitive for detecting colon polyps, although few studies have evaluated the impact of this screening method on CRC incidence or mortality rates.

Colonoscopy permits a full structural evaluation and simultaneously provides the opportunity to perform a polypectomy if needed. However, controlled studies have demonstrated colonoscopy false-negative rates ("miss rates") of approximately 5% for CRCs and 6% to 12% for advanced adenomas. CT colonography is emerging as another viable option for primary CRC screening, with sensitivity and specificity estimates of 90% and 86%, respectively, for large (>1 cm) lesions. Unexpected, extracolonic findings that require additional diagnostic evaluation may be detected in about 6% of patients who undergo screening by CT colonography.

Recommendations

Individuals with documented or suspected FAP should begin screening at age 10 to 12 years. Screening of HPNCC kindreds should begin at age 20 to 25 years or 10 years younger than the earliest colon cancer diagnosis in the family, whichever occurs first. Genetic counseling with the option of targeted genetic testing should be offered to patients with a family history suggestive of a heritable syndrome. Persons with a strong family history of CRC but no identifiable syndrome should begin screening by age 40 years or 10 years younger than the earliest diagnosis in the family, whichever occurs first. Patients with chronic inflammatory bowel disease should begin colonoscopy screening after 8 to 10 years of disease. Any abnormal CRC screening result should prompt performance of a diagnostic colonoscopy. Patients with confirmed adenoma or adenocarcinoma are at increased risk for recurrent neoplasia and should undergo routine surveillance (Box).

An algorithm for CRC screening is shown in Figure 3. With the exception of FOBT, each CRC screening test carries a small but real risk of procedure-related complications. Colonoscopy has the highest direct risk, with death or hospitalization in up to 2.5% of patients. Given that potential harms might outweigh benefits for some population subgroups, the USPSTF recommends discontinuing screening after age 85 years, with a case-by-case CRC screening approach advised for patients aged 76 to 85 years.

- Survival of colorectal cancer (CRC) is inversely associated with presentation stage, and the 5-year survival rate among patients with localized CRC is 90%.
- Effective screening tests can identify and remove adenomas and thereby truly prevent subsequent malignancy.

Box Surveillance Recommendations for Colorectal Cancer

1. Patients with small, hyperplastic, rectal polyps should be considered normal, and the subsequent colonoscopy should be in 10 y; however, patients with a hyperplastic polyposis syndrome have increased risk of adenomas and colorectal cancer and need to have more frequent follow-up evaluation

2. Patients with only 1 or 2 small (<1 cm) tubular adenomas with only low-grade dysplasia should have their next follow-up colonoscopy in 5-10 y; the precise timing within this interval should consider other clinical factors such as prior colonoscopy findings, family history, and the preferences of the patient and physician

3. Patients with 3-10 adenomas, at least 1 adenoma ≥1 cm or with villous features, or high-grade dysplasia should have their next follow-up colonoscopy in 3 y if the adenoma(s) were removed completely and without morcellation; if the follow-up colonoscopy is normal or shows only 1 or 2 small tubular adenomas with low-grade dysplasia, the interval until the next examination should be 5 y

4. Patients who have 10 adenomas identified during 1 colonoscopy should be examined frequently (<3 y between examinations), as established by clinical judgment; the clinician should consider the possibility of an underlying familial syndrome

5. Patients with sessile adenomas that are removed piecemeal should be considered for follow-up evaluation at short intervals (2-6 mo) to verify complete removal; after complete removal is established, subsequent surveillance needs to be individualized on the basis of the endoscopist's judgment; completeness of removal should be assessed by endoscopic and pathologic findings

6. More intensive surveillance is indicated when the family history is suggestive of hereditary nonpolyposis cancer syndrome

Adapted from Winawer SJ, Zauber AG, Fletcher RH, Stillman JS, O'Brien MJ, Levin B, et al. Guidelines for colonoscopy surveillance after polypectomy: a consensus update by the US Multi-Society Task Force on Colorectal Cancer and the American Cancer Society. Gastroenterology. 2006 May;130(6):1872-85. Used with permission.

• Only the fecal occult blood test (FOBT) has been shown to reduce CRC mortality rates (by 15%-33%) in randomized, controlled trials.
• Genetic counseling with the option of targeted genetic testing should be offered to patients with a family history suggestive of a heritable syndrome.

Endometrial Cancer

Endometrial cancer is the most common gynecologic cancer diagnosed in the United States, accounting for 6% of cancers in women. The incidence is higher in white women, but the mortality rate in blacks is nearly twice that of whites (7.1 vs 3.9 per 100,000). This difference has been attributed to disparities in health care and the aggressive nature of certain subtypes of endometrial cancer. Although endometrial cancer can develop in younger women, the average age at diagnosis is the early 60s.

Obesity is associated with increased incidence and mortality rates for premenopausal and postmenopausal women who have endometrial cancer. The relative risk of an endometrial cancer death is 6.25 times higher in women with a body mass index exceeding 40 kg/m^2 compared with those of normal weight. Women with a family history of HNPCC also have a markedly increased risk for endometrial cancer (40%-60% lifetime risk).

Endometrial cancers basically are categorized as 1 of 2 subtypes, distinguished by the response to estrogen stimulation. Type I (80% of endometrial cancers) is estrogen related and tends to be of low-grade malignancy. This endometrioid form is associated with endometrial hyperplasia. Risk factors include estrogen exposure without the protection of progestin. This typically occurs in a postmenopausal woman with an intact uterus who takes systemic estrogen replacement but not progesterone. Additional risk factors include anovulatory menstrual cycles (for premenopausal women), diabetes mellitus, or exposure to estrogen-like hormones such as tamoxifen. Type II (20% of endometrial cancers) is not associated with estrogen stimulation. This tumor type is often a high-grade malignancy and includes papillary-serous and clear-cell subtypes.

Endometrial cancer screening is not recommended for the asymptomatic, average-risk woman. The ACS recommends annual endometrial biopsy, starting at age 35, for women with known or suspected HNPCC, but this recommendation is not supported by the USPSTF. About 90% of endometrial cancers cause abnormal uterine bleeding. Thus, appropriate diagnostic evaluation of dysfunctional uterine bleeding is highly recommended, particularly if additional risk factors are present (eg, risk factors described above or personal or family history of ovarian, breast, colon, or endometrial cancer). For most patients (70%), early diagnostic evaluation results in a diagnosis of stage I endometrial cancer. Surgery is often curative for early stage disease. The 5-year survival rate is 95% for women with localized, treated endometrial cancer.

• Although endometrial cancer can develop in younger women, the average age at diagnosis is the early 60s.
• Endometrial cancer screening is not recommended for the asymptomatic, average-risk woman.

Gastric Cancer

Screening for gastric cancer currently is not recommended in countries such as the United States, where the population risk is low. However, the incidence and death rates are 2 times higher for Pacific Islanders and Asian Americans compared with those of European descent. Mass screening programs are currently conducted in Japan, Chile, and

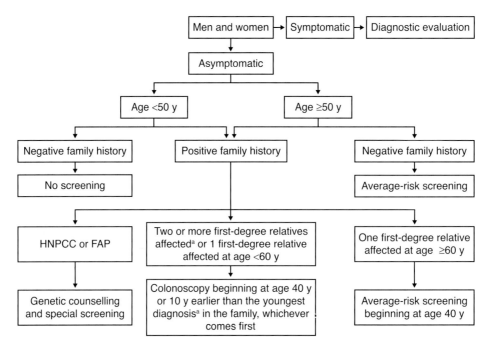

Figure 3 Algorithm for Colorectal Cancer Screening. FAP indicates familial adenomatous polyposis; HNPCC, hereditary nonpolyposis colorectal cancer. [a]Either colorectal cancer or adenomatous polyp. (Adapted from Winawer et al [2003]. Used with permission.)

Venezuela, where the incidence of gastric cancer is high. The overall effectiveness of screening programs on gastric cancer mortality rates is supported by some but not all studies; possibly, lead-time, length-time, and selection biases affect data interpretation. Cost-effectiveness of gastric cancer screening was evident in a Chinese population, for whom the incidence of gastric cancer was 25 per 100,000.

Chronic **Helicobacter pylori** infection has been associated with increased risk of gastric cancer and gastric mucosa-associated-lymphoid-tissue lymphoma of the stomach. *H pylori* eradication is associated with a decrease in precursor lesions of gastric cancer. The risk of gastric cancer developing in persons with *H pylori* and precursor lesions, atrophic gastritis, pernicious anemia, or a history of partial gastrectomy is 5 to 61 times greater than that of the general population. Additional risk factors associated with an increased incidence of gastric cancer include a diet high in salted fish or meat, pickled vegetables, and smoked foods. Thus, periodic surveillance could be advocated for select patients with 1 or more gastric cancer risk factors.

- Screening for gastric cancer currently is not recommended in countries such as the United States, where the population risk is low.
- *Helicobacter pylori* eradication is associated with a decrease in precursor lesions of gastric cancer.

Leukemia

Leukemia is the leading fatal malignancy for persons younger than 20 years. Fortunately, improved treatment regimens have increased the 5-year survival rate for acute lymphocytic leukemia (from 58% to 88%) and for acute myeloid leukemia (from 19% to 55%) from 1975 to 2004. Although leukemia incidence and mortality rates drop considerably in the adult population, acute myelogenous leukemia and chronic lymphocytic leukemia are more common in adults. Risk factors in the adult population include exposure to radiation, previous chemotherapy, benzene exposure, or a history of myelodysplastic or myeloproliferative syndromes. Population screening of the asymptomatic population currently is not recommended.

- Leukemia is the leading fatal malignancy for persons younger than 20 years.
- Acute myelogenous leukemia and chronic lymphocytic leukemia are more common in adults.

Liver Cancer

Primary liver cancer is the fifth-leading cause of cancer deaths worldwide, with 85% to 90% of these cases arising from hepatocytes. In the United States, hepatocellular and intrahepatic bile duct cancers together account for 2% of annual cancer deaths for women and 4% for men. Incidence and death rates are 2 times higher in Asian Americans and Pacific Islanders. Established risk factors for liver cancer include chronic infection with hepatitis B virus or hepatitis C virus, hemochromatosis, cirrhosis, and aflatoxin exposure.

Although definitive evidence is lacking, annual surveillance with serum α-fetoprotein level and liver ultrasonography is often used for hepatocellular cancer screening of high-risk populations. General population screening currently is not endorsed. Primary prevention strategies include immunization and education to reduce viral hepatitis transmission rates. Encouragingly, in global regions where such strategies have been widely implemented, an appreciable decline in liver cancer has been observed.

- Annual surveillance with serum α-fetoprotein level and liver ultrasonography is often used for hepatocellular cancer screening of high-risk populations.
- Primary prevention strategies include immunization and education to reduce viral hepatitis transmission rates.

Lymphoma

Non-Hodgkin lymphoma ranks fifth and sixth in terms of cancer incidence among US women and men, respectively. High-grade, non-Hodgkin lymphomas have a higher potential for cure than low-grade lymphomas, but the survival rate is lower if remission is not achieved. Paradoxically, low-grade non-Hodgkin lymphomas typically remain indolent but are not curable; they are associated with an average survival of 8 years.

Incidence rates of Hodgkin lymphoma have a bimodal distribution, with peak incidence at 25 and 60 years. The 5-year survival rate is greater than 80%. Major risk factors for lymphoma remain poorly understood, and population screening currently is not recommended.

- Major risk factors for lymphoma remain poorly understood.
- Population screening currently is not recommended.

Lung Cancer

Lung cancer has the second-highest incidence rate and the highest mortality rate among men and women in the United States. The incidence and mortality rates of lung cancer for men rose steadily from the 1930s, peaked during the late 1980s, and has declined since. The incidence and mortality rates of lung cancer for women have risen steadily since the 1960s but have plateaued since the late 1990s. Established risk factors include age, smoking, and environmental or occupational exposures (radon, asbestos, hydrocarbons, beryllium, chromium, methyl ethyl ether, nickel, arsenic, vinyl chloride, uranium). Lung cancer risk is 10 to 25 times greater for smokers than nonsmokers, and 90% of all lung cancer cases are attributable to smoking.

Approximately 75% of lung cancers have regional or distant metastases at the time of diagnosis. Thus, the 5-year survival rate for all lung cancers is less than 15%. Screening strategies of periodic chest radiography and sputum analysis did not show a reduction in mortality rates in the Mayo Lung Project, despite the detection of lung cancers in the screened population during more than 20 years of follow-up. However, many of the control subjects also had interval chest radiographs; this crossover of subjects could have lessened the potential difference between the groups.

A strategy of periodic chest CT scans in people with a clinically significant history of smoking has shown mixed results. The International Early Lung Cancer Action Program, an observational cohort study, published a report in 2006 showing that annual CT scans in asymptomatic, at-risk patients could identify lung cancers. Seventy-seven percent of those diagnosed had stage I cancer (surgically staged); they were projected to have a 10-year, lung cancer–specific survival rate of 88% after resection. In contrast, no decline in population-expected lung cancer deaths was observed in a prospective, observational, 3-center study of CT screening (published in 2007). Lung cancer was diagnosed 3 times more frequently than the expected rate of diagnosis when annual chest CT scans were performed in an at-risk population. This screening protocol resulted in 10 times the number of population-expected lung resections. Of the cancers diagnosed during annual surveillance, 61% were stage I and 33% were stage III or IV. The follow-up period averaged 4 years. The lack of apparent decline in lung cancer deaths, despite scheduled screening, has been attributed to lead-time, length-time, and overdiagnosis screening biases.

Additional randomized controlled trials are in process to evaluate the benefit and risks of CT screening. Other strategies under investigation include combined CT scan and positron emission tomographic evaluation of indeterminate pulmonary nodules for high-risk individuals. Because indeterminate pulmonary nodules identified during screening CT scans have a prevalence rate exceeding 50%, periodic surveillance and perhaps invasive diagnostic procedures are often pursued. The potential risks and patient anxiety associated with this screening strategy must be considered. A 2003 study estimated that the cost-effectiveness of lung cancer CT screening, in US dollars per quality-adjusted life-year, ranged from $116,300 in smokers to $2,322,700 in former smokers.

Smoking is the leading cause of preventable cancer in the United States. Physician advice to quit smoking, prescription of medication to facilitate quitting, and referral to smoking cessation programs are cost-effective strategies to reduce smoking and associated cancer risk. A former smoker is estimated to accrue a 20% to 90% reduction in lung cancer risk over time. Population-based strategies, including cigarette tax and restriction of smoking in public places, have clearly reduced the population smoking rate.

- Ninety percent of all lung cancer cases are attributable to smoking.
- No screening strategy to date has been associated with clearly reduced lung cancer mortality rates.
- Physician advice to quit smoking, prescription of medication to facilitate quitting, and referral to smoking cessation programs are cost-effective strategies to reduce smoking and associated cancer risk.

Oral Cancer

Oral cancers account for 3% of cancers diagnosed in men annually. Risk factors include tobacco and alcohol use. Screening for oral cancer is not recommended by the USPSTF. Data from small randomized controlled trials studying the impact of treatment of oral leukoplakia, considered a premalignant lesion, indicate increased remission rates, but a reduction in mortality rates has not been observed. However the number of relevant randomized controlled trials, size of the populations studied, and duration of follow-up have been limited.

The 2000 Kerala Trial, a cluster-randomized, controlled-setting study is an ongoing investigation of the impact of screening examinations at 3-year intervals. At the completion of the first screening cycle, the case-fatality rates were 14.9% in the intervention group and 56.3% in the control group. However, after completing 2 rounds of screening, no significant differences in the oral cancer rates were observed.

- Screening for oral cancer is not recommended by the United States Preventive Services Task Force (USPSTF).

Ovarian Cancer

Ovarian cancer is the fifth-leading cause of cancer death in women and the leading cause of gynecologic cancer death. Unfortunately, 68% of ovarian cancers are diagnosed at a relatively late stage. Five-year survival rates are 90% for stage I disease, 80% for regional disease, and 25% for metastatic disease. Risk factors for ovarian cancer include early menarche, late menopause, nulliparity, age, and family history.

A woman's lifetime risk can increase up to 5% with a family history of ovarian cancer, up to 25% with a BRCA2 mutation, and up to 50% with a BRCA1 mutation. Familial ovarian cancer syndromes are associated with 5% to 10% of ovarian cancer cases. Greater than 10 years of postmenopausal hormone replacement therapy was associated with an increased risk of ovarian cancer (hazard ratio, 1.58) in the Women's Health Initiative Trial. The use of oral contraceptives is associated with a reduction in ovarian cancer risk (up to 40%). Currently, routine ovarian cancer screening is not recommended by the USPSTF.

Bimanual pelvic examination is insensitive for ovarian cancer screening. The **cancer antigen CA 125** has a sensitivity of 70% to 80% for detecting preclinical disease, but it has a positive predictive value of 3% in the average-risk population. Testing strategies using serial measurements or measurement in conjunction with other tumor markers show promise in preliminary trials. The positive predictive value of pelvic transvaginal ultrasound in identifying early stage ovarian cancer in the average-risk population is 3%. Studies of a screening strategy that uses pelvic ultrasonography to evaluate women with elevated CA 125 levels have reported positive predictive values ranging from 3% to 20%. Several large population screening trials are in process.

The dilemma of false-positive results leading to invasive procedures remains. The report of surgical exploration in 3 to 4 women for every case of ovarian cancer detected is noted. The cost-effectiveness of a multimodal screening strategy, based on initial CA 125 screening results, was estimated at $100,000 per year of life saved in 1997. The apparent limited screening benefit for women with high risk of ovarian cancer has prompted some to advocate prophylactic oophorectomy at the completion of childbearing or by age 35 for those with greatest risk.

- Sixty-eight percent of ovarian cancers are diagnosed at a relatively late stage.
- Familial ovarian cancer syndromes are associated with 5% to 10% of ovarian cancer cases.
- Because of false-positive screening results, up to 4 women undergo surgical exploration for every case of ovarian cancer detected. Thus, routine ovarian cancer screening currently is not recommended by the USPSTF.

Pancreatic Cancer

Pancreatic cancer is the fourth-leading cause of cancer death in the United States. Unfortunately, 52% of patients with pancreatic cancer present with advanced-stage disease; for these patients, the 5-year survival rate is approximately 2%. For localized disease, the 5-year survival rate is only slightly better (20%). Risk factors for pancreatic cancer include age, smoking, obesity, diabetes mellitus, cystic fibrosis, chronic or hereditary pancreatitis, and family history of pancreatic cancer or other heritable syndromes (atypical multiple mole melanoma, Peutz-Jeghers syndrome, BRCA1 or BRCA2 mutations, FAP, and HNPCC).

Although the tumor marker CA 19-9 may be elevated in patients with known pancreatic cancer, the positive predictive value of this marker was less than 1% in an asymptomatic population and 71% in a symptomatic population (in which 49% were shown to have pancreatic cancer). Thus, screening of asymptomatic individuals currently is not recommended. Periodic screening of patients with very high risk of pancreatic cancer, in conjunction with appropriately targeted testing for genetic markers that confer risk, can be considered on the basis of consensus statement recommendations, but this has not been supported by data from clinical trials.

- Fifty-two percent of patients with pancreatic cancer present with advanced-stage disease.
- Screening of asymptomatic individuals currently is not recommended.

Prostate Cancer

Prostate cancer is the second-leading cancer diagnosis in men (the first is nonmelanoma skin cancer), accounting for 25% of new male cancer diagnoses annually. Prostate cancer is also the second-leading cause of cancer death in men, accounting for 9% of male cancer deaths annually in the United States. The decline in mortality rate, from 38 to 25 per 100,000 between 1990 and 2005, has been associated with earlier diagnosis and more effective treatment. The incidence of diagnosed prostate cancer peaked in 1992, attributed to the use of prostate-specific antigen (PSA) testing beginning in 1987, and then declined to a plateau above the 1985 level. Prostate cancer is estimated to affect 1 in 6 men, but only 1 of 34 (3%) of US men will die of the disease. The 5-year survival rate is 32% for men with distant metastasis at the time of diagnosis, but it approaches 100% for men with localized cancer at the time of diagnosis (91% have local disease at diagnosis). Seventy percent of new prostate cancer diagnoses are for men older than age 65, and 71% of prostate cancer deaths occur in men older than age 75.

Risk factors include age, family history (prostate cancer, *BRCA1* or *BRCA2* germline mutation in a first-degree relative), and African American heritage. Blacks have almost twice the risk of prostate cancer compared with whites, who have almost twice the risk compared with Asian Americans and Pacific Islanders. Blacks also have more than twice the prostate cancer mortality rate of whites, and they typically have an earlier age of onset and more advanced disease at diagnosis. A family history of prostate, breast, or ovarian cancer in a first-degree relative doubles the risk of prostate cancer. Forty-two percent of prostate cancers diagnosed before age 55 are thought to be due to genetic predisposition.

Screening for prostate cancer is a subject of debate. A review of autopsy findings identified a prostate cancer prevalence rate of up to 46% for men in their 50s, up to 70% for men in their 60s, and up to 83% for men in their 70s (all died of other causes). The sensitivity of a PSA test (PSA >4 ng/mL) ranges from 56% to 91% and the specificity is 91%. Other causes of elevated PSA include prostatic hypertrophy and prostatitis. Conversely, the use of 5-α-reductase inhibitors (finasteride and dutasteride) can lower the PSA value by up to 50%. The positive predictive value of a PSA test (PSA >4 ng/mL) is 30%. Use of PSA velocity

(measuring change in PSA over time), PSA doubling time, or the ratio of free PSA to total PSA may improve screening accuracy, but further data on the efficacy of these tests is needed. A digital rectal examination has a sensitivity of approximately 59% and a specificity of 94% for prostate nodule detection. The positive predictive value ranges from 5% to 30%. This examination technique limits evaluation to the posterior lateral aspects of the prostate.

Results from population-based, randomized controlled trials are conflicting about the effect of early detection and treatment on survival. Thus, recommendations for screening also vary. Aggressive screening for prostate cancer will uncover many new cases and result in many additional treatments. However, screening may have minimal effect on decreasing the number of prostate cancer deaths because the disease in many cases is slow to progress. The risks of prostate cancer treatment include those associated with surgery or radiotherapy, posttreatment risk of urinary incontinence, and risk of erectile dysfunction. After radiotherapy, patients have the risk of late radiation cystitis or proctitis.

The ACS recommends that a digital rectal examination and a PSA test be offered annually to men older than 50 years who have a life expectancy of at least 10 years. Prostate cancer screening can begin for men in their 40s if risk factors are present (prostate cancer in a first-degree relative, patient is black).

The USPSTF "concludes that the current evidence is insufficient to assess the balance of benefits and harms of prostate cancer screening in men younger than age 75 years" (grade I statement). The USPSTF also "recommends against screening for prostate cancer in men age 75 or older" (grade D recommendation) and recommends against screening men with an estimated life expectancy less than 10 years. Prostate cancer screening should be performed after describing to the patient the potential benefits and harms of screening and treatment of asymptomatic disease.

- Prostate cancer is estimated to affect 1 in 6 men, but only 1 of 34 (3%) of US men will die of the disease.
- Screening may have minimal effect on decreasing the number of prostate cancer deaths because the disease in many cases is slow to progress.
- Prostate cancer screening should be performed after describing to the patient the potential benefits and harms of screening and treatment of asymptomatic disease.

Renal Cancer

Renal cancer accounts for 3% to 5% of the annual cancer incidence rate in US women and men, respectively. Of primary renal cancers, 80% to 85% are renal cell carcinomas. Risk factors include age, male sex, smoking, obesity, occupational exposure (cadmium, asbestos, and gasoline), and acquired polycystic kidney disease for patients undergoing long-term dialysis. American Indians and Alaskan Natives have a higher mortality rate from renal cancer. Because of the low prevalence of this cancer and the low positive predictive value of screening tests, screening of the asymptomatic general population is not recommended.

- The low prevalence of renal cancer and low positive predictive value of screening tests preclude screening of asymptomatic individuals.

Skin Cancer

Basal and squamous cell carcinomas are the most common malignancy in the United States. Fortunately, early treatment is curative for at least 90% of cases. **Melanoma** accounts for 4% to 5% of the annual cancer incidence rate. The estimated 5-year survival rate has increased from 40% in the 1940s. Currently, the 5-year survival is highly correlated with the thickness of the tumor; it ranges from above 95% for patients with tumors thinner than 1 mm to 67% for patients with tumors thicker than 4 mm. Risk factors for melanoma include sun exposure, human immunodeficiency virus infection, immunosuppression, multiple nevi, or a personal or family history of atypical nevi or melanoma.

Wearing sun-protective clothing, applying sunscreen (sun protection factor of 30 or higher and with UVA protection), and limiting sun exposure are highly recommended methods of primary prevention. The USPSTF "concludes that the current evidence is insufficient to assess the balance of benefits and harms of using a whole-body skin examination by a primary care clinician or patient skin self-examination for the early detection of cutaneous melanoma, basal cell cancer, or squamous cell skin cancer in the adult general population" (grade I statement). However, noting risk factors associated with the development of skin cancer, education about strategies to reduce risk, and diagnostic evaluation of atypical skin lesions (lesions that are asymmetric or have irregular borders, variation in color, or diameter >6 mm) are recommended.

- Early treatment is curative for at least 90% of patients with basal or squamous cell carcinoma. The 5-year survival is highly correlated with the thickness of the tumor.
- Wearing sun-protective clothing, applying sunscreen (sun protection factor of 30 or higher and with UVA protection), and limiting sun exposure are highly recommended methods of primary prevention.

Testicular Cancer

Testicular cancer is the leading cancer diagnosed in males aged 15 to 35 years. Risk factors include cryptorchidism and Klinefelter syndrome. For patients with **seminoma testicular cancer**, the 5-year, disease-free survival rate ranges from 95% for those diagnosed and treated for stage I disease to 85% for those diagnosed and treated for stage

III disease. For patients with **nonseminoma testicular cancer**, the 5-year, disease-free survival rates are 90% to 95% for stage II disease and 50% for stage III disease. No published clinical data indicate that screening for testicular cancer decreases morbidity or mortality. Currently, population screening is not recommended.

- No published clinical data indicate that screening for testicular cancer decreases morbidity or mortality.

Thyroid Cancer

Papillary and follicular thyroid cancers account for approximately 85% and 10% of thyroid cancers, respectively. The 20-year mortality rate for these cancers ranges from 5% to 15%. Conversely, undifferentiated anaplastic thyroid cancer carries an extremely poor prognosis, with a 50% mortality rate within 3 months after diagnosis. Because most thyroid cancers have a relatively benign course after treatment, population screening is not recommended.

- Differentiated thyroid cancer has a 20-year mortality rate of 5% to 15%. Undifferentiated thyroid cancer has a 3-month mortality rate of 50%.
- Population screening is not recommended.

Implementation Tools for Ensuring High-Quality Screening and Follow-up

Various measures can be used to monitor compliance with existing cancer screening recommendations at the organizational level. For example, the National Committee for Quality Assurance has developed the Healthcare Effectiveness Data and Information Set, which is used by most US health care organizations and insurance plans to track group performance with respect to a broad range of conditions and services, including breast, cervical, and CRC screening. In addition, the Centers for Medicare and Medicaid Services provide financial incentives to eligible professionals who participate in the Physician Quality Reporting Initiative. Clinical tools have also been created to facilitate high-quality cancer screening; such tools include the risk assessment tool for breast cancer (www.cancer.gov/bcrisktool) and the Primary Care Clinician's Evidence-Based Toolbox and Guide for CRC screening (www.nccrt.org). Widespread dissemination and application of these and other standardized instruments help reduce variability and increase quality in cancer screening.

Manual and Automated Reminder Systems

Automated and manual chart audits and patient interview strategies implemented in primary care practices have improved completion of cancer screening protocols for at-risk populations. Although individualized patient counseling about cancer screening can markedly affect patient behavior, systematic organizational strategies to enhance population screening typically improve practice efficiency. Automated and manual patient reminder systems can improve screening rates for breast, cervical, and CRC in higher-risk groups and the general population.

In general, e-mail or Web-based strategies are more effective than mailed reminders. Telephone reminders are typically the most effective. However, the feasibility of each of these strategies must consider resource utilization, including information technology design and implementation, the use of designated personnel to implement the strategy, and financial resources to fund the intervention.

- Compliance with existing cancer screening recommendations is monitored.
- To facilitate high-quality cancer screening, widespread dissemination of risk assessment tools and other standardized instruments is recommended.
- Automated and manual chart audits and patient interview strategies at the primary care level can be used to improve cancer screening of at-risk populations.

SUGGESTED READING

Centers for Disease Control and Prevention [Internet]. Atlanta (GA): The Centers; [cited 2009 Sep 13]. Available from: http://www.cdc.gov/cancer/.

Jemal A, Siegel R, Ward E, Hao Y, Xu J, Thun MJ. Cancer statistics, 2009. CA Cancer J Clin. 2009 Jul-Aug; 59(4):225-49. Epub 2009 May 27.

Lindor NM, McMaster ML, Lindor CJ, Greene MH; National Cancer Institute, Division of Cancer Prevention, Community Oncology and Prevention Trials Research Group. Concise handbook of familial cancer susceptibility syndromes, 2nd ed. J Natl Cancer Inst Monogr. 2008;(38):1-93.

National Cancer Institute [Internet]. Bethesda (MD): US National Institutes of Health; [cited 2009 Sep 13]. Available from: http://www.cancer.gov.

Smith RA, Cokkinides V, Brawley OW. Cancer screening in the United States, 2009: a review of current American Cancer Society guidelines and issues in cancer screening. CA Cancer J Clin. 2009 Jan-Feb;59(1):27-41.

US Preventive Services Task Force (USPSTF) [Internet]. Rockville (MD): Agency for Healthcare Research and Quality; [cited 2009 Sep 13]. Available from: http://www.ahrq.gov/clinic/prevenix.htm.

Winawer SJ, Zauber AG, Fletcher RH, Stillman JS, O'Brien MJ, Levin B, et al; US Multi-Society Task Force on Colorectal Cancer; American Cancer Society. Guidelines for colonoscopy surveillance after polypectomy: a consensus update by the US Multi-Society Task Force on Colorectal Cancer and the American Cancer Society. Gastroenterology. 2006 May;130(6):1872-85.

Questions and Answers

Questions

1. A 29-year-old man presents for a general medical evaluation. He is in excellent health and has an unremarkable medical history. He attributes his 10-pound weight loss during the past 6 months to a recently instituted diet and exercise program. His family history includes a maternal grandmother with colorectal cancer diagnosed at age 54 years and a maternal uncle with "kidney cancer" diagnosed at age 47 years. The patient's mother also underwent hysterectomy for endometrial cancer at age 42 years. With respect to colorectal cancer screening, which of the following options is most appropriate for this patient?
   a. Begin colorectal cancer screening now
   b. Begin colorectal cancer screening at age 32 years
   c. Begin colorectal cancer screening at age 40 years
   d. Begin colorectal cancer screening at age 50 years
   e. Begin colorectal cancer screening at age 60 years

2. A 31-year-old woman visits your office to renew her prescriptions for thyroid replacement medication and oral contraception, which were last written 12 months earlier when she had a pelvic examination and cervical cytologic evaluation (Papanicolaou test). She has tolerated these medications without apparent complications. During your conversation, she asks about when to repeat cervical cancer screening. Her medical history is significant for 2 vaginal deliveries and hypothyroidism. She reports no new sex partners and has been compliant with cervical cancer screening since age 21, with normal cytology findings every year. Which of the following options is most appropriate?
   a. Repeat pelvic examination and cervical cytology now
   b. Repeat pelvic examination and cervical cytology in 1 year
   c. Repeat pelvic examination and cervical cytology in 2 years
   d. Repeat pelvic examination and cervical cytology in 4 years
   e. Recommend human papillomavirus (HPV) testing now; if negative, repeat pelvic examination and cervical cytology in 3 years

3. Which of the following patients does not meet usual criteria for increased breast cancer risk?
   a. A woman whose mother has a documented germline mutation in *BRCA1*
   b. A woman who received radiotherapy to the upper chest wall for a thyroid goiter at age 15 years
   c. A woman whose paternal cousin had colorectal cancer diagnosed at age 55 years
   d. A woman with a medical history of atypical ductal hyperplasia on breast biopsy
   e. A woman whose sister had ovarian cancer

4. Which of the following statements is correct?
   a. Annual screening with digital rectal examination has been shown to reduce prostate cancer deaths in prospective, randomized, controlled trials
   b. Annual screening with serum prostate-specific antigen (PSA) testing has been shown to reduce prostate cancer mortality in prospective, randomized, controlled trials
   c. Prostate cancer is the second-leading cause of cancer death among US men
   d. Prostate cancer mortality rates are higher for Asian Americans and Pacific Islanders than for blacks
   e. Prostate cancer risk is higher in a man with cryptorchidism

5. A screening test is proposed that is reported to have a sensitivity of 60% and a specificity of 90%. If the prevalence of the disease being tested is 10% in the screened population, what is the positive predictive value of this test?
   a. 40%
   b. 60%
   c. 80%
   d. 90%
   e. 95%

6. Which of following about lead-time bias is true?
   a. Reflects the variable duration of disease in a population according to disease severity factors
   b. Reflects pathology that would not have been clinically significant to the patient
   c. Reflects the time between early detection of disease through screening and the time of disease diagnosis on the basis of clinical symptoms
   d. Reflects a statistical challenge resulting from an inadequate sample size
   e. Reflects knowledge of the staff regarding which patients are in the treatment group

Answers

1. Answer a.

The patient's family history fulfills Amsterdam II criteria for hereditary nonpolyposis colorectal cancer syndrome. In this context, colorectal cancer screening should be initiated by age 20 to 25 years, or 10 years younger than the earliest cancer diagnosis in the family, whichever comes first.

2. Answer c.

Because the patient had a history of normal cervical cytology evaluations, repeat screening could be performed 3 years after the most recent evaluation. Current evidence is insufficient to support routine HPV testing. HPV testing is used as an adjunct to stratify risk when cervical cytologic (Papanicolaou test) findings are abnormal.

3. Answer c.

Family history of a germline mutation in *BRCA1* or *BRCA2*, previous radiotherapy to the chest wall (particularly during adolescence), and personal history of benign breast disease (including atypical ductal hyperplasia) are established breast cancer risk factors. Existing data do not support an increased breast cancer risk if a third-degree relative had colorectal cancer.

4. Answer c.

Among US men, prostate cancer is the most common incident cancer (other than skin cancer) and is the second-leading cause of cancer death overall. Blacks have the highest prostate cancer mortality rates and Asian Americans and Pacific Islanders have the lowest rates in the United States. Neither digital rectal examination nor serum PSA testing have strong evidence of reducing prostate cancer deaths, although annual performance of both tests may lead to diagnosis at an earlier stage. Cryptorchidism is associated with testicular cancer risk.

5. Answer a.

The positive predictive value is calculated using the formula

$$\frac{a}{a+b} = \frac{60}{60+90} = 40\%$$

		Target Disorder		
		Disease Present	Disease Absent	
Diagnostic Test Results	Positive	60 a	90 b	150 a+b
	Negative	c 40	d 810	c+d 850
		a+c 100	b+d 900	a+b+c+d 1,000

6. Answer c.

Lead-time bias is the time between early detection of disease through screening and the time of disease diagnosis on the basis of clinical symptoms. Length-time bias reflects the variable duration of disease in a population according to disease severity factors. Overdiagnosis bias because of detection of pseudodisease reflects pathology that would not have been clinically significant to the patient.

11

SECONDARY PREVENTION 2: COMMON CLINICAL AND CHRONIC DISEASES

Warren G. Thompson, MD; and Darryl S. Chutka, MD

Chronic diseases are responsible for 6 of the 7 leading causes of death in the United States. Heart disease and cancer account for about half of all deaths. Cerebrovascular disease, chronic lower respiratory tract diseases, diabetes mellitus, and Alzheimer disease account for an additional 16% of deaths. Chronic liver disease, cirrhosis, hypertension, and hypertensive renal disease account for 2% of all deaths in the United States. A substantial portion of these deaths is preventable; here, we provide a concise review of these common clinical diseases with an emphasis on prevention. In the first part of this chapter, we address cardiovascular disease (including coronary artery disease and cerebrovascular disease) and related risk factors (including diabetes mellitus, hyperlipidemia, and hypertension). In the second part of the chapter, we address other common clinical and chronic diseases; these are arranged in alphabetical order.

Coronary Artery Disease

Ninety percent of coronary artery disease (CAD) in the United States is preventable. The power of prevention was observed in a recent Centers for Disease Control and Prevention (CDC) study, which reported 309,000 fewer deaths from CAD than expected between 1980 and 2000. Medical intervention (eg, treatment of myocardial infarction, angina, and heart failure) accounted for 83,000 fewer deaths, secondary prevention (eg, treatment after myocardial infarction or bypass surgery)

accounted for 36,000 fewer deaths, and prevention (eg, treating hypertension, stopping smoking, cholesterol reduction) accounted for 190,000 fewer deaths. Had the increase in diabetes mellitus and weight been avoided in the population during this period, an additional 59,000 deaths would have been averted.

CAD Risk Factors

The global INTERHEART study was a case-control study of risk factors associated with acute myocardial infarction. Worldwide, 15,000 patients were enrolled. In 2004, INTERHEART researchers reported identification of 9 potentially modifiable risk factors that accounted for 90% of CAD (Box 1).

Apolipoprotein B and Apolipoprotein AI

The **ratio of apolipoprotein B to apolipoprotein AI** was the most important modifiable risk factor identified by the INTERHEART study, with a population-attributable risk of 49%. Recent studies with large numbers of cases have further reinforced that apolipoprotein B and apolipoprotein AI are superior to low-density lipoprotein (LDL) cholesterol and high-density lipoprotein (HDL) cholesterol for predicting risk. These tests can be performed in the nonfasting state. The Treating to New Targets study showed that an LDL cholesterol level of 70 mg/dL is the preferred target for patients with clinically significant CAD; this

Box 1 Risk Factors and Beneficial Factors in Coronary
Artery Disease

Risk factors for coronary artery disease

  Apo B–to–Apo AI ratio

  Smoking

  Waist-to-hip ratio

  Diabetes mellitus

  Psychosocial factors

  Hypertension

Beneficial factors for coronary artery disease

  Moderate alcohol consumption

  Exercise

  Consumption of fruits and vegetables

Abbreviations: Apo AI, apolipoprotein AI; Apo B, apolipoprotein B.
Data from Yusuf et al (2004).

target should be replaced with an apolipoprotein B goal
of 80 mg/dL. The National Cholesterol Education Program
recommends **screening adults 20 years or older every
5 years with a (fasting state) lipid profile**, although apolipoprotein B and apolipoprotein AI now may be preferred.

A number of authorities have recommended against
screening young adults because the number needed to treat
to prevent 1 death is high. However, it should be remembered that the number needed to treat is usually determined for a 5-year period. Given that every statin trial has
shown greater effects with longer treatment, it is highly
likely that the number needed to treat for a 10- or 20-year
period is considerably lower than that for 5 years.

Smoking

Smoking was the second-leading risk factor in the
INTERHEART study, with a population-attributable risk of
36%. After a myocardial infarction, continuing to smoke is
one of the important risk factors for recurrent myocardial
infarction. Two studies have shown that smoking cessation
rates exceeding 50% can be achieved with effective counseling for patients in the coronary care unit. This opportunity for counseling is unique compared with primary care,
where smoking cessation rates are considerably lower.
Quitting smoking reduces risk of heart attack to the level of
a nonsmoker within 3 years.

Waist-to-Hip Ratio

The waist-to-hip ratio had a population-attributable risk of
24% in the INTERHEART study. In INTERHEART, the
waist-to-hip ratio was a better predictor of CAD than body
mass index (BMI), which had a population-attributable
risk of 8%. Some but not all studies find waist-to-hip ratio
superior to waist circumference alone (ie, large hips are

protective). In the INTERHEART study, the **waist-to-hip
ratio was important for all BMI categories**, including the
very thin. Thus, clinicians would be wise to incorporate
measurement of waist-to-hip ratio into their practice. The
suggested target waist circumference for men is 100 cm,
but the INTERHEART study reported increased risk above
90 cm. Waist circumference for women should be no more
than 86 cm. The waist-to-hip ratio should be less than 0.93
for men and less than 0.86 for women.

Diabetes Mellitus

Diabetes mellitus had a population-attributable risk of 10%
in the INTERHEART study. Diabetes mellitus increases the
risk of CAD by 2- to 6-fold. Women with diabetes mellitus
have as great a risk of CAD as men with diabetes mellitus,
completely eliminating the 10-year advantage (ie, difference in age at presentation) that women usually have
compared with men. **Aggressive treatment** of risk factors
considerably reduces risk; however, it is less clear whether
good control of blood sugar will reduce risk.

Risk Factors. Type 2 diabetes mellitus has a strong genetic
component, but substantive evidence from randomized
trials indicates that it can be prevented or at least considerably delayed. Preventive efforts should be directed to those
with higher risk. Factors associated with type 2 diabetes
mellitus are listed in Box 2.

The importance of BMI for the development of diabetes
mellitus cannot be overemphasized. Those with a BMI of
22 to 24.9 kg/m^2 have double the relative risk of diabetes
mellitus compared with those with a BMI 20 to 21.9 kg/m^2.
Women and men who have a BMI exceeding 35 kg/m^2 have
a 30-fold or 40-fold higher relative risk of diabetes mellitus, respectively, when compared with those who are lean
(BMI, 20-22 kg/m^2). A recent, 12-year study of young Israeli
men showed that fasting glucose levels from 87 through
94 mg/dL were associated with double the risk of diabetes
mellitus development compared with those with glucose
levels less than 82 mg/dL; glucose levels from 95 through
99 mg/dL were associated with triple the risk. Elevated
triglycerides also heightened risk. Several large, randomized studies have shown a higher risk of developing diabetes mellitus with the use of β-blockers, compared with
other agents, for the treatment of hypertension.

Multiple prospective studies show that improved
fitness and increased activity reduce the risk of developing
diabetes mellitus. As little as 40 minutes of walking per
week appears to confer some protection. In the CARDIA
(Coronary Artery Risk Development in Young Adults)
study, young adults in the lowest-fitness quintile had
3.5 times the risk of diabetes mellitus and 4 times the risk
of metabolic syndrome as those in the 2 highest quintiles.
Those in the moderate-fitness quintiles had double the
risk of diabetes mellitus and triple the risk of metabolic

Box 2 Risk Factors and Protective Factors for Development of Type 2 Diabetes Mellitus

Risk factors

Age

Body mass index

Waist-to-hip ratio

Weight gain as an adult

Family history

Hypertriglyceridemia

Tobacco smoking

Low birth weight

Low high-density lipoprotein cholesterol

Hypertension

Elevated glucose and elevated hemoglobin A_{1c}

High ratio of saturated-to-polyunsaturated fat in the diet

History of gestational diabetes mellitus or delivery of an infant >4,100 g

Polycystic ovary syndrome

Protective factors

Exercise

Moderate alcohol consumption

Whole grain, fruits and vegetables, magnesium, and fiber intake

Low glycemic-index or glycemic-load diet (controversial)

Table 1 Treatment Goals for Type 2 Diabetes Mellitus

Variable	Goal
Plasma glucose, mg/dL	
Fasting	90-130
Bedtime	110-150
Hemoglobin A_{1c}, %	<7
Blood pressure, mm Hg	<130/80
Serum lipids, mg/dL	
Low-density lipoprotein cholesterol	<100 (<70 for patients with coronary artery disease)
High-density lipoprotein cholesterol	>45
Triglycerides, fasting	<200
Aspirin therapy	81 mg/d, unless contraindicated
Nicotine dependence	No nicotine use

syndrome compared with those in the highest quintiles. Prospective studies consistently show a reduced risk of diabetes mellitus for those who consume more whole grains.

Treatment. The Finnish Diabetes Prevention Study and the study conducted by the Diabetes Prevention Program Research Group were large, randomized trials that reported a 58% reduction in the incidence of diabetes mellitus in at-risk patients after a program of **weight reduction and increased exercise**. Both studies were halted early because the results were so dramatic. In the Diabetes Prevention Program Study, metformin was also an effective intervention, but it was not as successful as lifestyle change. For obese diabetic patients, metformin is superior to sulfonylurea agents with regard to reduced mortality rate, less weight gain, and lower risk for hypoglycemia. A randomized trial examining the diet of patients with metabolic syndrome showed that a Mediterranean diet, which consists mostly of fruits, vegetables, nuts, whole grains, and olive oil, was superior to a standard (Western) diet in reducing fasting glucose levels and the incidence of metabolic syndrome.

The goals of treatment in patients with type 2 diabetes mellitus are listed in Table 1. Achievement of these goals is associated with lower morbidity and mortality. Data indicate that a reduction in blood sugar decreases the incidence of microvascular events (nephropathy, retinopathy, and neuropathy). A target hemoglobin A_{1c} (HgbA$_{1c}$) of 7% is considered a reasonable goal. In an Israeli study, patients were given written targets for LDL, HgbA$_{1c}$, blood pressure, and weight; they were told that they were responsible for reaching these targets and were encouraged to make changes. These patients ultimately had lower levels of LDL cholesterol and HgbA$_{1c}$, lower blood pressure, and fewer vascular events during 4 years of follow-up. The United Kingdom Prospective Diabetes Study showed that tight control of blood pressure reduced mortality and complications of diabetes mellitus. Several randomized trials have also shown that statins reduce rates of death and cardiovascular events for diabetic patients. Aspirin also reduces risk in this population.

The major controversy is whether a reduction in blood sugar decreases mortality rates. Two recent, randomized trials (ACCORD and ADVANCE) studied intensive treatment and standard treatment of hyperglycemia. The ACCORD (Action to Control Cardiovascular Risk in Diabetes) trial randomized 10,251 patients and achieved a mean HgbA$_{1c}$ of 6.4% in the intensively treated group compared with 7.5% in the standard group. The intensive-therapy group had a higher mortality rate (but a lower rate of nonfatal myocardial infarction). The intensive-therapy group also had a mean weight gain of 3.5 kg (28% gained 10 kg or more). The intensive therapy group was much more likely to be receiving thiazolidinedione medications and insulin therapy; however, the authors did not believe these caused excess mortality, even though other studies have suggested that thiazolidinediones increase the risk of congestive heart failure and possibly also increase the risk of death. The increased incidence of hypoglycemia in the intensive-therapy group may have contributed to the excess mortality.

The ADVANCE (Action in Diabetes and Vascular Disease: Preterax and Diamicron Modified Release Controlled Evaluation) trial randomized 11,140 patients to receive intensive or standard treatment and achieved a mean $HgbA_{1c}$ of 6.4% versus 7.0%, primarily with a sulfonylurea. Weight gain did not occur, and hypoglycemia was less common than that reported by the ACCORD study. ADVANCE trial participants had a considerable reduction in nephropathy with intensive treatment, but no difference was observed in cardiovascular disease or mortality rates. If an $HgbA_{1c}$ level of 6.5% can be achieved without clinically significant hypoglycemia or weight gain, then 6.5% is a reasonable goal. If insulin or thiazolidinediones are being considered for therapy, a target $HgbA_{1c}$ level of 7% is reasonable.

A recent study randomized 160 diabetic patients with microalbuminuria to receive standard therapy or intensive combination therapy (stricter control of blood pressure, diet, cholesterol, and blood sugar, plus more exercise). The target $HgbA_{1c}$ was 6.5% (insulin and thiazolidinedione therapy were similar between groups). The study monitored patients for 13 years. The control group had a 50% mortality rate and the intensive-therapy group had a 30% mortality rate.

Data from prospective studies indicates that **exercise** is associated with major benefits for diabetic patients. In one study, patients who walked at least 4 hours a week had 50% fewer deaths (2 hours per week yielded a 33% benefit). The Cooper Clinic reported that fitness was an important predictor of mortality in diabetes mellitus, with patients in the lowest fitness quartile having a 4.5-fold increased relative risk and the second-lowest fitness quartile having a 2.8-fold increased risk relative to the highest-fitness quartile. Better heart rate recovery time also predicted better outcome for diabetic patients.

Data from the prospective EPIC (European Prospective Investigation of Cancer) study indicate that a **diet high in vegetables and legumes** is associated with a lower risk of overall mortality and cardiovascular mortality for patients with diabetes mellitus. Another prospective study showed that fish intake conferred a mortality benefit. Angiotensin-converting enzyme (ACE) inhibitors are indicated for renal protection for all diabetic patients with albuminuria, and they are a good choice for patients with hypertension. Other important preventive measures for diabetic patients include pneumococcal vaccine and annual vaccination for influenza.

Psychosocial Factors

Psychosocial factors had a population-attributable risk of 33% in the INTERHEART study. Depression, stressful life events, high stress at work or at home, and substantial financial stress were all more common in cases than controls. Some studies—but not all—have suggested that treating depression and type A personality traits (decreasing the sense of time urgency and easing hostility) can reduce the subsequent incidence of myocardial infarction. The largest study of depression and CAD (the ENRICHD [Enhancing Recovery in Coronary Heart Disease] study) showed improvement in depression but no improvement in coronary events. Dr Dean Ornish has shown that a combination of a very-low-fat diet, exercise, and stress reduction techniques reduces subsequent heart disease, but the effect of the stress reduction techniques is unclear. More research is needed in this area.

Hyperlipidemia

A healthy diet in childhood results in a lower risk of hyperlipidemia as an adult. A recent study from Finland compared 2 dietary patterns in children aged 3 to 18 years; they compared a diet consisting mainly of potatoes, butter, and sausage with a diet of fruits, legumes, vegetables, and nuts. The latter pattern was associated with lower cholesterol, lower blood pressure, and lower insulin levels 21 years later.

Dietary treatment of hypercholesterolemia is more problematic. The American Heart Association (AHA) Step I diet reduces LDL cholesterol by about 5% and lowers HDL cholesterol by 5% as well. A Mediterranean diet is somewhat better; one study showed a reduction in LDL cholesterol by 10% without a reduction in HDL cholesterol. The Toronto diet (combining plant sterols, vegetable proteins, and viscous fibers in a low-fat, low-cholesterol diet) can decrease cholesterol levels by as much as 20%, but maintaining compliance is problematic. Dr Dean Ornish's very-low-fat diet can decrease LDL cholesterol by 30% and markedly reduce HDL cholesterol, but patients in Western societies rarely adhere to this diet. Consumption of almonds, walnuts, and pecans has been shown to reduce LDL cholesterol by about 5% in small, randomized trials. Psyllium fiber can also cause a small reduction in cholesterol. Results with garlic are mixed. Plant stanol esters lower LDL cholesterol by as much as 10% to 15%, but they must be administered twice daily before meals, which is hard for patients to remember. Certain margarines, other food products, and several over-the-counter medications now contain plant stanol esters. Red yeast rice can lower cholesterol levels, but it essentially is a statin and has all the adverse effects of statins. However, red yeast rice is sold as a nutrition supplement; thus, it does not have the government oversight for product safety required for manufacture of pharmaceutical agents. Policosanol has not consistently lowered cholesterol levels in randomized trials and is not recommended.

For patients who require a substantial reduction in LDL cholesterol, the treatment of choice is a **statin**. It should be noted that many patients who begin a heart-healthy diet are discouraged by unchanging cholesterol levels. However, even when cholesterol levels do not improve, studies suggest that their risk of CAD is still considerably reduced. Heart-healthy diets should always be strongly encouraged.

Hypertension

Hypertension had a population-attributable risk of 18% in the INTERHEART study. Some authors have postulated that a plot of mortality rates and blood pressure would form a J-shaped curve, with higher mortality rates when the blood pressure is too low; however, the Prospective Studies Collaboration, which examined data from 1 million patients, showed no evidence of this. Systolic hypertension is at least as important as diastolic hypertension when predicting CAD. A recent study demonstrated the benefits of treating systolic hypertension in octogenarians. The association between blood pressure and risk of CAD is continuous, with a blood pressure of 115/75 mm Hg associated with half the risk compared with a blood pressure of 135/75 mm Hg.

Hypertension is a preventable condition. As noted above, Finnish children consuming a healthy diet were less likely to have hyperlipidemia as adults; they also were less likely to have hypertension. BMI, waist-to-hip ratio, and weight gain as an adult are all associated with the development of hypertension (Box 3). Less time sleeping and more time viewing television are associated with obesity and hypertension in children, adolescents, and adults. In the CARDIA study, the 15-year risk of hypertension was 2.5-fold higher in the low-fitness group and nearly 2-fold higher in the moderate-fitness group when compared with that of

the high-fitness group. Blacks have a higher incidence of hypertension, but this difference mostly is explained by risk factors. Even modest alcohol consumption is associated with increased blood pressure in men; however, for women, only heavy consumption is associated with hypertension. In societies where sodium intake is very low, the incidence of hypertension also is very low. However, salt restriction within the usual range of sodium intake in Western societies has fairly minimal effects on blood pressure.

Screening for hypertension is recommended every 2 years for adults (annual screening is recommended if systolic blood pressure is 120-140 mm Hg and diastolic pressure is 80-90 mm Hg). Ambulatory blood pressure is a better predictor of long-term outcomes than traditional office measurement. Automatic blood pressure measuring devices such as the BPTru (Smiths Medical PM, Inc, Waukesha, Wisconsin) have improved office measurement of blood pressure by checking the blood pressure 6 times in a quiet room, away from the physician. Severity of hypertension can be classified into 4 stages (Table 2). Patients should be cautioned to avoid coffee before blood pressure is measured. Secondary causes of hypertension (eg, renal artery stenosis, chronic renal disease, pheochromocytoma, hyperaldosteronism, Cushing disease, coarctation of the aorta) are uncommon (<5% of patients). Certain medications can raise blood pressure, including nonsteroidal antiinflammatory drugs (NSAIDs), corticosteroids, estrogen, appetite suppressants, and sympathomimetics.

All hypertensive patients should be examined for **renal artery bruit**, and blood pressure should be checked in both arms. Routine evaluation should include a complete blood count, fasting glucose level and lipid profile, potassium,

---

Box 3 Risk Factors for Hypertension

Age

Body mass index

Waist-to-hip ratio

Weight gain

Sedentary lifestyle

Poor fitness

Television viewing

High-salt diet

Diet reduced in vegetables, fruit, and low-fat dairy products

Diet increased in red meat

Alcohol (for women, only heavy consumption is associated with hypertension)

Time urgency and hostility (type A personality)

Cigarette smoking

Fasting insulin level

Table 2 Blood Pressure Stages for Evaluation of Hypertension

Stage	Definition		Comment
	Systolic Pressure, mm Hg	Diastolic Pressure, mm Hg	
Normal	<120	<80	. . .
Prehypertension	120-139	80-89	. . .
Stage 1 hypertension	140-159	90-99	Use single-agent therapy (a thiazide diuretic generally is preferred)
Stage 2 hypertension	≥160	≥100	Combination therapy usually is necessary (typically includes a thiazide diuretic)

Adapted from JNC 7 Express. The Seventh Report of the Joint National Committee on Prevention, Detection, Evaluation, and Treatment of High Blood Pressure. NIH Publication No. 03-5233. Bethesda (MD): National Heart, Lung, and Blood Institute; c2003. p.3.

creatinine, urinalysis, and an electrocardiogram. Additional tests for secondary causes should be undertaken only if prompted by the medical history, physical examination findings, or results from basic tests or if the patient has a poor response to treatment.

Treatment. Nonpharmacologic methods of treating hypertension with demonstrated benefit include **exercise**, **weight reduction**, **and diet**. The DASH (Dietary Approaches to Stop Hypertension) diet consists of increased intake of fruits, vegetables, and nonfat dairy products. Reduction in alcohol intake probably helps but has not been tested in randomized trials.

The ALLHAT (Antihypertensive and Lipid-Lowering Treatment to Prevent Heart Attack Trial) study suggested that diuretics should be the first-line treatment for most patients, especially older patients, because of equal efficacy and lower cost compared with other antihypertensive agents. ACE inhibitors should be considered for diabetic patients and younger patients. β-Blockers are useful for patients who have had a myocardial infarction, but the ASCOT (Anglo-Scandinavian Cardiac Outcomes Trial) and others argue against the first-line use of atenolol.

As with other diseases, long-term compliance with medication may be as low as 50%. The most common reason for noncompliance is the failure to remember. Younger adults are less compliant than older adults; older adults are more likely to use a reminder system. Compliance can be improved by using pill boxes, linking the medication with something the patient does every day, and taking the medication at the same time each day. In the Diabetes Prevention Program, use of all 3 strategies nearly tripled the rate of compliance with medication. It is easier to remember to take medicine once a day than twice a day, and medications that must be administered more than twice daily should be avoided if possible. Cost can be an important barrier to compliance, and patients may be reluctant to discuss this with physicians. Another form of noncompliance is failure to return for follow-up. This problem can be reduced by mailed or telephone reminders of upcoming appointments.

Other Risk Factors

Age is the strongest risk factor for CAD. Male sex is a risk factor for premature CAD. Women die of CAD as frequently as men, but it typically occurs 10 years later in life. The risk factors in the INTERHEART study accounted for the difference between the sexes (men were more likely to smoke, have abnormal lipid profiles, etc). Family history had a population-attributable risk of 10% in the INTERHEART study. There are many other risk factors for CAD, including fibrinogen, activated factor VII, white blood count, small dense LDL particles, and others.

Lipoprotein(a) is a risk factor for CAD, especially in South Asia. It should be measured for patients with a personal or family history of premature atherosclerosis. If it is high, the best approach is aggressive treatment of LDL cholesterol. High-sensitivity C-reactive protein (hs-CRP) is a minor risk factor; it often is elevated in obese patients but can be reduced with weight loss. It remains to be seen whether measuring hs-CRP leads to better patient outcomes.

The JUPITER (Justification for the Use of Statins in Primary Prevention: an Intervention Trial Evaluating Rosuvastatin) trial randomized more than 17,000 patients (without known CAD; LDL cholesterol, <130 mg/dL; hs-CRP, >3 mg/L) to receive 20 mg rosuvastatin or placebo. Cardiovascular deaths and overall deaths were reduced with rosuvastatin. The study did not show the utility of hs-CRP, but it did suggest aggressive cholesterol reduction was appropriate, even in relatively low-risk patients.

Although the novel risk factors discussed above may be important in selected cases, more than 90% of CAD can be explained by conventional risk factors.

- The ratio of apolipoprotein B to apolipoprotein AI and cigarette smoking are the 2 most important modifiable risk factors for development of coronary artery disease (CAD). Quitting smoking reduces risk of heart attack to the level of a nonsmoker within 3 years.
- The waist-to-hip ratio should be incorporated into routine clinical practice because it is a better predictor of CAD than body mass index (BMI) or waist circumference alone.
- Diabetes mellitus is a risk factor for CAD, but the effect of well-controlled blood glucose on risk is unknown. BMI and other lifestyle factors are associated closely with the risk of type 2 disease development. Metformin is an effective intervention but not as successful as lifestyle change.
- Depression, stressful life events, high stress at work or at home, and substantial financial stress are more common in patients with CAD.
- Therapy for elevated cholesterol should begin with more intensive efforts to change lifestyle habits and reduce the risk of heart disease and heart attacks. Patients who require a substantial reduction in low-density lipoprotein (LDL) cholesterol should be treated with a statin.
- Screening for hypertension is recommended every 2 years for most adults. Nonpharmacologic methods of treating hypertension include exercise, weight reduction, and diet. Long-term compliance with hypertension medication may be as low as 50%, usually because of failure to remember.
- Other risk factors for CAD include age, sex, family history of CAD, elevated lipoprotein(a), and elevated high-sensitivity C-reactive protein (hs-CRP).

CAD Protective Factors

Alcohol Consumption

Regular alcohol consumption conferred a population-attributable benefit of 7% in the INTERHEART study. More than 60 prospective studies have shown that moderate alcohol consumption is associated with a lower risk of CAD, with greater benefit for women than for men. **Red wine is not superior** to other forms of alcohol, despite the widespread belief otherwise.

The benefits of alcohol consumption likely are due to 2 effects: raising HDL cholesterol and decreasing risk of thrombosis. Most of the studies showing benefit have been of white populations. The ARIC (Atherosclerosis Risk in Communities) study has not shown benefit of alcohol in the black population. Binge drinking is associated with increased risk of CAD and calcification. Although people who consume moderate amounts of alcohol do not need to stop for health reasons, advising alcohol consumption to people who do not currently drink has not been shown to be beneficial and thus is not recommended.

Fruit and Vegetable Consumption

Daily consumption of fruits and vegetables had a population-attributable benefit of 14% in the INTERHEART study. The association between diet and risk of myocardial infarction has been difficult to study because it is hard to control diet in randomized trials.

The Lyon Diet Heart Study randomized 600 patients to a **Mediterranean diet** or to a standard (American) diet and reported a remarkable 65% reduction in subsequent cardiovascular death for those eating a Mediterranean diet. This occurred with no improvement in lipoproteins, weight, or blood pressure. Observational studies have also shown the potential benefit of a Mediterranean diet. A recent randomized trial patterned after a Step II AHA diet (55% carbohydrate, 15% protein, 30% fat [of which 7% is saturated]) showed no benefit for CAD.

Exercise

Regular exercise conferred a population-attributable benefit of 12% in the INTERHEART study. The benefit was greater for women than for men. It is important to distinguish between activity and fitness. Both confer benefit, independent of each other, although they are obviously related. Fitness is a better predictor of cardiac disease and death than activity (INTERHEART studied activity, not fitness).

The St. James Women's Heart Study determined that women in their 50s had an average fitness of 8 metabolic equivalent tasks (METs) on treadmill exercise testing. Compared with women with average or better than average fitness levels (>8 METs), women with a fitness level between 5 and 8 METs had twice the mortality risk, and women with fitness levels less than 5 METs had triple the mortality risk during the 8-year follow-up period. In another study, the 30% of women who had below-average maximum time on a treadmill and below-average heart rate recovery time (another fitness measure) accounted for 60% of total deaths and 70% of cardiovascular deaths during the ensuing 20 years. The Cooper Clinic study (Aerobics Center Longitudinal Study) showed that of conventional risk factors, fitness had the highest population-attributable risk for total mortality in the female population (fitness was equal to cholesterol and family history in men). The Honolulu Heart Program reported a 15% reduction in heart disease for every half-mile walked each day for men aged 70 to 90 years.

- Moderate alcohol consumption likely is beneficial because it raises high-density lipoprotein (HDL) cholesterol and decreases risk of thrombosis.
- The Mediterranean diet, which consists mostly of fruits, vegetables, nuts, whole grains, and olive oil, is believed to greatly reduce risk of CAD.
- Regular activity and higher fitness levels are associated with decreased risk of CAD and cardiovascular death.

Diagnosis and Treatment

The role of electron beam computed tomography (to measure coronary calcium) in the diagnosis of early CAD remains controversial. A positive scan is associated with increased likelihood of a subsequent event and is a risk factor for patients with otherwise low or intermediate risk. No evidence suggests that serial scans to monitor progression are beneficial, and the scan has no role in patients with established disease.

The power of aggressive risk factor intervention is illustrated by the COURAGE (Clinical Outcomes Utilizing Revascularization and Aggressive Drug Evaluation) trial, which randomized 2,287 stable patients with documented ischemia and CAD to optimal medical management or percutaneous coronary intervention. Both groups had similar outcomes. Patients receiving optimal medical management met regularly with trial staff to get assistance with stopping smoking, lowering blood pressure, increasing exercise, reducing weight, and following a more heart-healthy diet. LDL cholesterol was treated aggressively, and an attempt was made to raise HDL to above 40 mg/dL. Aspirin, medications to reduce ischemia, and ACE inhibitors were also prescribed. Equivalent results were observed in multiple subgroups (eg, those with multivessel disease, older than 65 years, decreased ejection fraction).

The point of the COURAGE trial is that **optimal medical management is an intensive intervention**. Treatment of CAD can be approached with the alphabetical mnemonic **ABCDEF**.

A Is for Aspirin and ACE Inhibitors

Aspirin reduces the risk of cardiovascular disease and should be prescribed to patients with known cardiovascular disease, diabetes mellitus, and other important risk factors. However, most healthy women younger than 65 years and most healthy men younger than 50 years do not fit into this category and should not be prescribed aspirin because the risk of gastrointestinal tract bleeding outweighs the cardiovascular benefit. Aspirin is beneficial for those with a Framingham 10-year risk score of 6% or greater. A study comparing different aspirin doses showed the effects of an 81-mg dose were equivalent to a 325-mg dose and superior to higher doses. Others have argued that aspirin resistance is common and that 162 mg should be prescribed, but data supporting this position currently are insufficient. ACE inhibitors lower risk in patients with CAD and especially should be prescribed to patients with reduced left ventricular function.

B Is for β-Blockers

β-Blockers lower the risk of subsequent myocardial infarction.

C Is for Cholesterol

Eighty percent of people with ischemic heart disease die of ischemic heart disease. Meta-analyses have shown that statins reduce both cardiac and total mortality rates, with a relative risk reduction exceeding 30%. The Treating to New Targets study showed that for high-risk patients, a target LDL of 70 mg/dL resulted in reduced risk of cardiac events relative to a target LDL of 100 mg/dL. Bile acid sequestrants have been shown to reduce cardiac events but not total mortality rates, probably because LDL cholesterol is not sufficiently lowered with these agents. Niacin may reduce cardiac and total mortality rates. Fibrates reduce cardiac events but do not reduce overall mortality rates, and meta-analysis showed an increase in noncardiovascular mortality rates with fibrates. Ezetimibe has not been shown to reduce either events or mortality. Every 1 mg/dL reduction in LDL cholesterol is associated with a 1% to 2% reduction in cardiac risk.

D Is for Diet

Observational studies suggest that either a Mediterranean (substituting monounsaturated fat for saturated fat) or an Asian diet (substituting high-quality carbohydrate for fat) will reduce risk of CAD. Fruits, vegetables, whole grains, and nuts have all been associated with a reduced risk of CAD in good-quality prospective studies. Trans fats should be avoided because they have been associated consistently with a higher risk of heart disease. The data are less consistent regarding the harmful effects of saturated fat and dietary cholesterol when studied in isolation. However, the Nurses' Health Study and the Health Professionals Follow-Up Study both showed that a prudent diet (fruits and vegetables, whole grains, fish, chicken, nuts, olive oil), which is lower in saturated fat, dietary cholesterol, and trans fats, is associated with better outcomes than a Western diet (red meat, cheese, french fries, butter, margarine, donuts, cookies, pastries, and other desserts).

E Is for Exercise

Comprehensive cardiac rehabilitation programs (with exercise being the main component) can reduce total mortality rates after myocardial infarction. All patients with myocardial infarction should undergo cardiac rehabilitation because prospective studies have shown that such patients who increase their physical activity have a better prognosis. A recent study showed that men who markedly increased their walking distance 12 months after myocardial infarction had half the risk of a recurrent event compared with those whose walking distance did not improve.

F Is for Fish Oil

The GISSI (Gruppo Italiano per lo Studio della Sopravvivenza nell'Infarto Miocardico)–Prevenzione trial (11,324 study subjects) showed a significant reduction in cardiac deaths after myocardial infarction for patients who consumed 1,000 mg/d of fish oil (they also showed that vitamin E was ineffective). The primary benefit was a 25% reduction in sudden cardiac deaths. Observational studies have also suggested an antiarrhythmic benefit with fish oil.

- The COURAGE trial found that optimal medical management resulted in outcomes equal to that of percutaneous angioplasty in patients with stable angina.
- Angiotensin-converting enzyme (ACE) inhibitors lower risk in patients with CAD and especially should be prescribed to patients with reduced left ventricular function.
- β-Blockers lower the risk of subsequent myocardial infarction.
- Every 1 mg/dL reduction in low-density lipoprotein (LDL) cholesterol is associated with a 1% to 2% reduction in cardiac risk.
- Fruits, vegetables, whole grains, and nuts are associated with reduced risk of CAD. Trans fats should be avoided because they are associated with a higher risk of heart disease.
- Patients who increase their physical activity after a myocardial infarction have better prognoses.
- One study of fish oil intake reported a 25% reduction in sudden cardiac death.

Cerebrovascular Disease

All causative factors discussed above for CAD are also important for stroke. **Hypertension** replaces cholesterol as the most important risk factor. Randomized trials of statins in patients with CAD show a reduced risk of stroke. Alcohol in moderation reduces the overall risk of stroke and the risk of ischemic stroke, but it increases the risk of hemorrhagic stroke. Some data suggest that psychological distress and depression are risk factors for stroke, but the evidence is inconsistent. Diabetes mellitus is an important risk factor. Aspirin is useful for primary and secondary prevention of stroke. Healthy diet and exercise are both associated with a reduced risk of stroke in large, prospective studies. Fish and fish oil have not been associated with a reduced risk of stroke.

The SPARCL (Stroke Prevention by Aggressive Reduction in Cholesterol Levels) trial, which randomized patients with stroke or transient ischemic attack to receive 80 mg/d of atorvastatin or a placebo, showed a marked reduction in ischemic strokes and overall strokes. Notably, the number of hemorrhagic strokes increased significantly; thus, statins should not be prescribed to patients after a hemorrhagic stroke. For most patients, however, the risk of hemorrhagic stroke is low and statins are indicated in secondary prevention of cerebrovascular disease.

- Hypertension is the most important risk factor for stroke.
- A healthy diet, exercise, aspirin, and statins can reduce risk of stroke.

Anemia

Iron Deficiency

Iron deficiency, diagnosed by the presence of low serum ferritin levels, is the most common nutritional deficiency worldwide. Iron deficiency can cause **hypochromic, microcytic anemia**. In the United States, iron-deficiency anemia affects 7% of children between the ages of 1 and 2 years. Iron-deficiency anemia in untreated pregnant women may be twice as prevalent.

Iron-deficiency anemia in pregnancy has been associated with low birth weight, preterm delivery, perinatal mortality, postpartum depression, and poor performance on mental and psychomotor testing in offspring. For most pregnant women with iron-deficiency anemia, 100 mg/d of iron is necessary. The CDC recommends administration of 40 mg/d of iron, starting early in pregnancy, to prevent iron-deficiency anemia. For women with severe iron deficiency in the third trimester, intravenous iron should be considered (particularly for women who refuse blood transfusions).

The US Preventive Services Task Force (USPSTF) "recommends routine screening for iron deficiency anemia in asymptomatic pregnant women" (grade B recommendation) but "concludes that evidence is insufficient to recommend for or against routine screening for iron deficiency anemia in asymptomatic children aged 6 to 12 months" (grade I statement). The American College of Obstetricians and Gynecologists recommends screening pregnant women at the first prenatal visit and early in the third trimester. The CDC recommends screening nonpregnant women of childbearing age, pregnant women, and high-risk infants and preschool children. The American Academy of Pediatricians recommends screening all infants between 9 and 12 months. Iron-deficiency anemia in children is associated with psychomotor and cognitive abnormalities. However, evidence of iron supplementation correcting these abnormalities is mixed.

Vitamin B$_{12}$ Deficiency

Vitamin B$_{12}$ (cobalamin) deficiency may cause **macrocytic anemia** and can cause a spectrum of neuropsychiatric disorders. Screening for vitamin B$_{12}$ deficiency is performed by measuring serum methylmalonic acid and homocysteine levels, which are increased early in vitamin B$_{12}$ deficiency. Use of the vitamin B$_{12}$ absorption test (Schilling test) for detection of pernicious anemia has been replaced largely by serologic testing for parietal cell and intrinsic factor antibodies. Supplementation with oral vitamin B$_{12}$ is a safe and effective treatment.

Folic Acid Deficiency

Folic acid deficiency is another cause of **macrocytic anemia**. Supplementing food with folic acid (400 mcg daily) during pregnancy has resulted in a marked reduction in **fetal neural tube defects** in the United States. It may also help reduce the incidence of low birth weight and other adverse consequences. This population approach is more cost-effective than screening pregnant women for folate deficiency.

- Pregnant women should be routinely screened for anemia. Iron-deficiency anemia can be prevented by administering iron (40 mg/d).
- Vitamin B$_{12}$ deficiency is a cause of macrocytic anemia. Supplementation with oral vitamin B$_{12}$ is safe and effective.
- Folic acid deficiency is another cause of macrocytic anemia and fetal neural tube defects. Requiring pregnant women to supplement their diet with folic acid (400 mcg daily) is more cost-effective than screening for folate deficiency.

Asthma

The prevalence of asthma is estimated at 300 million worldwide, and 250,000 asthma-related deaths occur each year. It is a substantial cause of disability and morbidity. The Global Initiative for Asthma provides guidelines on prevention and management of asthma.

Exposure to **tobacco smoke** in utero and after birth increases the risk of asthma and reduces lung function for children without asthma. Practitioners must counsel pregnant women to stop smoking because the likelihood of quitting is substantial during pregnancy. Parents of young children also should know that they are putting their children at risk by smoking.

Asthma should be suspected in patients with variable respiratory symptoms that often are aggravated by exercise, exposure to smoke, or exposure to fumes and if they have symptoms that typically worsen at night. Diagnosis is confirmed by observing a forced expiratory volume in 1 second (FEV_1) improvement of 12% or more with a bronchodilator. The ratio of FEV_1 to forced vital capacity (FVC) should be at least 0.80 (if not, emphysema may either coexist or be the diagnosis).

Much can be done to prevent exacerbations of asthma. Active and passive smoking should be avoided. Active smoking reduces the efficacy of inhaled corticosteroids, which are the mainstay of asthma treatment. The benefits of reducing **indoor allergens** (eg, controlling dust mites, using high efficiency particulate air filters, etc) are unclear but may be helpful when used in combination. Asthma can be aggravated by increases in certain outdoor pollutants (eg, ozone, particulates, nitric oxides), increases in respiratory allergens, and changes in weather (thunderstorms, changes in temperature and humidity). Staying indoors may be necessary when asthma is not well controlled.

Other factors may influence asthma. Obesity is associated with an increased prevalence of asthma for unclear reasons. Emotional stress can lead to airway narrowing and trigger an attack, but asthma is no longer considered a psychosomatic illness. Rhinitis and sinusitis are associated with asthma, and treatment may reduce the frequency and severity of asthma.

All adults with newly diagnosed asthma should be asked about their job. It is critical to ask patients whether symptoms improve when away from work. **Occupational asthma** accounts for at least 10% of new-onset adult asthma cases; it may be caused by isocyanates, laboratory animal allergens, flour and grain dust, crab and salmon, acid anhydrides, platinum salts, latex, and wood dust. More details can be found in the chapter on occupational medicine (Chapter 14).

Prevention of asthma exacerbations is facilitated by physician-guided self-management because strong evidence indicates that this approach reduces morbidity in children and adults. Physician-guided self-management consists of patient education, monitoring of symptoms and peak flow by the patient, regular physician review, and a written self-management action plan when symptoms or a decrease in peak flow occur. Examples of such plans are available from the United Kingdom National Asthma Campaign. These plans are more likely to be successful with good doctor-patient communication. Physicians should encourage their patients to ask questions, and they should ensure that patients understand physician instructions. Better outcomes (eg, improved satisfaction, reduced use of health care, and better health) have been documented when these techniques are used. Nonadherence to long-term therapy is common in asthma. The best approach is to ask about adherence while acknowledging that adherence is difficult.

- Asthma is confirmed by observing a forced expiratory volume in 1 second (FEV_1) improvement of 12% or more with a bronchodilator.
- Inhaled corticosteroids are the mainstay of asthma treatment.
- At least 10% of new-onset adult asthma cases can be attributed to occupational exposure.
- Nonadherence to long-term therapy is common in asthma.

Chronic Obstructive Pulmonary Disease

Chronic obstructive pulmonary disease (COPD) is defined by the Global Initiative for Chronic Obstructive Lung Disease as "a preventable and treatable disease. . . . Its pulmonary component is characterized by airflow limitation that is not fully reversible. The airflow limitation is usually progressive and associated with an abnormal inflammatory response of the lung to noxious particles and gases." COPD is expected to be the third-leading cause of death worldwide by 2020. Currently, it affects at least 16 million people in the United States and is the fourth-leading cause of death. In contrast to cardiovascular diseases, the mortality rate of COPD is increasing considerably.

Cigarette smoke is the most important risk factor for COPD. Pipe and cigar smokers have a higher rate of COPD than nonsmokers but a lower rate than cigarette smokers. Women may be more susceptible than men. Passive smoking can also contribute to COPD. Smoking cessation is the most effective way to prevent the development of COPD and to stop its progression, but only 50% of smokers report that they have been advised to stop smoking by their physician. Although the likelihood of stopping smoking after a brief counseling session is low, some smokers will quit, and the public health benefit of every health care provider advising every smoker to stop would be enormous. A detailed discussion of strategies to help patients stop smoking can be found in the chapter on behavioral medicine (Chapter 5).

The second-leading cause of COPD worldwide is **indoor pollution** from cooking and heating in poorly ventilated areas. This is the primary cause of COPD for women in developing countries. Efficient, nonpolluting cookstoves are a major intervention that could reduce the development of COPD. Unfortunately, they are relatively expensive, and adoption is likely to be low unless the price decreases.

Occupational dusts and chemicals can also contribute to COPD. Reducing inhaled particles and gases in the workplace can reduce the incidence of occupationally induced COPD. The role of outdoor air pollution in causing COPD is unclear, but it is harmful to those who already have the disorder.

The USPSTF "recommends against screening adults for chronic obstructive pulmonary disease (COPD) using spirometry" (grade D recommendation). However, patients with cough, chronic sputum production, or dyspnea should be screened for COPD. The test of choice is spirometry. An FEV_1/FVC ratio less than 0.70 after a bronchodilator is diagnostic of COPD.

Medications for COPD help symptoms and may reduce exacerbations, but **medications do not stop progression** of the disorder. For patients with COPD, influenza vaccine reduces morbidity. Pneumococcal vaccine is also recommended. All patients should be encouraged to join an **exercise training program** because good evidence supports exercise training to reduce dyspnea and fatigue and increase exercise tolerance. Supplemental oxygen reduces mortality rates of patients with advanced COPD and respiratory failure. For further details on medical management, refer to guidelines from the Global Initiative for Chronic Obstructive Lung Disease (www.goldcopd.org).

- Cigarette smoke is the most important risk factor for chronic obstructive pulmonary disease (COPD). The second-leading cause of COPD worldwide is indoor pollution from cooking and heating in poorly ventilated areas (often affecting women in developing countries).
- Occupational dusts, chemicals, and outdoor air pollution can contribute to COPD.
- Medications help symptoms and may reduce exacerbations but do not stop progression of the disorder.

Dementia

Dementia is an extremely common disorder that primarily affects elderly patients. The prevalence increases dramatically for patients older than 75 years. **Alzheimer disease** (AD) is the most common type of dementia, making up approximately three-fourths of all cases. In addition to AD, other types of dementia include vascular (multistroke) dementia, Pick disease, frontotemporal dementia, Jakob-Kreuztfeld disease, and dementia associated with Parkinson disease. The available treatments for dementia have been disappointing. At best, they are able to slow or delay the

progression of the disease. Unfortunately, there are also no highly effective, proven prevention strategies. Nevertheless, some evidence suggests that dementia due to AD can be delayed or prevented through the strategies detailed below.

Nutrition

Oxidative trauma and inflammation influence the development of AD. β-**Amyloid** has been implicated as a toxic substance; it is thought to participate in the destruction of neurons by generating free radicals. Studies have attempted to evaluate the effect of antioxidants in preventing the disease, but the results have been somewhat conflicting.

Observational studies have shown a reduced risk of AD development for those taking antioxidant supplements or those with diets containing generous amounts of antioxidants. The Rotterdam Study showed that those taking large amounts of vitamins C or E had a reduced risk of AD development. The Chicago Health and Aging Project showed similar results with vitamin E supplementation. However, other studies have not reported the association between antioxidant intake and AD prevention. The Washington Heights–Inwood Columbia Aging Project showed no benefits for the prevention of AD with an increased intake of vitamin C, vitamin E, or carotene. The effect of vitamin E on the progression of AD was evaluated by the Alzheimer's Disease Cooperative Study; their clinical trial studied the effects of vitamin E supplementation (400 IU/d) in patients with mild cognitive impairment. The results indicated that treatment with vitamin E did not slow the progression of mild cognitive impairment to AD. Similarly, the Women's Health Study monitored healthy women aged 65 years and older for nearly 10 years and observed no benefit of vitamin E supplementation for cognitive function. Recently published data suggest that vitamin E supplementation increases the risk of all-cause mortality. Consequently, this and the conflicting results of the vitamin E studies have dampened the enthusiasm about vitamin E supplementation for those with AD. No consistent evidence indicates that dietary antioxidants prevent or slow the progression of AD.

Homocysteine can be neurotoxic, and excess amounts are associated with vascular dementia and rapidly progressive AD. Low levels of folate, vitamin B_6, and vitamin B_{12} are associated with cognitive impairment and increased risk of AD, but studies have not consistently shown that supplementation prevents or slows the progression of AD. A study of 276 elderly individuals with elevated homocysteine levels showed no evidence of cognitive improvement after folate and vitamin B_{12} supplementation, even though homocysteine levels decreased in the treatment group. Another study reported that diets high in total fat, saturated fat, and cholesterol increased the risk of developing AD. Animal studies showed that diets high in saturated fat increase the deposition of β-amyloid within the central nervous system. High-fat diets, including those with saturated fats and hydrogenated (trans) fats, are associated with an increased risk of AD.

Some evidence suggests that a diet high in **fish and omega-3 fatty acids** decreases the risk of AD development. Although the data are conflicting, several large, longitudinal studies have shown that individuals with a generous dietary fish intake have a lower risk of AD development. The Framingham Heart Study showed that those in the top quartile of docosahexaenoic acid (an omega-3 fatty acid) ingestion had a lower incidence of dementia during 9 years of follow-up.

Several studies have examined the effects of a diet high in **fruits and vegetables** on the incidence of dementia. Again, the evidence is conflicting. Some studies suggest that diets containing generous amounts of fruits and vegetables are associated with a decreased incidence of dementia. Similarly, several studies have shown that those following a Mediterranean diet, which typically contains little red meat and high amounts of vegetables, fruits, whole grains, and olive oil, had a lower incidence of AD.

The effects of alcohol on cognitive function are complex. Several case-control studies have shown that moderate alcohol consumption is associated with a markedly reduced risk of dementia. Some studies suggest that this effect holds true, regardless of the type of alcohol ingested, whereas others have shown benefits only with wine. Chronic, heavy alcohol intake, however, has been associated with an increased incidence of dementia. Individuals who drink in moderation may be encouraged to continue to do so, but those who do not drink alcohol should not be encouraged to start drinking for the purpose of reducing their risk of dementia.

Caffeine is associated with reduced incidence of cerebral ischemia in animal studies, and it may provide some protection against the development of AD. The Canadian Study of Health and Aging showed a lower risk of AD in those who drank coffee.

Physical Activity and Lifestyle

Some evidence suggests that those with increased levels of physical activity have a reduced incidence of dementia, but the results have been inconsistent. The Canadian Study of Health and Aging showed a decreased risk of AD for those who had regular physical activity; apparently, **vigorous physical activity was not required**. Cognitive benefits accrued even with a regular walking program. Unfortunately, not all studies have shown that exercise reduces the progression or incidence of dementia. Several longitudinal, observational studies have indicated that **active social interactions** may have somewhat protective effects (reduced development of dementia). Similar findings have been shown for those who are physically active throughout life.

Pharmacologic Treatment

AD is associated with reduced production of choline acetyl transferase in the brain and a consequent reduction of the neurotransmitter acetylcholine. **Cholinesterase inhibitors** such as tacrine, donepezil, galantamine, and rivastigmine slow degradation of acetylcholine and increase its transmission across the synapse.

Cholinesterase inhibitors have been used in the treatment of AD for some time. They are indicated and approved for use in early AD. When effective, they temporarily delay the progression of the disease. More recently, they have been used to treat those with mild cognitive impairment. **Memantine**, an antagonist of the N-methyl-D-aspartate receptor, protects the receptor from excessive stimulation by the amino acid neurotransmitter glutamate. Unlike cholinesterase inhibitors, memantine may be a disease-modifying treatment for AD and may slow progression of the disease.

Early prospective and case-control studies showed a reduced risk of dementia in women who took estrogen-replacement therapy. Several small trials also indicated that estrogen slowed the progression of dementia. However, more recent evidence, including data from the Women's Health Initiative and the Women's Health Initiative Memory Study, observed no benefit of hormone-replacement therapy on the prevention of dementia; furthermore, they concluded that it may actually increase the risk.

Inflammation appears to have a role in the development of AD; this prompted evaluation of NSAIDs in the prevention of the disease. Some animal studies and several epidemiologic studies indicated some benefit after NSAID use in prevention of AD, but subsequent studies showed conflicting results. A large study of subjects taking low-dose aspirin showed no effect on the prevention of AD. Long-term use of NSAIDs is associated with clinically significant risks, which may exceed any potential benefit in the prevention of AD; thus, **chronic use of NSAIDs is not recommended** for the prevention of AD.

Several retrospective studies have shown that 3-hydroxy-3-methylglutaryl coenzyme A reductase inhibitors provide some benefit in the prevention of dementia, whereas prospective studies have shown variable results. *Ginkgo biloba* extract, a nutritional supplement, has been promoted as a treatment to improve cognitive function. Several trials have evaluated its effects on the progression of dementia. Some showed benefit, but the study designs and analyses of many of these studies have been criticized. A meta-analysis did not identify any benefit from *G biloba* supplementation.

- Alzheimer disease (AD) is the most common type of dementia (about 75% of all cases).
- Oxidative trauma and inflammation influence the development of AD. However, no consistent evidence

indicates that substantial levels of antioxidants (through diet or supplements) prevent or slow the progression of AD.

- High-fat diets, including those with saturated fats and hydrogenated (trans) fats, are associated with an increased risk of AD.
- Physical activity (moderate) and social interactions may reduce the risk of dementia.
- Cholinesterase inhibitors typically are used in the treatment of AD.

Hearing Disorders

Hearing loss can occur in 1 of 3 forms: sensorineural, conductive, or mixed. **Sensorineural loss** is caused by disorders of the inner ear, cochlea, or auditory nerve. **Conductive loss** occurs with disorders of the ear canal or middle ear or by abnormalities of the bones of the middle ear. **Mixed hearing loss** is a combination of sensorineural and conductive hearing loss.

Sensorineural hearing loss may be congenital and may be caused by various maternal viral infections during pregnancy, including rubella, cytomegalovirus, toxoplasmosis, human immunodeficiency virus infection, syphilis, or hepatitis. Substances such as alcohol, quinine, and various recreational drugs taken during pregnancy also may cause congenital hearing loss. Inherited disorders may be responsible for some cases of congenital sensorineural hearing loss.

Presbycusis is a sensorineural hearing loss that occurs in adults and becomes more common with advancing age. It is typically symmetric and involves decreased perception of higher frequencies. It is often associated with tinnitus. Previous exposure to loud noises tends to produce a similar, bilateral, high-frequency hearing loss. This may occur after very brief exposure to an extremely loud noise or, more commonly, after chronic exposure to a noisy environment. Infection of the cochlea may result in an acquired sensorineural hearing loss. The cause is usually a viral infection, typically meningitis in children. Various medications can also cause hearing loss, including antibiotics (aminoglycosides, tetracycline, erythromycin, or vancomycin) and chemotherapy agents (cisplatin, 5-fluorouracil, nitrogen mustard, or bleomycin).

High-dose aspirin or use of quinine or chloroquine may produce a reversible, high-frequency hearing loss. Other acquired causes include demyelinating disorders (eg, multiple sclerosis), Meniere disease, acoustic neuroma, head trauma, or an ischemic vascular event. Malignancies of the inner ear rarely are responsible for sensorineural hearing loss. Autoimmune conditions that can cause sensorineural hearing loss include rheumatoid arthritis, systemic lupus, Wegener granulomatosis, or polyarteritis nodosa. Asymmetric sensorineural hearing loss should not be assumed to be due to presbycusis; other causes should be investigated.

Conductive hearing loss can have **congenital and acquired causes**. Developmental abnormalities can result in stenosis of the external auditory canal or absence or malformation of the auricle. Atresia (a deformity of the bony ossicles) can cause conductive hearing loss. Acquired causes of conductive hearing loss include infection of the external auditory canal (external otitis), debris within the canal, or swelling because of inflammation. Otitis media can also cause conductive hearing loss due to the fluid accumulating in the middle ear space. Perforation of the tympanic membrane can result in conductive hearing loss, the degree of which depends on the location and extent of the perforation. The external auditory canal can be affected by squamous cell carcinoma, basal cell carcinoma, or (rarely) melanoma. Occlusion of the canal by excessive bony growths due to exostosis or an osteoma can produce conductive hearing loss. Benign polyps of the external canal are uncommon but can occlude the auditory canal. The 2 most common causes of conductive hearing loss are cerumen impaction of the external auditory canal and eustachian tube dysfunction.

Cholesteatoma, excessive squamous cells within the middle ear space, can destroy the ossicles and eventually erode into bone, sinuses, or even the brain. Otosclerosis produces an overgrowth of bone involving the stapes, resulting in impaired function of the ossicle and hearing loss.

Although guidelines regarding hearing testing are not well established, a simple but reasonably sensitive indicator of potential hearing loss is to ask patients whether they have any difficulty with their hearing. A very effective office screening test for hearing loss is the **whispered voice test**. It has a fairly high sensitivity and specificity for hearing loss. Although the Rinne and Weber tuning fork tests can also be performed in the office, many providers find the results somewhat difficult to interpret. It is appropriate to pursue formal audiometric testing for patients with routine occupational exposure to loud noise, patients who have participated in activities involving loud noise exposure (eg, firearm use), and patients who indicate some difficulty with their hearing. More formal screening tests for hearing loss include pure-tone audiometric testing and tests for speech discrimination. Additional, more sophisticated testing is also available if screening tests suggest a hearing problem.

- Sensorineural loss is caused by disorders of the inner ear, cochlea, or auditory nerve. Conductive loss occurs with disorders of the ear canal or middle ear or by abnormalities of the bones of the middle ear. Mixed hearing loss is a combination of sensorineural and conductive hearing loss.
- Very brief exposure to an extremely loud noise or, more commonly, chronic exposure to a noisy

environment can produce a bilateral, high-frequency hearing loss.

- The most common causes of conductive hearing loss are cerumen impaction of the external auditory canal and eustachian tube dysfunction.
- A reasonably sensitive indicator of potential hearing loss is to ask patients if they have any difficulty with their hearing. A very effective office screening test for hearing loss is the whispered voice test.

Osteoporosis

Hip fracture after age 50 years has a 1-year mortality rate of 20%. It results in substantial morbidity and is a frequent cause for nursing home admission (20% of patients). Six months after a hip fracture, only 15% of people are able to walk across a room without help. The main risk factor for hip fracture is osteoporosis. The cost of osteoporosis-related fractures is estimated to be $25 billion by 2025. The Surgeon General's report on bone health indicates that 10 million Americans (8 million women and 2 million men) have osteoporosis and 44 million have **osteopenia**. Forty percent of white women and 13% of white men will have an osteoporosis-related fracture after age 50 years.

All women 65 years and older and women aged 60 to 64 years with risk factors for osteoporosis should be screened. Rescreening should take place no more than every 2 years; for younger women, it probably can be done at 5-year intervals. The USPSTF "makes no recommendation for or against routine osteoporosis screening in postmenopausal women who are younger than 60 or in women aged 60-64 who are not at increased risk for osteoporotic fractures" (grade C recommendation). Other organizations recommend screening all postmenopausal women, except for those taking hormone-replacement therapy. Box 4 shows risk factors for osteoporosis.

Guidelines for screening men have not been established. Men who have had **fragility fractures** (fracture after a fall from standing height or less) should be screened for osteoporosis. Generally, screening men with a history of hypogonadism or prolonged corticosteroid use seems prudent; consideration should also be given to screening men older than 75 years and those with a family history of osteoporosis.

Bone mineral density testing with dual energy x-ray absorptiometry is the screening test of choice. Bone density is expressed as T scores and Z scores. The T score is the difference in number of standard deviations between the patient and the average value for young women with peak bone mass. The Z score is the difference in number of standard deviations between the individual and age-matched controls. Osteoporosis is defined as a **T score of −2.5 or lower**. Osteopenia is defined as a T score between −1.0 and −2.4. For patients with a Z score of −1.0 or lower

Box 4 Risk Factors for Osteoporosis

Low body weight (<57 kg or body mass index <20 kg/m²)

Family history of fracture or osteoporosis

Current smoker

Menopause before age 40 y

Glucocorticoid therapy (dosage, 7.5 mg/d or higher)

Prolonged immobilization (bedrest or wheelchair, >1 y)

Transplant recipient

Chemotherapy

Men with hypogonadism >5 y

Personal history of fragility fracture

Radiographic evidence of osteopenia or vertebral fracture

European or Asian heritage

Excessive vitamin A intake OR insufficient calcium or vitamin D intake

Excessive alcohol consumption

Specific medications (heparin, anticonvulsant agents, lithium)

(which will include premenopausal women and most men), other causes of osteoporosis should be considered. Diagnostic tests may include parathyroid hormone and thyroid-stimulating hormone (TSH) for hyperthyroidism, vitamin D for deficiency, serum protein electrophoresis for myeloma, transglutaminase antibodies for celiac disease, free cortisol in a 24-hour urine sample for Cushing disease, and testosterone levels in men for hypogonadism. It is also important to avoid overreplacement of thyroid hormone because this can increase bone loss.

Prevention of osteoporosis should begin in childhood because bone mass peaks in late adolescence; the higher the peak bone mass, the lower the risk of osteoporosis. Exercise in childhood and early adolescence results in higher peak bone mass.

Studies suggest that **dietary calcium** (1,200 mg/d or more) and vitamin D (800 U/d) may help prevent the development of osteoporosis and subsequent hip fracture. However, excessive calcium intake is not more effective; similarly, insufficient intake of vitamin D (eg, 400 U) also is not effective. Patients with osteoporosis should also consume at least 1,200 mg/d of calcium and 800 U/d of vitamin D. Calcium carbonate is less expensive than calcium citrate, but it is associated with a higher risk of kidney stones and stomach upset. Caffeine causes **urinary calcium excretion** and may increase the risk of hip fracture. Vitamin D also appears to have a beneficial effect on muscle strength and seems to reduce the risk of falls. Circumstantial evidence indicates that vitamin D may decrease the risk of colon cancer, multiple sclerosis, and possibly other cancers and heart disease. Calcium and vitamin D recommendations from the National Osteoporosis Foundation are shown in Table 3.

Table 3 Dietary Calcium and Vitamin D
Recommendations of the National Osteoporosis
Foundation

Population and Age	Calcium, mg/d	Vitamin D, IU/d
Children and adolescents		
1-3 y	500	400[a]
4-8 y	800	400[a]
9-18 y	1,300	400[a]
Adult women and men		
19-49 y	1,000	400-800
≥50 y	1,200	800-1,000
Pregnant and breastfeeding women		
≤18 y	1,300	400-800
>18 y	1,000	400-800

[a] The National Osteoporosis Foundation does not have specific vitamin D recommendations for these age groups. These are the recommendations of the American Academy of Pediatrics.
Adapted from the National Osteoporosis Foundation [Internet]. Washington, DC: the Foundation. What you should know about calcium; 2008 [cited Sep 2009]. Available from: http://www.nof.org/prevention/calcium2.htm. Used with permission.

Exercise slightly improves bone density of the spine. Regular walking can help prevent hip fractures by reducing the risk of falling, but only high-impact aerobic exercise improves hip bone density. Exercise has a greater benefit on bone density when calcium intake is adequate (1,000 mg/d or more). The main reason to recommend exercise to patients with osteopenia and osteoporosis is because it reduces the risk of falls and therefore the risk of hip fracture. In the Nurse's Health Study, walking 4 hours or more per week reduced the incidence of hip fracture by 40% compared with walking for 1 hour or less.

The National Osteoporosis Foundation has recently released the *Clinician's Guide to Prevention and Treatment of Osteoprosis*, which includes an algorithm for when to begin medical therapy for osteoporosis. If the 10-year risk of hip fracture is greater than 3% or if the 10-year risk of total fracture is greater than 20%, then medication is warranted. First-line treatment usually is with **bisphosphonates** or **estrogen** (in selected patients); both can reduce subsequent risk of fracture, especially for patients who consume adequate calcium and vitamin D. Parathyroid hormone therapy is reserved for patients who do not respond to first-line therapy. Thiazide diuretics are not prescribed for osteoporosis, but they do reduce urinary calcium excretion, improve bone density, and are associated with a lower risk of hip fracture. For older patients with hypertension, thiazides are a good choice because they also benefit bone health. Calcitonin is a third-line treatment that is most helpful for patients with painful spinal vertebral fractures. Hip pads reduce the risk of hip fracture with falls and should be considered for those with high risk. All patients with osteoporosis should be advised to stop smoking and to limit alcohol use.

Follow-up bone-density testing for patients with osteoporosis should be performed no more than every 2 years, with the possible exception of those taking corticosteroids and those who have recently stopped hormone-replacement therapy. Routine measurement of markers of bone turnover is not recommended.

- Prevention of osteoporosis should begin in childhood because bone mass peaks in late adolescence; the higher the peak bone mass, the lower the risk of osteoporosis. Exercise in childhood and early adolescence results in higher peak bone mass.
- The main risk factor for hip fracture is osteoporosis. Exercise reduces the risk of falls and therefore reduces the risk of hip fracture.
- All women 65 years and older, women aged 60 to 64 years with risk factors for osteoporosis, men with fragility fractures, and possibly all men 75 years and older should be screened every other year.
- Bone mineral density testing with dual energy x-ray absorptiometry is the screening test of choice.
- First-line treatment of osteoporosis usually is with bisphosphonates or estrogen.

Psychiatric Illnesses and Stress

Depression and Suicide

The World Health Organization rated depression as the fourth-leading cause of disease in the world, ahead of ischemic heart disease. Depression occurs in 5% to 9% of US adults. The risk is higher for women, persons with a family history of depression, unemployed persons, and patients with chronic disease. Depression results in considerable disability ($17 billion annually) and is a leading risk factor for suicide.

Screening for depression can be done with various formal instruments, including the Zung Self-Rating Depression Scale, the Beck Depression Inventory, the General Health Questionnaire, and the Center for Epidemiologic Studies Depression Scale. The best questions are 1) "Over the past 2 weeks, have you felt down, depressed, or hopeless?" and 2) "Over the past 2 weeks, have you felt little interest or pleasure in doing things?" The USPSTF "recommends screening adults for depression in clinical practices that have systems in place to assure accurate diagnosis, effective treatment, and followup" (grade B recommendation) but "concludes the evidence is insufficient to recommend for or against routine screening of children or adolescents for depression" (grade I statement). The American Academy of Pediatrics recommends screening all adolescents for depression and suicidal ideation.

Approximately one-third of patients with a positive screening test result will have major depression. Other patients may have a dysthymic disorder, minor depression, anxiety disorder, grief reaction, substance abuse, panic disorder, or posttraumatic stress disorder. Further questioning is necessary using the Diagnostic and Statistical Manual of Mental Disorders (fourth edition) criteria for depression (Box 5) to determine if a patient has major depression.

Depression often is treated inadequately. Major depression warrants treatment with antidepressant medication or cognitive-behavioral therapy (or preferably both). Patients should know that the adverse effects of medications often resolve with continued use. Medications generally take 4 to 6 weeks to help with depression, and it is important to **continue medication for at least 1 year**. Psychiatric consultation is indicated if a patient has psychotic features, the possibility of bipolar disorder, or a significant suicide risk. Depression may be treated in several ways (Box 6).

Suicide is the eighth-leading cause of death in the United States. Eighteen percent of patients with major depression will attempt suicide (24% of patients with bipolar disorder attempt suicide), whereas 1% of patients without mental disorders will attempt suicide. Depression is thought to contribute to 60% of completed suicides. Other risk factors include substance abuse, schizophrenia, psychotic depression, recent panic attacks, rapid switching from depression to anxiety to anger, and severe hopelessness.

The suicide rate among American adolescents is the highest in the world. The best strategy for suicide prevention is early identification and treatment of depression. The great majority of those who attempt suicide remain alive, but about 20% of those who complete suicide have made previous attempts. Physicians have an important role because 75% of persons who completed suicide saw a physician (usually in primary care) in the 6 months before suicide, and 50% saw a physician in the month before suicide.

Bipolar Disorder

Bipolar disorder affects about 1% of US adults. In addition to the **depression** (described above), patients have episodes of **mania** (type 1 bipolar disorder) or **hypomania** (type 2 bipolar disorder). Symptoms of mania include euphoria, restlessness, irritability, racing thoughts (jumping from one idea to another), lack of sleep, poor concentration, spending sprees, promiscuity, unrealistic beliefs about one's abilities, drug abuse, and aggressive behavior. A manic episode is defined by elevated mood plus 3 other above symptoms that lasts for most of each day and for longer than a week. It is important to recognize bipolar disorder because treatment of depressive episodes with antidepressants can trigger a manic episode. **Mood stabilizers**

Box 5 Criteria for Major Depression

A. Five (or more) of the following symptoms have been present during the same 2-week period and represent a change from previous functioning; at least one of the symptoms is either 1) depressed mood or 2) loss of interest or pleasure.[a]

   1) Depressed mood most of the day, nearly every day, as indicated by either subjective report (eg, feels sad or empty) or observation made by others (eg, appears tearful). For children and adolescents, consider irritable mood.

   2) Markedly diminished interest or pleasure in all or almost all activities most of the day, nearly every day, as indicated by subjective account or observation by others.

   3) Marked weight loss when not dieting, weight gain (eg, a change of more than 5% of body weight in a month), or decrease or increase in appetite nearly every day. For children, consider failure to make expected weight gain.

   4) Insomnia or hypersomnia nearly every day.

   5) Psychomotor agitation or retardation nearly every day (observable by others, not just subjective feelings of restlessness or being slowed down).

   6) Fatigue or loss of energy nearly every day.

   7) Feelings of worthlessness or excessive or inappropriate guilt nearly every day (may be delusional; not just self-reproach or guilt about being sick).

   8) Diminished ability to think or concentrate, or indecisiveness, nearly every day (either by subjective account or as observed by others).

   9) Recurrent thoughts of death (not just fear of dying), recurrent suicidal ideation without a specific plan, a specific plan for committing suicide or a suicide attempt.

B. The symptoms do not meet criteria for a mixed episode (no evidence of bipolar disorder).

C. The symptoms cause clinically significant distress or impairment in social, occupational, or other important areas of functioning.

D. The symptoms are not due to the direct physiological effects of a substance (eg, a drug of abuse, a medication) or a general medical condition (eg, hypothyroidism).

E. The symptoms are not likely to be due to bereavement (eg, after the loss of a loved one). Symptoms persist for longer than 2 months or are characterized by marked functional impairment, morbid preoccupation with worthlessness, suicidal ideation, psychotic symptoms, or psychomotor retardation.

---

[a] Do not include symptoms that are clearly due to a general medical condition, mood-incongruent delusions, or hallucinations.

Adapted from the Diagnostic and Statistical Manual of Mental Disorders: DSM-IV. Washington, DC: American Psychiatric Association; c1994. Used with permission.

such as lithium or valproate should be prescribed for most patients with bipolar disorder because they can prevent manic episodes from occurring. Suicide risk is increased, and recognition and early treatment may prevent this outcome.

Box 6 Treatments for Depression

Antidepressants

    Selective serotonin-reuptake inhibitors

    Tricyclic antidepressants

    Heterocyclics

    Monoamine oxidase inhibitors

Other treatments

    Psychotherapy (individual, group, and family therapy)

    Light therapy (increased exposure to natural or artificial light)

    Electroconvulsive therapy for severe and prolonged depression

Stress

It is intuitively obvious but empirically difficult to demonstrate that stress affects mortality. Multiple aspects of stress have been measured and correlated with outcome. Among the best studied aspects are hostility (a component of the type A personality), depression, and job strain (defined as a job with high demands but low levels of control). These constructs appear to be associated with higher total and cardiovascular deaths (although not all studies agree).

Job strain has been associated with recurrent events for patients with known cardiac disease and also has been linked to a higher risk of depression. One aspect of job strain may be perceived injustice (perceived unfair treatment by supervisors). This has been related to psychiatric and cardiac morbidity, independent of job strain, in the Whitehall Study. Job strain also appears to be a risk factor for the development of depression and hypertension.

Another source of stress is marital relationship difficulties. The Stockholm Female Coronary Risk Study and the Whitehall II Study both showed increased incidence of coronary events that was concurrent with marital relationship difficulties. Marital difficulties also increase the risk of depression. Physical exercise, cognitive-behavioral therapy, rational emotive therapy, meditation, and social support (including self-help groups) can all combat stress. Recognizing that one has control over how one responds to environmental stimuli is helpful. Type A patients usually find this approach to be the most helpful suggestion for dealing with stress.

- Depression is thought to contribute to 60% of completed suicides. The best strategy for suicide prevention is early identification and treatment of depression.
- Major depression should be treated with antidepressant medication or cognitive-behavioral therapy (preferably both).
- Patients with bipolar disorder must be recognized because treatment of depressive episodes with antidepressants can trigger a manic episode.

- Hostility, depression, and job strain may be associated with higher total and cardiovascular deaths. Marital relationship difficulties are associated with increased incidence of coronary events and increased risk of depression.

Thyroid Disorders

For thyroid disease, the most important preventive measure worldwide is dietary **iodine supplementation**. Iodine is necessary for the synthesis of thyroid hormones, which are essential for brain development. Thus, iodine deficiency is the most common cause of intellectual deficiency worldwide.

Iodine deficiency generally is not a problem in the United States, where iodized salt commonly is used. The benefits of screening adults for thyroid disease are unclear. The USPSTF "concludes the evidence is insufficient to recommend for or against routine screening for thyroid disease in adults" (grade I statement). The American Thyroid Association recommends checking TSH levels every 5 years, beginning at age 35, whereas the American College of Physicians recommends screening women older than 50 years who have any general symptoms that could be attributable to thyroid disease. Patients should be screened if they have Down syndrome, Turner syndrome, type 1 diabetes mellitus, a history of radiotherapy to the neck or thyroid surgery, or are taking lithium, interferon, or amiodarone.

The screening test of choice measures **TSH levels**. Generally, patients with a TSH level exceeding 10 mU/L should be treated; such patients usually report feeling better with treatment. For patients with subclinical hypothyroidism or mild thyroid failure, treatment is more controversial. If **antibodies to thyroid peroxidase** are present, the patient has a 5% chance of converting to overt hypothyroidism during the next 20 years (if no thyroid peroxidase antibodies are detected, the patient has a 2% chance). Pregnant women or women trying to conceive should be treated if TSH levels are between 5 and 10 mU/L. In a Dutch study of 558 adults aged 85 to 89 years, low TSH was associated with a higher mortality rate, and elevated TSH was associated with a reduced mortality rate. Thus, in the oldest patients, treatment is not indicated for TSH levels between 5 and 10 mU/L. A useful algorithm for treating nonpregnant adults younger than 80 years is shown in the Figure.

Treatment is with **levothyroxine**, which should be taken on an empty stomach. Levothyroxine cannot be taken concurrently with calcium, iron, or aluminum (antacids). A TSH goal of 1 to 3 mU/L is recommended; overtreatment (TSH <0.3 mU/L) should be avoided because of increased risk of osteoporosis and atrial fibrillation. TSH should be checked 8 weeks after initiating or changing therapy and then at 1-year intervals.

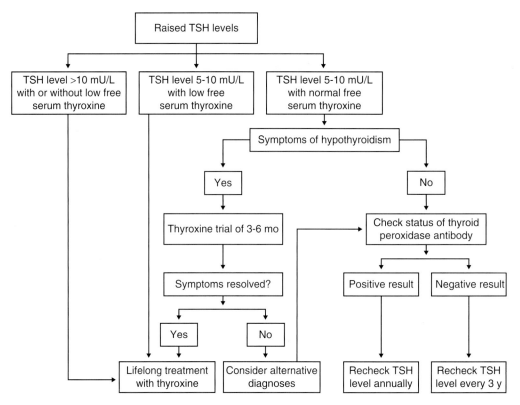

Figure Algorithm for Management of Primary Hypothyroidism in Nonpregnant Adults. TSH denotes thyroid-stimulating hormone. (Adapted from Vaidya B, Pearce SHS. Management of hypothyroidism in adults. BMJ. 2008;337:a801;doi.10.1136.bmj.a801. Used with permission.)

Radiotherapy to the neck during childhood is a major risk factor for the development of thyroid cancer. Such high-risk patients should be monitored yearly. Some experts suggest ultrasonographic follow-up as well, but this is controversial. Radiotherapy to the neck as an adult is a risk factor for hypothyroidism but not for thyroid cancer. Potassium iodide will prevent development of thyroid cancer if it is administered promptly after radiation exposure. **Medullary carcinoma** of the thyroid is a rare familial cancer. All first-degree relatives of such patients should be screened for mutations in the *RET* proto-oncogene. If a mutation is identified, annual screening starting at age 6 years is indicated, and prophylactic thyroidectomy should be considered because the risk of cancer development is 90%.

Patients with thyroid nodules should be referred for possible aspiration. Imaging is rarely useful in such settings. Patients with hyperthyroidism should have an iodine uptake scan to determine whether hyperthyroidism is due to Graves autoimmune disease or thyroiditis.

- Iodine is necessary for the synthesis of thyroid hormones, which are essential for brain development. Thus, iodine deficiency is the most common cause of intellectual deficiency worldwide.

- Generally, patients with a thyroid-stimulating hormone (TSH) level exceeding 10 mU/L should be treated with levothyroxine. Patients with thyroid nodules should be referred for possible aspiration.

Visual Impairment

Impaired vision is very common with advancing age; it has numerous social implications and influences the quality of life and independence of affected individuals. The most common causes of clinically significant visual impairment are macular degeneration, glaucoma, and cataracts.

Age-Related Macular Degeneration

Age-related macular degeneration affects the portion of the retina associated with central vision and causes considerable difficulty in reading and driving. It is the **leading cause of blindness in US adults**. The incidence increases dramatically after age 65 years. Macular degeneration exists in 2 forms, neovascular (wet) and atrophic (dry). Although the atrophic form is more common, those with severe vision loss from macular degeneration more commonly have the neovascular form. The neovascular form has greater potential for treatment. Although the development of macular degeneration has a genetic component, some evidence suggests that smoking increases the risk. Diet, hypertension, and cardiovascular disease also may have a role.

The Age-Related Eye Disease Study examined the effect of consuming high levels of antioxidants (vitamin C, vitamin E, β-carotene) and zinc. It showed reduced progression for individuals with advanced, unilateral macular degeneration but no benefit for those with mild disease or advanced, bilateral disease. However, β-carotene supplementation may be associated with an increased risk of lung cancer in smokers and possibly an increased risk of CAD. Vitamin E supplementation may increase all-cause mortality and the risk of heart failure. These findings limit the recommendations for the use of β-carotene and vitamin E for those with macular degeneration.

Intravenous administration of a photosensitive dye, followed by treatment with a photo-activating laser, has been used with some success in the management of wet macular degeneration. However, it has no role in the treatment of dry macular degeneration.

Glaucoma

The term "glaucoma" is used to describe various diseases that ultimately damage the optic nerve. Glaucoma generally is diagnosed by findings of a funduscopic examination (eg, **damage to the optic nerve**) and visual field loss in the setting of **elevated intraocular pressure**. Untreated glaucoma eventually results in blindness. There are 4 major types of glaucoma: 1) primary open-angle glaucoma, 2) acute angle-closure glaucoma, 3) secondary glaucoma, and 4) congenital glaucoma.

Primary open-angle glaucoma is the most common type of glaucoma and the most common cause of irreversible blindness worldwide. Primary open-angle glaucoma generally is not associated with external ocular findings. Risk factors include older age, African American heritage, elevated intraocular pressure, and a family history of glaucoma. Other suspected risk factors include hypertension, diabetes mellitus, hypothyroidism, cardiovascular disease, and myopia. Those who use corticosteroids (oral, inhaled, ophthalmic forms) also appear to have increased risk. The relationship between glaucoma and elevated intraocular pressure is somewhat controversial. Although most patients with glaucoma have elevated intraocular pressure, a considerable number do not, and some individuals with elevated intraocular pressure never have clinical features of glaucoma.

Acute angle-closure glaucoma accounts for about 10% of all glaucoma cases in the United States. It is caused by the narrowing or closure of the anterior chamber angle, which prevents adequate drainage of the intraocular

aqueous humor. Without adequate drainage of the aqueous humor, subsequently increased intraocular pressure rapidly damages the optic nerve. Angle-closure glaucoma presents with symptoms such as eye pain, reduced vision, halos around lights, headache, nausea, and vomiting. Increasing intraocular pressure often is associated with conjunctival erythema, cloudiness of the cornea, a fixed, mildly dilated pupil, and a shallow anterior eye chamber. Risk factors for angle-closure glaucoma include age older than 40 years, a family history of angle-closure glaucoma, female sex, hyperopia, and Asian or Inuit heritage.

Secondary glaucoma is caused by an underlying disease or previous eye trauma. It may be associated with chronic corticosteroid use, uveitis, or vasoproliferative retinopathy. Treatment of secondary glaucoma should involve management of the underlying disease. Congenital glaucoma is associated with various causes.

The USPSTF "found insufficient evidence to recommend for or against screening adults for glaucoma" (grade I statement). Those with high risk of glaucoma should be referred to an ophthalmologist.

Cataracts

Cataracts reduce visual acuity and impair color discrimination by clouding and yellowing the crystalline lens. In most patients, cataracts are bilateral, although the cataract in one eye may be more advanced than the other. Cataracts are the most common cause of blindness worldwide, but in developed countries, they usually are treated before blindness occurs. Several types of cataracts exist; these may be classified by the cause of the cataract (congenital, age-related, medication-induced, or traumatic) or the anatomic location of the lens opacification (anterior, nuclear, or posterior).

A risk factor for the development of all cataract types is increased alcohol use. Some cataracts are associated with various disease states, including diabetes mellitus, increased exposure to solar ultraviolet radiation, and use of either systemic or inhaled corticosteroids. Smokers have a 2-fold higher risk of developing nuclear cataracts than nonsmokers (risk can be decreased by smoking cessation). No evidence supports use of any vitamin, nutritional supplement, or sunglasses to prevent cataract development or slow disease progression. The most effective treatment is resection of the cloudy lens and an intraocular lens insertion. The decision regarding timing of cataract surgery is not based purely on visual acuity but on the patient's perception of impaired lifestyle.

- Age-related macular degeneration is the leading cause of blindness in US adults.
- Smoking appears to increase risk of macular degeneration. Diet, hypertension, and cardiovascular disease also may have a role.

- Untreated glaucoma eventually results in irreversible blindness. It often occurs with high intraocular pressure.
- Primary open-angle glaucoma is not associated with specific symptoms, but angle-closure glaucoma presents with eye pain, reduced vision, halos around lights, headache, nausea, vomiting, or some combination of symptoms.
- Cataracts are the most common cause of blindness worldwide.
- A risk factor for the development of all cataract types is increased alcohol use. No evidence supports use of any vitamin, nutritional supplement, or sunglasses to prevent cataract development or slow disease progression.

SUGGESTED READING

Bateman ED, Hurd SS, Barnes PJ, Bousquet J, Drazen JM, FitzGerald M, et al. Global strategy for asthma management and prevention: GINA executive summary. Eur Respir J. 2008 Jan;31(1):143-78.

Boden WE, O'Rourke RA, Teo KK, Hartigan PM, Maron DJ, Kostuk WJ, et al; COURAGE Trial Research Group. Optimal medical therapy with or without PCI for stable coronary disease. N Engl J Med. 2007 Apr 12;356(15):1503-16. Epub 2007 Mar 26.

Congdon N, O'Colmain B, Klaver CC, Klein R, Munoz B, Friedman DS, et al; Eye Diseases Prevalence Research Group. Causes and prevalence of visual impairment among adults in the United States. Arch Ophthalmol. 2004 Apr;122(4):477-85.

GOLD, the Global initiative for chronic Obstructive Lung Disease [Internet]. Portland (OR): GOLD; Executive summary: global strategy for the diagnosis, management and prevention of chronic obstructive pulmonary disease [cited Feb 2008]. Available from: http://www.gold-copd.org.

Knowler WC, Barrett-Connor E, Fowler SE, Hamman RF, Lachin JM, Walker EA, et al; Diabetes Prevention Program Research Group. Reduction in the incidence of type 2 diabetes with lifestyle intervention or metformin. N Engl J Med. 2002 Feb 7;346(6):393-403.

National Osteoporosis Foundation [Internet]. Washington, DC: NOF; c2008. Clinician's guide to the prevention and treatment of osteoporosis [cited 2 Mar 2009]. Available from: http://www.nof.org/professionals/Clinicians_Guide.htm.

Raina P, Santaguida P, Ismaila A, Patterson C, Cowan D, Levine M, et al. Effectiveness of cholinesterase inhibitors and memantine for treating dementia: evidence review for a clinical practice guideline. Ann Intern Med. 2008 Mar 4;148(5):379-97.

U.S. Preventive Services Task Force. Screening for dementia: recommendation and rationale. Ann Intern Med. 2003 Jun 3;138(11):925-6.

Yusuf S, Hawken S, Ounpuu S, Dans T, Avezum A, Lanas F, et al; INTERHEART Study Investigators. Effect of potentially modifiable risk factors associated with myocardial infarction in 52 countries (the INTERHEART study): case-control study. Lancet. 2004 Sep 11-17; 364(9438):937-52.

Questions and Answers

Questions

1. Which of the following statements about risk for coronary artery disease is true?
   a. Only 50% of coronary disease is explained by conventional risk factors.
   b. Body mass index is a better predictor of risk than waist-to-hip ratio.
   c. Activity levels and fitness levels are independent predictors of coronary disease.
   d. Low-density lipoprotein (LDL) cholesterol and high-density lipoprotein (HDL) cholesterol are equal to or better than apolipoprotein B (Apo B) and apolipoprotein AI (Apo AI) for predicting coronary disease.
   e. Diastolic hypertension is a better predictor of coronary disease than systolic hypertension.

2. Which of the following statements about primary prevention of coronary disease is true?
   a. Aspirin should be recommended to all patients aged 50 years and older.
   b. The American Heart Association Step II Diet is more effective at improving the LDL-to-HDL ratio than the Mediterranean diet.
   c. Nuts should be avoided because they are high in fat.
   d. Stress reduction programs have proven benefit in preventing heart disease.
   e. Although moderate alcohol consumption has been associated with less coronary disease in many studies, little evidence indicates that red wine is associated with greater risk reduction than other forms of alcohol.

3. Which of the following statements concerning diabetes mellitus is *false*?
   a. The relative risk of diabetes mellitus in patients with a body mass index (BMI) of 22 to 25 kg/m^2 is double that of patients with a BMI of 20 to 22 kg/m^2.
   b. Although lifestyle changes can help prevent diabetes mellitus, metformin is more effective than lifestyle change.
   c. Aggressive treatment of hypertension and hyperlipidemia has proven benefit in diabetes mellitus, but aggressive treatment of hyperglycemia is not associated with improved mortality rates.
   d. Diabetic patients who walk 4 hours or more every week reduce their risk of cardiac death by greater than 50%.
   e. Diets high in fruit and vegetables, whole grains, and magnesium are associated with a lower risk of diabetes mellitus.

4. Which of the following statements concerning osteoporosis is true?
   a. Studies show that 800 U of vitamin D is effective in preventing fractures, whereas 400 U is ineffective.
   b. Screening for osteoporosis in women should begin at menopause.
   c. All patients with osteoporosis should be screened for secondary causes such as multiple myeloma and hyperparathyroidism.
   d. Patients with osteoporosis should be monitored by dual energy x-ray absorptiometry scanning every year.
   e. Walking improves hip bone density.

5. Which of the following occupations is *not* associated with an increased risk of occupational asthma?
   a. Baker
   b. Nurse
   c. Painter
   d. Professional athlete
   e. Farmer

6. Which of the following statements about glaucoma is true?
   a. Acute angle-closure glaucoma is the most common form of the disease.
   b. Elevated intraocular pressure is required for a diagnosis of primary open-angle glaucoma.

c. A risk factor for primary open-angle glaucoma is being of African American heritage.

d. Most patients with glaucoma have a family history of disease.

e. Classic visual abnormalities resulting from glaucoma include a loss of central vision.

7. Which of the following statements about cataracts is true?

a. Cataracts are the most common cause of blindness for adults in the United States.

b. Smoking increases the risk of developing cataracts.

c. The use of sunglasses will decrease the likelihood of developing cataracts.

d. Cataract formation is usually unilateral.

e. Cataract surgery should be performed when a patient's vision is 20/100 or worse.

8. Which of the following statements about age-related macular degeneration is true?

a. It is the leading cause of blindness for adults in developed countries.

b. The classic symptom is peripheral vision loss.

c. The wet form of age-related macular degeneration is more common than the dry form.

d. High-dose antioxidants can reverse some of the pathology associated with age-related macular degeneration.

e. Laser therapy is effective for most patients with the dry form of age-related macular degeneration.

9. Which of the following statements regarding Alzheimer disease (AD) is true?

a. High-dose vitamin E has consistently been shown to reduce the risk of AD development.

b. Cholinesterase inhibitors are indicated only for those with advanced AD.

c. Data from the Women's Health Initiative showed that hormone-replacement therapy reduced the risk of AD development.

d. *Ginkgo biloba* extracts have not been shown to reduce the risk of AD development.

e. Some evidence suggests that nonsteroidal antiinflammatory drugs are somewhat protective against dementia. They are recommended for patients with increased risk of AD development.

Answers

1. Answer c.

Activity and fitness predict outcome independent of each other (ie, they are both important). The INTERHEART study found that greater than 90% of coronary artery disease can be explained by common risk factors. Waist-to-hip ratio was considerably better than obesity when predicting coronary disease in this study. Apo B and Apo AI are better predictors than LDL and HDL and should be used to monitor patients with known coronary disease. Systolic hypertension is of equal importance to diastolic hypertension and more important in the elderly when predicting coronary disease.

2. Answer e.

The 2 largest studies of alcohol and heart disease (from the American Cancer Society [Alcohol Consumption and Mortality Among Middle-Aged and Elderly Adults] and Kaiser-Permanente [Relationships Between Alcoholic Beverage Use and Other Traits To Blood Pressure]) found no difference between red wine and other forms of alcohol. Most healthy women do not have sufficiently high risk of heart disease (6% or higher) to warrant aspirin therapy until age 65. The Step II diet replaces fat with carbohydrate, which results in small reductions of LDL and HDL cholesterol levels. A Mediterranean diet is preferred because it replaces saturated fat with monounsaturated fat, lowering LDL without changing HDL. Nuts (especially walnuts and almonds) are high in unsaturated fats and appear to have beneficial effects on cholesterol levels and heart disease. Although stress, depression, and type A personality traits appear to increase the risk of heart disease, the studies of treatment have reported mixed results.

3. Answer b.

In the Diabetes Prevention Program study, lifestyle changes were more effective than metformin for preventing the development of diabetes mellitus.

4. Answer a.

Randomized trials have not shown any benefit from regular doses of vitamin D, but intake of 800 U/day appears to reduce the risk of fracture. Screening for osteoporosis is recommended for women age 65 years and older (select women should be screened starting at age 60 to 64 years). Only patients with a Z score of −1.0 or lower should be evaluated for secondary causes of osteoporosis. Bone densitometry measurement is recommended no more frequently than every other year. Although walking reduces the risk of hip fracture by reducing the risk of falling, only high-impact aerobic exercise improves hip bone density.

5. Answer d.

Bakers can become sensitive to flour dust, nurses and painters to latex, and farmers to grain dust.

6. Answer c.

Individuals of African American descent have an increased risk for the development of primary open-angle glaucoma. The prevalence exceeds 11% in those older than age 80. Glaucoma is also the leading cause of irreversible blindness in those of African American descent. Primary open-angle glaucoma is the most common form of glaucoma; angle-closure glaucoma accounts for only 10% of all glaucoma cases. Although most patients with open-angle glaucoma have elevated intraocular pressure, some have normal intraocular pressure. A small percentage of patients with primary open-angle glaucoma have genetic risk factors (ie, family history of glaucoma). These individuals often show signs of disease by age 40 years. Glaucoma typically affects peripheral vision, not central vision.

7. Answer b.

Smoking increases the risk of cataract development by a factor of 2. There is a dose-response relationship between smoking and cataracts. Although cataracts are the most common cause of blindness worldwide, in developed countries, cataracts usually are treated before blindness occurs. Exposure to ultraviolet light is considered a risk factor for the development of cataracts; however, use of sunglasses has not been shown to prevent or slow the progression of cataracts. Cataracts are usually bilateral, although it is not unusual for a cataract to be worse in one eye. Cataract surgery is performed on the basis of perceived impairment of the individual patient's lifestyle; no recommendations on the basis of visual acuity have been made.

8. Answer a.

Age-related macular degeneration is the most common cause of blindness in developed countries. The most common symptom is a loss of central vision. Although the dry form is more common, those with severe vision loss more often have the wet form. High-dose antioxidants plus zinc reduced the risk of macular degeneration progression for individuals with advanced, unilateral disease but did not benefit those with mild disease or advanced, bilateral disease. Although several early trials of laser therapy showed some benefit in the treatment of age-related macular degeneration, more recent studies have not supported those findings. It currently is not recommended for the treatment of macular degeneration.

9. Answer d.

Ginkgo biloba supplementation does not appear to reduce the risk of AD development. Although some evidence suggests that antioxidants can reduce the risk and slow the progression of AD, studies have not consistently shown that vitamin E prevents or improves cognitive function. Cholinesterase inhibitors, which prolong the activity of the neurotransmitter acetylcholine, are best for patients with early manifestations of AD. In late-stage disease, very little acetylcholine is present and the medications lose their effectiveness. The Women's Health Initiative study showed no benefits from hormone-replacement therapy in reducing the risk of developing AD. Although some studies suggested the chronic use of nonsteroidal antiinflammatory drugs prevent AD, more recent randomized clinical trials have not shown this; due to their potential for clinically significant adverse effects, they are not recommended for use in preventing AD.

INJURY PREVENTION AND CONTROL

Kodjo M. Bossou, MD, MPH; and Philip T. Hagen, MD

In its most basic definition, **human injury** is the result of a transfer of energy of sufficient magnitude to damage tissues of the human recipient. Adoption of the infectious disease model of an agent (energy), a carrier (living or inanimate; a vector), and the affected person (host) has proved helpful in analyzing **the chain of causation that leads to injury** (see Chapter 3 for more details on this model). For the inclusion of important injuries, the definition of causation is often modified to include exposures that prevent needed energy from reaching a host—for example, a lack of thermal energy (heat) that results in frostbite.

The US Bureau of Labor Statistics operationalizes this definition for traumatic injury at work:

A **traumatic injury** is defined as any wound or damage to the body resulting from acute exposure to energy, such as heat, electricity, or impact from a crash or fall; or from the absence of such essentials as heat or oxygen, caused by a specific event or incident within a single workday or shift. Included in traumatic injuries are open wounds, intracranial and internal injuries, heatstroke, hypothermia, asphyxiation, acute poisonings resulting from short-term exposures limited to the worker's shift, suicides and homicides, and work injuries listed as underlying or contributory causes of death. Heart attacks and strokes are considered illnesses and therefore excluded from CFOI [Census of Fatal and Occupational Injuries] unless a traumatic injury contributed to the death.

Epidemiologic Factors of Injury

Injury is the public health threat that is perhaps the most diverse in its etiologic characteristics, and it is prevalent in all age groups. In fact, injury is both morbid and fatal in its effects, and across all age groups, it is the fifth-leading cause of death.

Although more than 161,000 persons in the United States die each year of injury, nearly 30 million are injured badly enough to seek emergency department evaluation, and nearly 2 million are injured badly enough to require hospitalization. For persons younger than 45 years, injury is the number 1 cause of death (Table 1).

Another important measure of the impact of injury on a population is the **years of potential life lost** (YPLL; also referred to as years of productive life lost) before age 65 years. This measure is useful because it may better represent the cost and health burden on society of a category of diseases or a specific disease. When people die of a disease at a young age—typically considered before the common retirement age of 65—their death not only represents an early death but also has a societal impact of **lost productive years**. Because injury disproportionately affects younger people, it is the leading cause of YPLL (Figure 1).

Health costs due to injuries are also high. The amount is estimated to be about **10% of the total US health care spending**, which is $1.8 trillion. Because the cost both in dollars and YPLL to the country is high, the emphasis by the US Centers for Disease Control and Prevention (CDC) on safety has become critical. **Many injuries are preventable**, and

Table 1 Ten Causes of Death and the Number of Total Deaths per Cause for All Races and Both Sexes by Age, 2006

Rank	Age Group, y										Total
	<1	1-4	5-9	10-14	15-24	25-34	35-44	45-54	55-64	65+	
1	Congenital anomalies, 5,819	Unintentional injury, 1,610	Unintentional injury, 1,044	Unintentional injury, 1,214	Unintentional injury, 16,229	Unintentional injury, 14,954	Unintentional injury, 17,534	Malignant neoplasms, 50,334	Malignant neoplasms, 101,454	Heart disease, 510,542	Heart disease, 631,636
2	Short gestation, 4,841	Congenital anomalies, 515	Malignant neoplasms, 459	Malignant neoplasms, 448	Homicide, 5,717	Suicide, 4,885	Malignant neoplasms, 13,917	Heart disease, 38,095	Heart disease, 65,477	Malignant neoplasms, 387,515	Malignant neoplasms, 559,888
3	SIDS, 2,323	Malignant neoplasms, 377	Congenital anomalies, 182	Homicide, 241	Suicide, 4,189	Homicide, 4,725	Heart disease, 12,339	Unintentional injury, 19,675	Chronic lower respiratory disease, 12,375	Cerebrovascular, 117,010	Cerebrovascular, 137,119
4	Maternal pregnancy complications, 1,683	Homicide, 366	Homicide, 149	Suicide, 216	Malignant neoplasms, 1,644	Malignant neoplasms, 3,656	Suicide, 6,591	Liver disease, 7,712	Unintentional injury, 11,446	Chronic lower respiratory disease, 106,845	Chronic lower respiratory disease, 124,583
5	Unintentional injury, 1,147	Heart disease, 161	Heart disease, 90	Heart disease, 163	Heart disease, 1,076	Heart disease, 3,307	HIV, 4,010	Suicide, 7,426	Diabetes mellitus, 11,432	Alzheimer disease, 71,660	Unintentional injury, 121,599
6	Placenta cord membranes, 1,140	Influenza and pneumonia, 125	Chronic lower respiratory disease, 52	Congenital anomalies, 162	Congenital anomalies, 460	HIV, 1,182	Homicide, 3,020	Cerebrovascular, 6,341	Cerebrovascular, 10,518	Diabetes mellitus, 52,351	Diabetes mellitus, 72,449
7	Respiratory distress, 825	Septicemia, 88	Cerebrovascular, 45	Chronic low respiratory disease, 63	Cerebrovascular, 210	Diabetes mellitus, 673	Liver disease, 2,551	Diabetes mellitus, 5,692	Liver disease, 7,217	Influenza and pneumonia, 49,346	Alzheimer disease, 72,432
8	Bacterial sepsis, 807	Perirratal period, 65	Influenza and pneumonia, 40	Cerebrovascular, 50	HIV, 206	Cerebrovascular, 527	Cerebrovascular, 2,221	HIV, 4,377	Suicide, 4,583	Nephritis, 37,377	Influenza and pneumonia, 56,326
9	Neonatal hemorrhage, 618	Benign neoplasms, 60	Septicemia, 40	Septicemia, 44	Influenza and pneumonia, 184	Congenital anomalies, 437	Diabetes mellitus, 2,094	Chronic lower respiratory disease, 3,924	Nephritis, 4,368	Unintentional injury, 36,689	Nephritis, 45,344
10	Circulatory system disease, 543	Cerebrovascular, 54	Benign neoplasms, 38	Benign neoplasms, 38	Complicated pregnancy, 179	Influenza and pneumonia, 335	Septicemia, 870	Viral hepatitis, 2,911	Septicemia, 4,032	Septicemia, 26,201	Septicemia, 34,234

Abbreviations: HIV, human immunodeficiency virus; SIDS, sudden infant death syndrome.
Adapted from the Office of Statistics and Programming, National Center for Injury Prevention and Control, Centers for Disease Control and Prevention [Internet]. Atlanta (GA): the CDC. 10 Leading Causes of Death, United States, 2006, All Races, All Sexes; [cited 09/21/2009]. Available from: http://webappa.cdc.gov/sasweb/ncipc/leadcaus10.html.

Cause of Death	YPLL	Percentage
Unintentional injury	2,292,894	19.4%
Malignant neoplasms	1,892,406	16.0%
Heart disease	1,422,345	12.0%
Perinatal period	943,945	8.0%
Suicide	679,282	5.7%
Homicide	595,553	5.0%
Congenital anomalies	482,051	4.1%
Cerebrovascular	246,386	2.1%
HIV	244,072	2.1%
Liver disease	232,733	2.0%
All others	2,791,274	23.6%

Figure 1 Years of Potential Life Lost (YPLL) Before Age 65 Years in the United States, 2005. All races, both sexes, and all deaths are included. HIV indicates human immunodeficiency virus. (From the National Center for Injury Prevention and Control. Available from: http://webappa.cdc.gov/sasweb/ncipc/ypll10.html)

substantial progress has been made in recent decades in most areas of injury prevention. Injuries may be classified as fatal, or directly resulting in or contributing to death, and nonfatal, or resulting in damage requiring self-care, first aid, or medical attention.

Further segmentation of injuries into 2 other groups is useful. **Intentional injuries** are those in which the carrier of the energy transfers it to the host with the intent of doing harm (eg, murder, domestic abuse). **Unintentional injuries** are those that are frequently referred to as *accidents*, though that term is often avoided because it lends a connotation of unavoidability, which does not apply to most injuries. Table 2 summarizes the distribution of types of fatal injuries in the United States in 2002.

Because of the diverse nature of injuries, their epidemiologic makeup is particularly important in identifying and tracking methods of prevention. Collecting injury-related information requires not only the tracking of the death certificate and medical diagnosis information but also reliance on sources of data less familiar to most clinicians.

Table 2 Causes of Fatal Injuries in the United States, 2002

Unintentional[a] (66%)	Intentional[a] (30%)
Motor vehicle	Suicide
Poisoning	Homicide
Fall	
Firearm	
Suffocation	

[a] Undetermined and legal interventions/war account for about 4%.
Data from Miniño AM, Anderson RN, Fingerhut LA, Boudreault MA, Warner M. Deaths: injuries, 2002. Natl Vital Stat Rep. 2006 Jan 31;54(10):1-124.

Box 1 Landmark Reports on Injury in the United States

US Department of Health, Education, and Welfare. 1979. *Healthy People: The Surgeon General's Report on Health Promotion and Disease Prevention.* Identified injury prevention as an area of focus for improving the nation's health.

National Research Council and Institute of Medicine. 1985. *Injury in America: A Continuing Public Health Problem.* Noted that funding was inadequate and identified priority areas.

Institute of Medicine. 1999. *Reducing the Burden of Injury: Advancing Prevention and Treatment.* Identified priority areas and encouraged both a coordinating body and improved data systems.

Centers for Disease Control and Prevention. 2006. *CDC Injury Fact Book.* Outlines data and public health methods to improve injury control.

Numerous influential groups over the years have recognized the importance and cost of injuries in the United States. They have published a number of landmark reports that encourage a coordinated approach to systematically collecting data in order to reduce injuries (Box 1).

In the past 20 years or so, cooperation and coordination have increased among organizations and agencies aimed at tracking, analyzing, and preventing injuries. The CDC has taken a leading role in this effort, especially in the area of applying the public health approach to the problem. It has helped coordinate broad-based injury data collection and made these data available on its Web site (http://www.cdc.gov). Sources used in the CDC's injury epidemiology effort are shown in Box 2.

- Injury is the public health threat that is perhaps the most diverse in its etiologic characteristics, and it is prevalent in all age-groups.
- Injuries may be classified as fatal or nonfatal and as intentional or unintentional.
- For persons younger than 45 years, injury is the most frequent cause of death.
- Years of potential life lost (YPLL) is an important measure of the cost and health burden of injuries on society.

Injury Prevention

The study of injury prevention began thousands of years ago with the development of armor as a protective barrier against the mechanical energy carried in a lance, arrow, or sword during warfare. The modern systematic study of injury prevention in public health began in the 1940s. An early example is a study by a World War II military surgeon, Hugh Cairns. He showed through accident analysis that military motorcycle deaths could be reduced by wearing crash helmets.

Box 2 Sources of Data Used by the Centers for Disease Control and Prevention (CDC) in Its Analysis of Injury in the United States

Behavioral Risk Factor Surveillance System (BRFSS)—Data on adults age 18 years and older. Assesses risk factors and allows analysis by age, sex, race, education, and ethnicity. Structured questionnaire administered nationally.

Central nervous system surveillance for traumatic brain injury (TBI)—State-collected data according to the CDC rubric. Designed to identify high-risk populations and guide resource use and prevention programs.

Fatality Analysis Reporting System (FARS)—Managed by the National Highway Traffic Safety Administration. Tracks fatal traffic crash information in United States.

National Crime Victimization Survey—Run by the Bureau of Justice Statistics. Tracks data on crime frequency and consequences, including domestic abuse and homicide.

National Electronic Injury Surveillance System All Injury Program (NEISS-AIP)—Operated by the Consumer Product Safety Commission. Collects data from hospitals on nonfatal injuries requiring emergency department evaluation.

National Hospital Discharge Survey—Managed by the CDC's National Center for Health Statistics (NCHS). Gathers information from a representative sample of about 500 hospitals nationwide on patients who survive injuries and are discharged from the hospital.

Uniform Crime Reports—Managed by the Federal Bureau of Investigation (FBI). Collects data from law enforcement agencies nationwide and allows analysis of information on violent crimes nationwide.

For injury prevention, the CDC applies its systematic model, called public health approach to injury prevention, which involves 4 steps:

1. Define the problem. Data gathering and analysis are performed to define the size and extent of the problem and who is affected by it and to allow tracking of change over time.
2. Identify risk and protective factors. Research is pursued into what factors put people at risk or protect them from injury.
3. Develop and test preventive strategies. On the basis of the research findings, preventive interventions are carried out, results are tracked, and interventions are modified.
4. Ensure widespread adoption. Successful strategies are identified and promulgated as broadly as possible.

This list is featured in the *CDC Injury Fact Book* (http://www.cdc.gov/ncipc/fact_book/InjuryBook2006.pdf).

Haddon Matrix

William Haddon Jr in the 1970s developed a model for systematic injury analysis in which he looked at host and energy factors over time as a method to define ways of intervening to reduce injury. He focused on automobile crash injuries using a matrix model, and the format is now called the **Haddon matrix**.

In this matrix model, columns represent causal agents and rows represent time in the sequence of events leading up to and following the injury. With systematic identification of these causal and contributing factors, a comprehensive intervention can be carried out to reduce injuries in various settings. In addition to the agent and the host, the environment in which injury occurs is important to understanding and preventing injury. The Haddon matrix divides these many factors into pre-event factors, in which intervention is primary prevention; event-associated factors, in which intervention is secondary; and postevent factors, in which the extent of injury or death is limited through tertiary preventive measures. Automobile-related injury and death reduction proved a good example of the effectiveness of this approach (Figure 2).

The work of Haddon and colleagues led to important legislation such as the National Traffic and Motor Vehicle Safety Act of 1966, which followed Haddon's rubric and introduced numerous measures to improve motor vehicle safety. For example, between 1993 and 2002, the rate of alcohol-related motor vehicle crashes decreased by 13%, from 6.9 per 100,000 population to 6.0 per 100,000 population. However, much work in the area of alcohol-related motor vehicle injury is still needed to prevent motor crashes because the goal for the Healthy People 2010 public health initiative is 4.0 per 100,000 population.

Christoffel and Gallagher outline Haddon's 10 ways to modify or prevent energy transfer that leads to injury in their book *Injury Prevention and Public Health: Practical Knowledge, Skills, and Strategies.*

1. Prevent the initial creation of the hazard by banning the manufacture and sale of inherently unsafe products or prohibiting inherently unsafe practices (eg, stop production of firecrackers, 3-wheeled all-terrain vehicles; eliminate spearing—the act of running into another football player with the top of the helmet).
2. Reduce the energy contained in the hazard (eg, limit the muzzle velocity of guns and the amount of gunpowder in firecrackers; limit the horsepower of motor vehicle engines; package toxic drugs in smaller, safer amounts).
3. Prevent the release of hazard that already exists (eg, store firearms in locked containers, close pools and beaches when no lifeguard is on duty).
4. Modify the rate or spatial distribution of the hazard (eg, require safety valves on boilers, use seat belts to control the deceleration of occupants in motor vehicle crashes, use short cleats on football shoes so the player's feet rotate rather than transmit sudden force to the knees).

Causal Agents

Time	Human	Vehicle/Equipment	Physical Environment	Social/Economic
Precrash	Poor vision or reaction time, alcohol, speeding, risk taking	Failed brakes, missing lights, lack of warning systems	Narrow shoulders, ill-timed signals	Cultural norms permitting speeding, red-light running, DUI
Crash	Failure to wear seat belt	Malfunctioning seat belts, poorly engineered air bags	Poorly designed guard rails	Lack of vehicle design regulation
Postcrash	High susceptibility alcohol	Poorly designed fuel tanks	Poorly emergency communication systems	Lack of support for EMS and trauma systems

Figure 2 Haddon Matrix for Automobile-Related Injuries. DUI indicates driving under the influence; EMS, emergency medical services. (Adapted from UC Berkeley Traffic Safety Center. A look at the Haddon Matrix: showing the need for depth and breadth. TSC Newsletter. 2005-06 Winter [cited 13 Mar 2009];30(1); ©UC Regents and the UC Berkeley Safe Transportation Research and Education Center. Available from: http://www.tsc.berkeley.edu/newsletter/. Used with permission.)

5. Separate in time and space the hazard from the object to be protected (eg, provide pedestrian overpasses at high-volume traffic crossings, avoid having play areas near unguarded bodies of water).

6. Separate the hazard from the object to be protected with a material barrier (og, install fencing to enclose all 4 sides of a swimming pool, insulate electrical cords, provide protective eyewear for racquet sports, build highway medians, use bulletproof barriers).

7. Modify relevant basic qualities of the hazard (eg, provide padded dashboards in motor vehicles, make crib slat spacing too narrow to allow the strangling of a child, adopt the use of safer baseballs and breakaway baseball bases, install nonslip surfacing in bathtubs).

8. Make the object to be protected more resistant to damage from the hazard (eg, encourage calcium intake to reduce osteoporosis and brittle bones, for protection in case of falls; encourage musculoskeletal conditioning for athletes; prohibit alcohol sales and consumption near recreational water areas).

9. Begin to counter the damage already done by the hazard (eg, provide emergency medical care on-site at car crashes, use systems to route injured persons to appropriately trained trauma care providers, develop school protocols to respond to injury emergencies).

10. Stabilize, repair, and rehabilitate the object of the damage (eg, develop rehabilitation plans at an early stage of injury treatment, make use of occupational rehabilitation for paraplegic persons).

Specific Injury Prevention Areas

The Healthy People 2000 initiative targeted 45 injury prevention objectives, 26 of which dealt with unintentional injuries and 19 with violence prevention. It is instructive to look at the Healthy People 2010 objectives related to injury prevention for the United States. These objectives make up Section 15 of the Healthy People 2010 report (available in print or online [http://www.healthypeople.gov/document/HTML/Volume2/15injury.htm]).

Six of the objectives are described in the following examples.

1. Decrease the number of firearm-related deaths. The baseline rate in 1998 was 11.3 deaths per 100,000 population, with a reduction target set at 4.3 deaths per 100,000 population by 2010. Suicide (6.5 deaths per 100,000 population) and homicide (4.3 deaths per 100,000 population) account for most of these deaths. The data source for tracking these deaths is the National Vital Statistics System (NVSS), maintained by the CDC and the National Center for Health Statistics (NCHS). Deaths related to firearms have a wide range of disparities related to sex, ethnicity, and education. For example, black and African American persons in the United States had a baseline rate of firearm-related deaths of 21.0 per 100,000 population, while Asian and Pacific Islanders had a rate of 4.2 per 100,000 population. Men have a baseline rate of 20.1 deaths per 100,000 population; women have a rate of 3.3 deaths per 100,000 population. People with less than a high school education are 3 times more likely to die of a firearm-related injury—a baseline rate of 21.4 deaths per 100,000 population—than people with at least some college education, whose baseline rate is 7.0 deaths per 100,000 population. The proper storage of firearms is a good example of a method to reduce firearm-related injury.

2. Reduce nonfatal poisonings. The baseline rate of nonfatal poisonings was 348.4 per 100,000 population in 1997. The target was set at "better than the best"

(a term typically used to set a goal at a rate better than that found in the best subgroup of a population). The data source for its tracking is the National Hospital Ambulatory Medical Care Survey (NHAMCS), maintained by the CDC through the NCHS. Since most poisonings are unintentional, about 90% occur in the home and nearly half occur in children younger than 4 years. A good mitigating strategy is the proper storage of potential home poisons, including cosmetics, cleaners, workshop products, plants, and medications. Reducing the death rate from poisoning is covered in Objective 15.8 of Healthy People 2010, which seeks to reduce the death rate from 6.8 deaths per 100,000 population to 1.5 deaths per 100,000 population. Again, significant racial (6 times higher) and educational (3 times higher) disparities exist.

3. Increase the number of states that collect data on external causes of injury through hospital discharge data systems. The baseline in 1998 was 23 states that collected information on external causes of injury through hospital discharge data systems. The target goal is to achieve total coverage. The data source for this information is the External Causes of Injury Survey, conducted by the American Public Health Association (APHA). This objective shows the importance of good data systems and the use of a data system from a respected professional organization and advocacy group. This goal may be achieved by passing a law requiring emergency departments to comply or by having advocacy and professional groups working to support nationwide efforts by hospitals.

4. Reduce deaths caused by motor vehicle crashes. The baseline 1998 death rate due to motor vehicle crashes was 15.6 per 100,000 population. The target rate by 2010 is 9.2 deaths per 100,000 population. A couple interesting features of these data and targets are worth noting. **Motor vehicle crashes are the leading cause of unintentional death in the United States**. In motor vehicle–related deaths, differences related to ethnicity (3 times higher), gender (2 times higher), and education level (3 times higher) are significant. Motorcycles result in a much higher death rate (21.0 per 1 million vehicle miles traveled) compared with cars. Protecting pedestrians, using child safety seats, and wearing helmets and seat belts are some of the prevention strategies advocated to reduce the morbidity and death associated with different types of motor vehicle crashes.

5. Reduce deaths from falls. The age-adjusted baseline rate in 1998 was 4.7 deaths per 100,000 population and the target for 2010 is 3.0 deaths per 100,000 population (source: NVSS of the NCHS). Subset analysis shows that the rate has a huge age differential; for persons age 65 to 84 years, the death rate is 3.6 times the baseline rate, and for persons age 85 years and older, it is 23 times as high.

6. Reduce homicides. The baseline age-adjusted homicide rate in 1998 was 6.5 deaths per 100,000 population and the target for 2010 is its reduction to 3.0 deaths per 100,000 population. This target is developed by using the better-than-the-best approach. A look at the subgroup analysis shows that the 3 "best" subgroups are Asian Americans and Pacific Islanders (3.5 per 100,000 population), whites (4.0 per 100,000 population), and girls and women (3.1 per 100,000 population).

Homicide is the second leading cause of death, behind motor vehicle accidents, for people age 15 to 24 years, and although its rate is decreasing, it is not doing so quickly. US boys and men in this age group are 10 times more likely to die of homicide than their peers in Canada and 15 times more likely than their peers in Australia. These data suggest the need for more intensive intervention and better understanding of the causal factors leading to homicide. To this end, the assessment of such objectives as "reduce the rate of physical assault by current or former intimate partners," "reduce physical fighting among adolescents," and "reduce weapon carrying by adolescents on school property" use data to create targets and focus interventions that should decrease violent injury and death in youth. In this regard, the Federal Bureau of Investigation Uniform Crime Reports (FBI-UCR) data showed that in 1995, almost 5,000 women were murdered in the United States, with about 85% of the murders committed by someone the woman knew and half of these murders committed by a husband, an ex-husband, or a boyfriend.

The Healthy People 2010 objectives also point out the interrelatedness of the causes of injury and other health conditions. For example, mental health issues such as depression have a clear role in suicide and suicide attempts in adolescents (Objectives 18-1 and 18-2). Poisoning deaths can be further reduced through such initiatives as the objectives of a single toll-free number for poison control centers and a reduction in pesticide exposure.

- With systematic identification of the causal and contributing factors of injury and the events leading up to and following injury, identified in the Haddon matrix, a comprehensive intervention can be carried out to reduce the occurrence of injury in various settings.
- The focus of Healthy People 2010 is wide ranging in regard to injury and includes reductions in firearm-related death, nonfatal poisonings, motor vehicle–related deaths, homicides, and death due to falls, as well as data collection from hospital discharge records.
- Disparities of ethnicity, sex, and education often exist among these injuries.

Injuries Due to Violence

Domestic Violence

The CDC defines domestic violence as "physical, sexual, or psychological harm by a current or former partner or spouse." Domestic violence, also called battery, partner abuse, spousal abuse, or intimate partner violence, is a serious public health problem around the world. The US Department of Justice (DOJ) estimated in 1998 that about 1 million violent crimes were committed against persons by their current or former intimate partners. Most (85%) of these crimes were committed against women. In 2005, more than 1,500 people in the United States died at the hands of an intimate partner. Of these deaths, 25% were men and 75% were women. The National Violence Against Women Survey (http://www.ncjrs.gov/pdffiles1/nij/181867.pdf) found that 22.1% of women and 7.4% of men in the United States had experienced physical forms of domestic abuse at some point in their life. Domestic violence is the most common cause of injury to girls and women age 15 to 44 years.

Domestic abuse can be classified as physical, sexual, emotional, psychological, and economic. Several factors contribute to abuse, but the **best single predictor of domestic violence is a history of abuse in a family member**. Other predictors of domestic violence include an environment where violence is either taught or accepted; poor self-esteem and anger; drug or alcohol abuse (or both); and loss of physical health or wage-earning power (or both).

Domestic Violence During Pregnancy

The CDC estimates that pregnant women are about 60% more likely to be beaten compared with women who are not pregnant. The violence is usually directed at the victim's breasts, abdomen, or genitals. This situation is likely due in part to the partner's stress over the impending birth or the unintended or unwanted nature of the pregnancy. In fact, women are 4 times more likely to experience increased abuse as a result of an unintended or unwanted pregnancy.

Diagnosis of Domestic Violence

The diagnosis of domestic violence is challenging due in part to a lack of clinical guidelines, wide variations in clinical presentation, and the victim's fear of retaliation from the abuser. Unfortunately, screening for domestic violence is not a routine part of most medical visits. Yet, the health care professional has a critical role in identifying domestic abuse of a patient through routine screening for domestic violence. Sherin and associates developed a domestic violence screening tool that can be used in the community (Figure 3).

The American College of Obstetrics and Gynecology recommends that physicians screen all female patients for domestic violence. For women who are not pregnant, screening should occur at routine gynecologic visits, family planning visits, or preconception visits. For pregnant women, screening should occur at the first prenatal visit, at least once per trimester, and at the postpartum visit.

Characteristics of Potential Abusers

A potential abuser does not consider himself or herself an abuser. Several characteristics are expressed by an abuser; however, none of these characteristics are specific to prompting domestic abuse. They can include extreme dependence on the relationship, impulsiveness in decision making, general possessiveness and jealousy that may reach a pathologic level, a focus on fear of losing the partner, and effort to isolate the partner from friends, family, and coworkers. An abuser may be extremely manipulative of the partner, become angry when drinking alcohol or using illicit drugs, or have witnessed or experienced family violence while growing up.

Please read each of the following activities and fill in the circle that best indicates the frequency with which your partner acts in the way depicted.

How often does your partner?	Never	Rarely	Sometimes	Fairly often	Frequently
1. Physically hurt you	O	O	O	O	O
2. Insult or talk down to you	O	O	O	O	O
3. Threaten you with harm	O	O	O	O	O
4. Scream or curse at you	O	O	O	O	O
	1	2	3	4	5

Each item is scored from 1 to 5. Thus, scores for this inventory range from 4 to 20. A score >10 is considered a positive result for intimate partner violence.

Figure 3 HITS Tool for Intimate Partner Violence Screening. HITS indicates hurt, insulted, threatened with harm, and screamed at. (Adapted from Sherin et al [1998]. Used with permission.)

Treatment of the Abuse Victim

The treatment of the abuse victim is multifactorial and includes both physical and psychological support. Health care professionals, social workers, and case managers are key caregivers for the abuse victim. The ultimate goals for the treatment are to provide immediate assistance to the victim, identify the risk factors that contribute to the abuse, and address these risk factors to prevent future abuse of the victim. The CDC and other agencies have developed several programs to assist in the care of the abuse victim.

Prevention of Domestic Violence

The CDC and various agencies have been actively involved in reducing the incidence of domestic violence. According to the CDC, all forms of domestic violence are preventable. Primary prevention by intervening before someone hurts an intimate partner for the first time is critical. The key strategy is the promotion of respectful, nonviolent, intimate-partner relationships through change at the individual, community, and societal levels. Another key strategy is to focus on the initial episode of abuse by offering emotional and psychological support to the abused person and assistance and counseling to the couple for future prevention. The Domestic Violence Prevention Enhancement and Leadership Through Alliances (DELTA) activities from the CDC are guided by a set of prevention principles. These principles include 1) prevention of first-time perpetration and first-time victimization, 2) reduction of risk factors associated with domestic violence perpetration or victimization, 3) promotion of protective factors that reduce the likelihood of domestic violence, 4) planning of evidence-based programs, 5) use of behavior and social change theories in prevention program planning and evaluation, and 6) the evaluation of prevention programs and use of these results to form future program plans.

Domestic violence continues to be underreported, which minimizes the problem and hampers prevention efforts. Underreporting is in large part due to the victim's shame and fear of retribution from the abuser.

Homicide

Homicide refers to the act of killing another human being. Different types of homicide have been described. Criminal homicide occurs when a person purposely, knowingly, recklessly, or negligently causes the death of another person. Noncriminal homicide is one of the most recognized forms of homicide, done through self-defense and committed to protect one's own life from a deadly threat. State-sanctioned homicide refers to capital punishment, in which the state determines that a person should die.

Criminal homicide is a significant public health concern in the United States. The DOJ notes that the rate of homicide has been decreasing during the past several years (Figure 4). However, a significant disparity exists among ethnic groups, between the sexes, and among age-groups. The following 4 examples from the Bureau of Justice Statistics are illustrative:

1. In 2005, homicide victimization rates for black persons were 6 times higher than for white persons
2. In 2005, offending rates for black persons were more than 7 times greater than for white persons
3. Boys and men were almost 10 times more likely than girls and women to commit murder in 2005
4. Young adults (age, 18-24 years) have had the highest offending rates historically

Homicide Prevention

The DOJ Office of Justice, in partnership with the RAND Corporation, identified 4 potential interventions that will help reduce the rate of homicide:

1. Direct patrol and field interrogations through increasing police patrol in targeted areas
2. Firearms law enforcement because of the high proportion of homicides that are committed with firearms
3. Enforcement of collective responsibility
4. Education and treatment, especially for individuals at risk for commiting crimes (eg, probationers, parolees, marginal students, unemployed persons) in the community (http://www.rand.org/pubs/working_papers/2005/RAND_WR284.pdf)

Suicide

In the United States, suicide is the 11th leading cause of death among all persons, the fifth leading cause of death among children age 5 to 14 years, and the third leading cause of death among persons age 15 to 24 years. It accounts for 1.3% of all deaths in the United States. A significant sex disparity exists in suicides, with boys and men taking their own life 4 times more often than girls and women. Elderly white men have the highest suicide rate. The CDC estimates that each year, more than 32,000 people kill themselves and more than 395,000 people with self-inflicted injuries are treated in emergency departments.

Several factors that contribute to suicide risk are noted in Figure 5. Other factors include a history of depression or other mental illness, drug abuse, a family history of suicide or violence, a history of abuse in childhood, physical illness, and feelings of aloneness.

Identifying Individuals at Risk for Suicide

Most suicides are related to some psychiatric illness, especially depression. Suicide can also occur in situations where

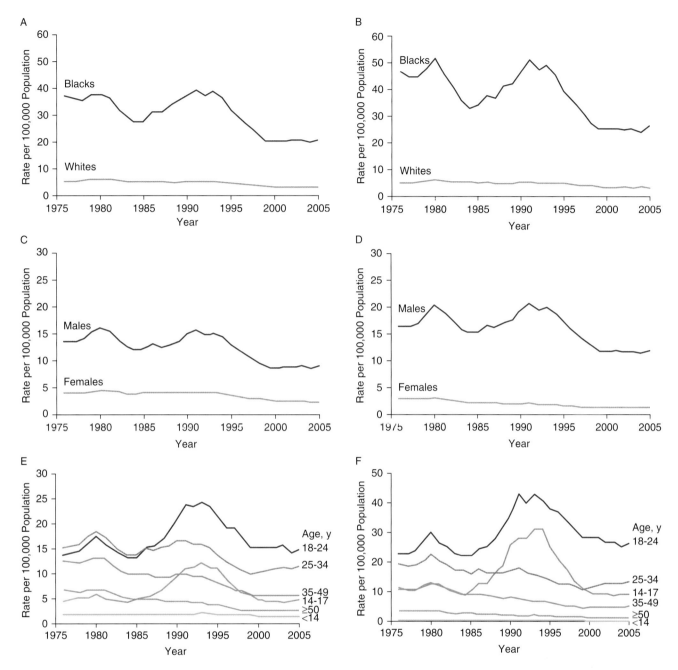

Figure 4 A, Homicide victimization rates by race, 1976-2005. B, Homicide offending by race, 1976-2005. C, Homicide victimization by sex, 1976-2005. D, Homicide offending by sex, 1976-2005. E, Homicide victimization by age, 1976-2005. F, Homicide offending by age, 1976-2005. G, Homicide by weapon type, 1976-2005. H, Violent crime rates by age of victim, 1973-2003. I, Violent crime rates by race of victim, 1973-2003. J, Homicide cases under selected circumstances in the United States, 2003 and 2004. Percentages may total >100% because certain incidents involve multiple circumstances. *Brawl* refers to a mutual physical fight involving 3 or more persons. *Jealousy* refers to a lovers' triangle (ie, perceived infidelity) and includes homicide of the intimate partner or a third party involved in a relationship. *Intimate partner conflict* includes separation, major argument, or violence. (Figures 4A through 4G adapted from Fox JA, Zawitz MW. Homicide trends in the United States [Internet]. Bureau of Justice Statistics, US Department of Justice, Office of Justice Programs [cited 13 Mar 2009]. Available from: http://www.ojp.usdoj.gov/bjs/homicide/homtrnd. htm#contents; Figures 4H and 4I adapted from Additional Crime Facts at a Glance [Internet]. Bureau of Justice Statistics, US Department of Justice, Office of Justice Programs [cited 13 Mar 2009]. Available from: http://www.ojp.usdoj.gov/bjs/gvc. htm#Victims; and Figure J adapted from Centers for Disease Control and Prevention [CDC]. Homicides and suicides: National Violent Death Reporting System, United States, 2003-2004. MMWR Morb Mortal Wkly Rep. 2006 Jul 7;55[26]:721-4. Erratum in: MMWR Morb Mortal Wkly Rep. 2006 Oct 6;55[39]:1074-5.)

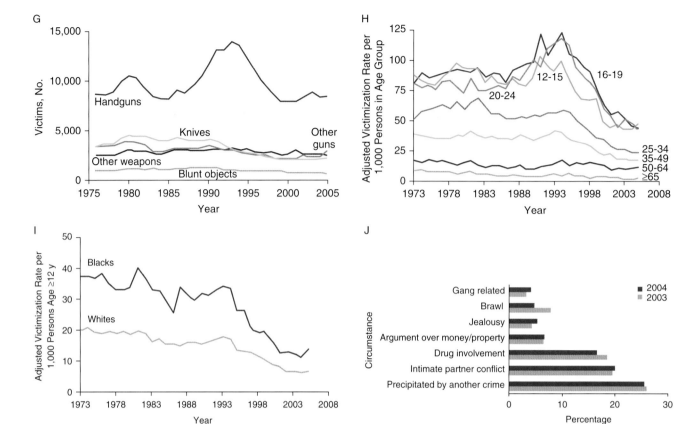

Figure 4 continued

the person feels that he or she either is not in control of the future or has a living situation that is overwhelming. **Any comment made by an individual about attempting suicide should be taken seriously**. In fact, many persons express their desire to commit suicide before making the attempt. Health care professionals have an important role in identifying the population at risk for committing suicide, especially persons with mental illness. In assessing a person for possible suicidal ideation, the health care professional might ask whether the person has had thoughts that he or she would be better off dead or of imposing physical self-hurt in some way. A positive answer to this question needs immediate attention and, possibly, referral for assistance. Treatment of this patient includes the involvement of a psychiatrist, a psychologist, a social worker, and case management.

Firearm-Related Injury

According to the CDC, firearm-related injury is the second leading cause of death from injury, ranked after motor vehicle crash. Firearm-related homicide is the second leading cause of death among US persons between 15 and 24 years of age. Of the firearm-related deaths in 2000, 57.9%

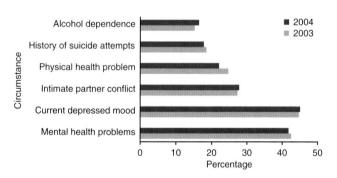

Figure 5 Percentage of Suicide Cases by Selected Circumstances, United States, 2003 and 2004. Percentages may total >100% because certain incidents involve multiple circumstances. *Intimate partner conflict* includes separation, major argument, or violence. Current depressed mood was based on the family's or friends' impression of the decedent's mood. *Mental health problems* includes any mental illness diagnosis of the decedent (eg, clinical depression, dysthymia, bipolar disorder, schizophrenia). (Adapted from Centers for Disease Control and Prevention [CDC] Homicides and suicides: National Violent Death Reporting System, United States, 2003-2004. MMWR Morb Mortal Wkly Rep. 2006 Jul 7;55[26]:721-4. Erratum in: MMWR Morb Mortal Wkly Rep. 2006 Oct 6;55[39]:1074-5.)

were suicides and 37.7% were homicides (http://www.cdc.gov/mmwr/preview/mmwrhtml/rr5214a2.htm).

Several research studies have showed that guns in the home are a significant risk to families. The CDC and other agencies identify several societal factors in the United States associated with firearm-related injury: poverty, illicit drug trade, lack of education or employment opportunity, substance abuse and mental health problems, fear or stress, income inequalities, and racial tension.

About 1 million violent crimes occurred in 2002 in which victims perceived the offender to have been drinking at the time of the offense. The state of Maine conducted research in 2004 in which the characteristics of gun crimes and offenders were analyzed. Based on the state's study, the common characteristics associated with the perpetrators were the following:

<25% of the offenders work full time
21% of cases were related to domestic violence
42% of cases were related to use of illicit drugs or alcohol
87% of offenders had a prior criminal record
34% of offenders had less than a high school education
43% of offenders had a history of mental illness

Firearm-Related Injury Prevention

The data source for tracking firearm-related injury is the NVSS. Prevention is multidisciplinary and involves local and federal government, community activists, health care professionals, and the CDC. It also includes individual and parental responsibilities for the prevention of firearm-related injury. The American College of Emergency Physicians, in its effort to prevent firearm-related injuries and deaths, endorses the following efforts:

1. Aggressively enforce current laws against illegal possession, purchase, sale, or use of firearms
2. Ensure that new firearms are rendered as safe as possible by treating them with safety regulations similar to those applied to any other consumer product
3. Limit the availability of firearms to persons whose ability to responsibly handle the weapons is ensured
4. Encourage the creation and evaluation of community and school-based education programs targeting the prevention of firearm injuries
5. Educate the public about the risks of improperly stored firearms, especially in the home
6. Devote tax revenue from the sale of firearms and ammunition to both provide care for victims of firearm violence and promote firearm safety

7. Hold adult individuals legally accountable for harm resulting from a child's access to firearms

Firearm-Related Injury of Children

Parental responsibility is critical to prevent childhood injury from firearms. Having guns in the house presents a significant risk to the family. According to the American Academy of Pediatrics, **the best way to keep children safe from firearm-related injury is to never have a gun in the house**. For persons who keep a gun in the home, the following actions are recommended: always keep the gun unloaded and locked up; lock and store ammunition in a separate place, and keep keys to these locked boxes out of reach of and hidden from children

- The ultimate goal for the treatment of an abuse victim is to provide immediate assistance, identify the risk factors that contribute to the abuse, and address these risk factors to prevent their recurrence.
- A notable disparity in homicide exists among ethnic groups, between the sexes, and among age groups.
- Any comment made by an individual regarding a suicide attempt should be taking seriously.
- Firearm-related injury is the second-leading cause of death from injury; firearm-related homicide is the second-leading cause of death among US persons between 15 and 24 years of age.

SUGGESTED READING

Centers for Disease Control and Prevention. Injury and violence prevention, chapter 15. In: Healthy People 2010. 2nd ed. With Understanding and Improving Health and Objectives for Improving Health. Vol. 2. Washington, DC: U.S. Government Printing Office, 2000.

Christoffel T, Scavo Gallagher S. Injury prevention and public health: practical knowledge, skills, and strategies. Sudbury (MA): Jones and Bartlett Publishers; c2006.

Doll LS, Bonzo SE, Sleet DA, Mercy JA, Haas EN, editors. Handbook of injury and violence prevention. New York (NY): Springer Science + Business Media, LLC; c2007.

National Center for Injury Prevention and Control. CDC Injury Fact book. Atlanta (GA): Centers for Disease Control and Prevention; c2006.

Peek-Asa C, Heiden EO. Injury control: the public health approach. In: Wallace RB, editor. Wallace/Maxcy-Rosenau-Last. Public health & preventive medicine. 15th ed. United States of America: The McGraw-Hill Companies, Inc; c2008. p. 1319-28.

Sherin KM, Sinacore JM, Li XQ, Zitter RE, Shakil A. HITS: a short domestic violence screening tool for use in a family practice setting. Fam Med. 1998 Jul-Aug;30(7): 508-12.

Questions and Answers

Questions

1. Which of the following statements about injury is *not* correct?
   a. Injury is the leading cause of death in people age 1 to 34 years in the United States
   b. Injury is the leading cause of death in infants <1 year old
   c. Injury is the leading cause of years of potential life lost in the United States
   d. Injury is the fifth-leading cause of death in the United States overall
   e. Injuries are responsible for 30 million emergency department visits per year

2. Although injury is different in many respects from other causes of morbidity and death in the United States, the traditional epidemiologic model of disease can be applied. Which of the following definitions does *not* apply to this model?
   a. The agent is energy
   b. The vector is the agent
   c. The host is the injured person
   d. The carrier is the transfer of energy to the host
   e. The traditional epidemiologic model works well for injury

3. The work of William Haddon Jr at the New York State Health Department resulted in a rubric for analyzing injuries and developing and tracking interventions. Which of the following was *not* characteristic of his rubric?
   a. A matrix of factors that analyzed the energy transfer from high to low energy states through a materials science grid

   b. A matrix of factors and phases that analyzed the time sequence of an injury and host and environment factors
   c. A prevention strategy to ban inherently unsafe products
   d. Recognition that, even after injury, tertiary prevention measures can be applied to reduce the morbidity and death due to injuries
   e. Rubric was developed in the 1970s

4. Regarding injuries, which statement is *not* true?
   a. Unintentional injuries cause about two-thirds of injury-related deaths
   b. Motor vehicle injury is the leading cause of unintentional injury
   c. Homicide and suicide are the second- and third-leading causes of death in people age 15 to 24 years
   d. Injury prevention is a new discipline implemented in the public health sphere with the Healthy People initiative of the Centers for Disease Control and Prevention in the late 1990s.
   e. Healthy People 2010 has objectives for injury reduction

5. Which of the following statements about injuries is *not* true?
   a. The Centers for Disease Control and Prevention (CDC) has an important coordinating role in data collection related to injury prevention
   b. Injuries have a diverse mix of types and causes
   c. A cooperative effort is ongoing to improve data collection and coordination
   d. The CDC is under local and regional governmental authority
   e. National Highway and Traffic Safety Administration (NHTSA), the US Department of Justice (DOJ), and the CDC's National Center for Health Statistics (NCHS) all participate in collecting injury-related data

Answers

1. Answer b.

The top 5 leading causes of death in the United States overall are heart disease, cancer, stroke, chronic lower respiratory disease, and unintentional injury, respectively. However, because unintentional injury is the leading cause of death for people age 1 to 34 years in the United States, it disproportionately affects the young and thus is the leading cause of years of potential life lost. Although injury imposes a high burden of death, the burden of medical cost and nonfatal impact on the population is borne out by the approximately 30 million emergency department visits—2 million of which result in hospitalization—due to injuries each year in the United States.

2. Answer b.

It has proved helpful to use the epidemiologic model of agent, carrier, and host to analyze injury as a cause of morbidity and death in the population. Similar to an infectious agent in the traditional epidemiologic model, energy is the agent of direct injury to human tissues. The energy is transferred to the host's tissues by a carrier (vector), which may be living (eg, an assailant) or inanimate (eg, a car). The host is the same in both models: the affected person. For inclusion of deaths due to such causes as drowning or exposure, carriers can also prevent needed energy (oxygen or heat) from reaching a tissue. Teasing apart this simple model into the true "web of causation" is often as difficult for injury as for other illnesses.

3. Answer a.

Haddon was essential in developing the discipline of injury prevention in the 1970s. He proposed using a matrix with such characteristics as host factors, agent factors, and environmental factors along 1 axis of a grid and temporal phases—pre-event, event, and postevent—along the other axis. This matrix became known as the Haddon matrix and proved highly effective for developing interventions in numerous injury areas. Haddon was particularly influential in the area of motor vehicle safety.

4. Answer d.

Unintentional injuries cause about two-thirds of injury-related deaths. Motor vehicle injuries are the single most important cause of unintentional injuries, followed by poisoning, falls, and suffocation. Unintentional injuries are often referred to as "accidental injuries," but this term should not be interpreted as meaning unavoidable. Understanding causal factors and intervening appropriately can substantially reduce unintentional injuries. Intentional injuries include homicide, suicide, and nonfatal assault. Homicide and suicide are the second- and third-leading causes of death for youth and for young adults age 15 to 24 years. Although the science of injury prevention as a study discipline is new relative to many medical disciplines, it has been in existence for 50 or more years. It was first included in the Centers for Disease Control and Prevention's original Healthy People initiative, Healthy People 2000, which proposed 45 injury prevention objectives—26 dealt with unintentional injuries and 19 dealt with violence prevention.

5. Answer d.

The Centers for Disease Control and Prevention (CDC) plays an important coordinating role in data collection related to injury prevention. It is under federal govermental control. However, injuries have such a diverse mix of types and cause that no one organization or database yet tracks all of the relevant data. Nevertheless, a cooperative effort is ongoing to improve data collection and coordination among diverse groups, including the National Highway and Traffic Safety Administration (NHTSA), the Department of Justice (DOJ), the CDC's National Center for Health Statistics (NCHS), and the American Public Health Association (APHA). The CDC draws on this diverse group of statistics in its Healthy People initiative to set targets for improvement in injury prevention and to track changes over time.

13

ENVIRONMENTAL HEALTH

Richard D. Newcomb, MD, MPH; Richard J. Vetter, PhD; and
Clayton T. Cowl, MD, MS

Environmental medicine is the broad discipline that focuses on environmental factors that cause or influence disease. These factors typically are components of 4 major categories: air, water, soil, and food. Often, an environmental toxin or agent may have numerous means by which it causes disease, such as a toxin primarily soil bound that is aerosolized as dust or is made soluble and then infiltrates water and plants.

The primary role of the clinician in environmental medicine is as a resource and risk communicator for patients. In circumstances where a patient has adverse health effects, the clinician's role is to determine how likely it is that an environmental toxin has contributed to the patient's symptoms or an underlying disease. When a hazard is recognized, the clinician helps control and reduce exposure, as well as treats any illness when effective treatment options are available.

Risk Assessment

Risk assessment is the process of determining the probability that an exposure to hazardous material will damage the health of individuals in a population. The process involves the determination of whether a particular chemical or mix of chemicals is a known risk to humans or animals, through reviewing medical and toxicology literature for known acute or long-term effects.

For many chemicals, little or no data are available about their effects on humans, and a risk assessment may require extrapolation where possible from animal toxicology and known tissue culture effects. International agencies have identified some chemicals of most concern for the risks they present, such as capacity to cause cancer.

The World Health Organization is such an agency, as is the International Agency for Research on Cancer (IARC), which provides a world literature review and ranks risks according to evidence in several categories. These categories include risk of carcinogenesis in humans, a category that contains chemicals with sufficient evidence, limited evidence, and inadequate evidence for carcinogenesis and those for which evidence suggests a lack of carcinogenicity. Additional categories remark on evidence for carcinogenicity in animals as well.

Other agencies are a resource on how chemicals may cause health effects for humans other than cancer. The Agency for Toxic Substances and Disease Registry in Atlanta, Georgia, and the US Environmental Protection Agency (EPA) are resources in this regard, in addition to their being a source of scientific and medical literature databases.

Dose-Response Assessment

After the determination that a chemical has the potential to cause health effects in an individual or a human population, the clinician or public health official needs to determine whether the toxin has a dose-response effect. With the assumption that no specific data are available about the chemical's effects on health in large human populations, this determination requires that the following assumptions hold true for carcinogenesis:

1. High-dose findings can be extrapolated to low or ambient doses
2. Dose-response gradients observed in experimental studies can be extrapolated to humans
3. Extrapolations from high to low doses follow a no-threshold model at low doses

The last point infers that some chemicals have a threshold at which either no health effect occurs or the body is able to safely neutralize the toxicity through normal mechanisms of metabolism and elimination.

The EPA and other agencies estimate excess risk from linearized, multistage models to predict excess lifetime risk. Other biostatistical models are used as well, intended to estimate risk from the known or experimental models to the unknown levels in individuals or populations. For health effects other than carcinogenesis, other models are used that are based primarily on the concept of either estimating the dose of a chemical at which no findings were detected or using the lowest dose at which findings were detected. When no adverse effects are observed, this absence of effect is called the no observed adverse effect level (NOAEL) and, similarly, the lowest observed adverse effect level (LOAEL).

Exposure Assessment

The next step in risk assessment is to obtain an estimate of chemical concentration in the environment and the potential for human exposure. This step is typically carried out by an industrial or environmental hygienist. This expert is specifically trained to provide reliable testing procedures for measuring levels of toxins in air, water, soil, plants, and animals and in humans exposed to the toxins. After determining that the entry route was through dermal exposure, inhalation, or ingestion, the hygienist presents the data, typically in milligrams per kilogram per day. Exposure data are often derived using techniques that range from biologic monitoring (such as samples of blood, hair, fat, or urine), which is most reliable, to ambient monitoring of plants, air, and water for indicator pollutants (such as the levels of pesticide in water supplies), which involves estimations when extrapolating to individuals or human populations.

Risk Characterization

The final step of risk assessment is providing an overall risk determination or characterization. In this step, risk is extrapolated from exposure data and models that provide cancer probability or, when cancer is not the main concern, risk is determined by comparison with a reference concentration or dose for the average individual or population. When risk is less than that for the average reference population, no regulatory action, control, or cleanup is warranted.

- In risk assessment, a process of determining the probability that an exposure to hazardous material will damage health, the clinician or public health official needs to determine whether the toxin has a dose-response effect.
- Risk assessment also requires an estimate of chemical concentration in the environment and the potential for human exposure.
- An overall risk determination or characterization is done, in which risk is extrapolated from exposure data and models that provide cancer probability.

Public Health Protection

Air Quality

Improved air quality in North America over the past several decades has generally prevented catastrophic episodes of concentrated outdoor air pollution. However, such pollutants as ozone and particulates may still be responsible for considerable respiratory illness. The US **Clean Air Act** of 1970 required the EPA to list those compounds present in the atmosphere for which scientific data support an increased potential risk to public health if ambient exposure is not regulated. The result is the **National Ambient Air Quality Standard** (NAAQS), which has been published for each criterion pollutant. The Clean Air Act amendments of 1990 served to regulate point-source, high-toxicity compounds ("air toxics") present in low ambient concentrations with unknown or limited pathologic effect to the respiratory tract.

The main types of outdoor air pollutants are emitted from stationary or mobile sources. Stationary pollutant sources consist primarily of large-scale manufacturing or power production industries; mobile pollutant sources include automotive and combustion engines. Air pollutants from these sources may be gases or aerosols, the latter type composed of liquid or particles suspended in a gaseous emulsion.

Water solubility is a key factor for determining the anatomical site of the deposition of air pollutants. Compounds that are highly water soluble, such as sulfur-based products and nitric acid vapors, are deposited, absorbed, and eliminated in the upper respiratory tract. By comparison, gases with limited water solubility (eg, oxides of nitrogen, ozone) tend to affect distal airways, including the alveoli.

Particulate Matter

Particulate matter consists of both solids and liquids and involves particles of diverse sizes and morphologic characteristics, usually including such organic substances as pollens and fungal elements. The distribution of particulate matter includes coarse particles (soil-based material) and fine particles (by-products of the combustion process) originating from heavy-industry sources, power generation facilities, fireplaces and stoves, and diesel-powered motor vehicles. The increased development of industries across the globe has resulted in increased concentrations of particulate matter in the atmosphere. Controlled studies have not showed a direct link between exposure to particulate matter and long-term human morbidity or death, although increased prevalence of respiratory symptoms and some association with cardiovascular disease and death have been reported.

Sulfur Dioxide

The burning of sulfur-based coal for energy production has resulted in substantial emissions of sulfur dioxide (SO_2), a major atmospheric pollutant in many urban environments. Construction of elevated towers and smokestacks to reduce local deposition of SO_2 has inadvertently resulted in dispersion of these products in the troposphere, where high-level winds carry the compounds across large geographic regions, resulting in what has been termed "**acid rain**." Regulatory efforts, including the Clean Air Act and its amendments of 1990, have resulted in marked reductions in SO_2 emissions. Currently, the highest concentration of SO_2 exposure occurs within a relatively close range of stationary emission sources. Individuals in these areas with asthma seem to have a greater prevalence of bronchoconstriction, especially during physical exertion.

Nitrogen Oxides

Oxides of nitrogen, some of the most common air pollutants, are produced as a by-product of the combustion of petroleum-based fuels. In this process, nitrogen reacts with oxygen to form nitrogen oxide, followed by rapid synthesis of nitrogen dioxide (NO_2) and various other oxides of nitrogen (NO_x). NO_2 is also present as an indoor air pollutant, with frequently high measured levels indoors compared with outdoors because of the combustion products of gas stoves, kerosene lights and heaters, and gas-fired furnaces.

In similarity with ozone, NO_2 is a strong oxidant. However, it is less cytotoxic than ozone because it does not typically develop free radicals and is less chemically reactive. Its water solubility is relatively low, so it tends to penetrate the pulmonary parenchyma. However, NO_2 may form acidic chemical compounds, such as nitric acid, when it contacts the moist upper respiratory mucosa at inspiration. These compounds may result in upper airway irritation.

Carbon Monoxide

Carbon monoxide (CO) is produced from the use of various fuels, most notably gasoline, propane, natural gas, oil, wood, coal, and tobacco. Automobiles produce the largest proportion of CO in the atmosphere. In general, ambient levels of CO are low, although increased levels have been reported in buildings with underground parking garages, businesses with drive-up windows, and enclosed ice rinks with propane-powered ice-resurfacing machines.

Deaths have been reported with accidental exposure to CO resulting from the use of stoves or outdoor grills in an indoor environment, malfunctioning furnaces, or fireplaces that have been installed incorrectly. Some jurisdictions have mandated the use of **CO detectors** inside homes and commercial buildings.

CO is odorless, colorless, and tasteless and results in hyphemic hypoxia because of its avid binding of hemoglobin, which causes tissue and brain hypoxia with insidious asphyxiation. The resulting bound carboxyhemoglobin (COHb) molecule is also thought to have direct toxic effects on tissues through its binding of heme proteins, such as cytochrome oxidase and myoglobin. **COHb is a valid biomarker of exposure dose** to CO. Levels have been measured at up to 0.5% in nonsmokers without environmental CO exposures and in the range of 4% to 10% in smokers. Acute CO poisoning is associated with COHb levels of 20% or more. It results in headaches, weakness, and eventually seizures or coma, or both, or even death.

Additional studies have focused on cardiovascular or neurocognitive changes due to chronic low-dose CO exposures. Treatment includes removal from exposure and the use of supportive therapy, including application of high-flow supplemental oxygen. For persistent neurocognitive abnormalities due to CO exposure, hyperbaric oxygen treatment is recommended.

Lead

Lead is a heavy metal that has been mined and processed for thousands of years, causing toxicity with resulting long-term morbidity and death. Exposures are most commonly through inhaled and oral routes, but lead also may be absorbed dermally. Today, most exposure reported in developed countries is the result of occupational hazards, leaded paint, and leaded gasoline. The production and use of leaded gasoline have been phased out in most countries. However, undeveloped countries commonly do not restrict its use, which allows improved performance of gas-powered engines.

Long-term lead toxicity may result in neurologic problems, such as reduced cognitive abilities, or nausea, abdominal pain, irritability, insomnia, a metallic taste in the oropharynx, excessive lethargy or hyperactivity, chest pain, headache, and, in extreme cases, seizure and coma. Peripheral neuropathy with painless wrist or foot drop may occur. Also, associated gastrointestinal problems, such as constipation, diarrhea, vomiting, poor appetite, and weight loss, are common in acute poisoning.

Other associated effects are anemia, kidney problems, and reproductive problems. Lead toxicity may result in a bluish line along the gums, known as **Burton's line**, although this finding is uncommon in young children. **Basophilic stippling of red blood cells**, as well as the changes normally associated with iron-deficiency anemia (ie, microcytosis and hypochromia), may be seen with lead toxicity.

Lead levels are most commonly measured from whole blood, and regulatory agencies set a level of 10 mcg/dL as an acceptable safe level, although neurocognitive development has been shown to be blunted at lesser levels. The most important part of treating lead poisoning is decreasing the exposure to lead. For substantially elevated lead levels with associated clinical findings, chelation therapy with meso-2,3 dimercaptosuccinic acid (DMSA), ethylene diaminetetraacetic acid (EDTA), and British anti-lewisite, also known as 2,3-dimercaptopropanol (BAL), has been used successfully.

Environmental Tobacco Smoke

Smoking prevalence has decreased in the United States over the past several decades. Nevertheless, tobacco abuse is prevalent and affects thousands of individuals who do not smoke but are in an environment where tobacco smoke is present. Environmental tobacco smoke (ETS) refers to the combination of sidestream smoke released from the tip of a burning cigarette and mainstream smoke exhaled by the smoker. More than 150 chemical compounds have been identified in cigarette smoke, including benzene, CO, and nicotine, and the term most commonly used to describe the presence of fine particulates in the smoking environment is "respirable suspended particles."

Several expert panels have performed detailed reviews of the medical literature in regard to ETS. They have established that ETS is associated with **increased risk of pulmonary malignancy** in nonsmokers, persistent irritation of the upper respiratory tract with underlying cellular inflammatory changes, and attenuated respiratory development, as well as an increased prevalence of respiratory symptoms and lower respiratory tract infections in children and adolescents.

Asbestos

Asbestos includes several fibrous inorganic materials with a crystalline structure and is grouped into serpentine, curved, and straight fibers. It was used for acoustical insulation and fire protection and has been incorporated into various building materials, including ceiling tiles, pipe wrap, tiles, insulation, and shingles.

Epidemiologic investigations support strong associations between the inhalation of asbestos fibers and the development of fibrotic change of the pulmonary parenchyma (asbestosis), pleural and peritoneal mesothelioma, bronchogenic carcinoma, laryngeal malignancies, and possibly gastrointestinal cancers. The EPA banned most applications of asbestos in 1973. However, as many as 20% of buildings (excluding schools and residences) in the United States still contain some asbestos material.

Formaldehyde

Formaldehyde is a relatively common chemical used as a preservative in the textile industry, as well as being a key component of resins used to manufacture such wood products as particle board, plywood, and fiberboard. Exposure to formaldehyde may occur in the manufacturing of either the chemical or the products in which it is used. Health effects of formaldehyde inhalation include upper respiratory tract irritation with conjunctival burning and oropharyngeal irritation.

Radon

Radon is a naturally occurring radioactive gas that cannot be seen, smelled, or tasted. The EPA has concluded that radon is the **leading cause of lung cancer among nonsmokers** and the second leading cause of lung cancer in the United States, claiming about 20,000 lives annually.

Radon occurs in the soil as a byproduct from the radioactive decay of uranium. Because radon is a gas, it is able to seep into a house through cracks, construction joints, sump holes, and holes in the foundation where utility lines enter the building. The house then traps the radon inside, where its concentration can build to levels higher than those in the soil.

Predicting which houses are likely to have elevated radon levels is difficult, but both old and new houses may have concentrations in excess of those in the soil around the structure. The only way to know the radon level of a house is to test for radon concentration. The EPA recommends a maximum acceptable concentration of 4 pCi/L.

Residents can test their homes for radon concentration or hire a professional to do the testing. Some county health departments have obtained the appropriate equipment to test homes for radon and will test houses in the county for free or for a nominal fee.

The radon testing process has 2 steps. First, a short-term test is taken. If the result is a radon concentration of 4 pCi/L or greater, a follow-up test is taken to ensure its accuracy. The follow-up test involves either a long-term test or a second short-term test. For a better understanding of the year-round average radon level, residents can do the long-term test. If results are needed quickly, they may choose to instead take a second short-term test.

Charcoal canisters, an alpha track detector, an electretion chamber, continuous monitors, and charcoal liquid scintillation detectors are most commonly used for short-term testing. Because radon levels tend to vary from day to day and season to season, a short-term test is less likely than a long-term test to provide the year-round average radon level. However, if results are needed quickly, a short-term test followed by a second short-term test may be used to decide whether to take action to lower the radon levels in the home. Actions needed to accomplish this decrease depend on the house's construction and its radon level. The EPA provides guidance on which actions to take.

Biologic Contaminants

Indoor air may be contaminated with various microbial organisms and antigenic proteins. Sampling technology improvements allow for measurements of these allergens, although airborne levels of specific microbial particles in indoor environments have not been well characterized, nor do they have threshold levels established. Growth of microorganisms in damp indoor environments has been associated with severe indoor biologic pollution. Dust mites, cat and dog dander, feces of domestic cockroaches, and spores of various fungi (eg, *Cladosporium*, *Penicillium*, *Alternaria*, *Aspergillus*) represent other common respiratory allergens and irritants.

Water Quality

In the United States, several laws regulate water quality, with the primary laws being the Clean Water Act (with subsequent amendments) and the Safe Drinking Water Act of 1974. Both laws enable the EPA to ensure compliance. The Clean Water Act primarily addresses protection of water for rivers and harbors and regulates point-source pollution. It requires permits for industries to discharge waste liquids into rivers and requires pretreatment to minimize water degradation at the point of discharge.

The Safe Drinking Water Act is aimed at ensuring that public water supplies are safe and valuable aquifers are protected. This legislation protects not only surface waters but also groundwater, regulating underground discharge of contaminants. The EPA Web site provides detailed information on the particular chemicals and microorganisms that are regulated, as well as a description of how safe levels are determined. Standards require zero levels of *Cryptosporidium*, *Giardia*, *Legionella*, coliform bacteria, and enteric viruses.

Of special note, some toxicants in water are of increased risk. Arsenic occurs naturally in the environment and has organic and inorganic forms. **Inorganic arsenic is the most toxic water toxicant** and causes increased incidence of cancers of the skin, bladder, liver, and lung. A lifetime cancer risk similar to that from radon exposure and secondhand cigarette smoke is associated with an arsenic level of 50 parts per billion.

Radon is another toxicant that can cause increased cancer through both direct ingestion of contaminated water and inhalation after radon has volatilized from tap water or from bedrock and seeped into a house. Of the estimated 40,000 deaths per year in the United States due to radon exposure, approximately 1% to 5% may be related to water sources.

In addition, nitrates and nitrites are common groundwater contaminants, especially in agricultural areas, from use of fertilizers. Nitrates can cause **methemoglobinemia** in infants. In the gut, nitrates convert to nitrites, which are absorbed into the bloodstream and form methemoglobin, thus decreasing the ability of the blood to absorb oxygen. This condition is also known as **blue baby syndrome**.

Mercury

Scientists and the general public are increasingly concerned about mercury exposure. News reports have highlighted potential exposures from gas meters, thermometers, industrial sites, and dental amalgams. The US Food and Drug Administration (FDA) has warned pregnant women and other vulnerable groups to limit consumption of certain large predator fish. Mercury exposure in humans is primarily through exposure to 1) elemental mercury (eg, gas meters, thermometers, dental amalgams) and 2) methylmercury (eg, fish).

Methylmercury is a by-product of manmade pollution, in which the sediment of lake and sea bottoms has been contaminated with elemental or metallic mercury and mercuric salts from industrial pollution. Mercury in lake and sea waters undergoes aerobic and anaerobic methylation by microorganisms. The resulting methylmercury is rapidly absorbed by aquatic microorganisms and gradually bioaccumulates in the food chain. Fish also concentrate methylmercury directly from aqueous intake through gills.

Large predator fish, such as tuna, shark, halibut, and freshwater pike, have been found to accumulate organic mercury to levels 3,000 to 10,000 times the concentration in water. Larger, older fish tend to have higher levels of methylmercury in their muscles. Humans absorb methylmercury from the intestines in a highly efficient manner after ingestion of these fish. Methylmercury enters the bloodstream and becomes distributed in tissues, with a high affinity for nerve and brain tissue.

The toxic effects of mercury were well dramatized in the epidemic known as Minamata disease. This outbreak occurred in Japan in the 1950s, when a chemical company dumped elemental mercury into Minamata Bay. The mercury was subsequently taken up in local sea life and eaten by the residents of this area. More than 100 people and many animals had debilitating and unusual neurologic disease. More than 50 fatalities occurred, along with multiple cases of cerebral palsy and mental retardation.

Other symptoms associated with mercury intake include nonspecific paresthesias, nausea, diarrhea, anorexia, sleep disturbances, and personality changes. Symptoms of chronic exposure include constriction of vision, ataxia, tremors, and dementia. These symptoms have been associated with estimates of a minimum daily intake of 300 mcg of methylmercury in the diet. The FDA and the EPA provide guidelines for US consumers regarding the amount and type of fish to eat to stay safely within recommended consumption guidelines to prevent mercury toxicity.

Exposure to elemental mercury and respiration of mercury vapors occur occasionally through spills and when uninformed persons bring elemental mercury home from medical equipment that has been disposed of improperly. Officials from local and state environmental agencies mitigate mercury spills larger than 2 tablespoons.

- Air quality can be compromised by many airborne pollutants, not the least of which are tobacco smoke, radon, particulates, and asbestos, which may cause respiratory irritation and disease, cancer, and gastrointestinal problems.
- Water quality laws cover chemicals and microorganisms in the water of harbors and rivers and in the public water supply, which includes lakes and aquifers.
- Toxicity from mercury, which has a high affinity for nerve and brain tissue, generally occurs from either exposure to elemental mercury or ingestion of methylmercury in fish.

Food Quality and Foodborne Illness

In the United States and much of the developed world, people have become accustomed to having food in varieties and abundance as never before, thanks to improvements in farming, industrialization, transportation, and storage. They assume that their food will be safe, affordable, fresh, and perfect in appearance. Generally, this assumption holds true, but health professionals know that there are exceptions to the assumption that food is always safe.

The US Centers for Disease Control and Prevention (CDC) estimates that each year, 76 million people get sick, more than 300,000 are hospitalized, and 5,000 die as a result of foodborne illnesses. Most, but not all, cases of foodborne illness have gastrointestinal tract symptoms. When determination of a specific pathogen is needed because of the severity, duration, or unusual nature of the illness, the clinician should obtain stool cultures and also recognize that testing for some pathogens may require special arrangements with the testing laboratory, such as tests for *Escherichia coli* O157:H7 and the *Vibrio* species.

When suspected cases of foodborne illness occur, consideration should be given to informing the appropriate public health officials and to addressing regulatory obligations of the local area. Many states have legislation in place that either requires the ordering physician to review the test result with state authorities or requires the testing laboratory to report results to public health officials when certain types of bacterial strains are identified in cultures and screening tests for genetic identification of pathogens.

When a case has been identified as having a suspicious association with a food source, the clinician should also be aware that the patient's condition may be a sentinel case of a more widespread outbreak. Clinicians need to talk with their patients about ways to prevent foodborne illness.

Recognizing Foodborne Illness

Symptoms of nausea, vomiting, diarrhea, or abdominal pain may be due to a foodborne illness. It is inherently important that the clinician keep a high index of suspicion for infections with foodborne etiologic characteristics. Important clues to determining a foodborne disease include a probable incubation period, the duration of the resulting illness, the predominant clinical symptoms, and the possible population involved in an outbreak.

Further information of importance includes a history of consumption of raw or undercooked foods (ie, eggs, meats, fish, or shellfish), unpasteurized milk or juices, fresh vegetables or fruit, or soft cheeses made from unpasteurized milk. The clinician should inquire whether acquaintances or family members have become ill and determine whether the patient lives on a farm, has pet contact, or has contact with children who attend day care. Also, consideration should be given to the individual's occupation, foreign travel, and camping excursions.

When a foodborne illness is suspected, the clinician should submit appropriate specimens for culture, with attention to request special cultures when unusual organisms are suspected. Table 1 summarizes important microbial pathogens and guides clinicians to the diagnosis and treatment of foodborne illness.

Infection With *Escherichia coli* O157:H7

The bacterial pathogen *E coli* O157:H7 has been associated with meats, and particularly hamburger, that have been undercooked, as well as unpasteurized milk and juices; raw fruits, vegetables, and seeds (such as alfalfa sprouts); salami; and contaminated water. During the processing of hamburgers, the bacteria, a surface contaminant, are mixed deeply with the meat. Individuals (especially young children, the elderly, and persons who are immunocompromised) may be susceptible to this pathogen when hamburger is not cooked to an internal temperature sufficient to kill

Table 1 Foodborne Illnesses Caused by Bacteria and Viruses

Etiologic Factor	Incubation Period	Signs and Symptoms	Duration of Illness	Associated Foods	Laboratory Testing	Treatment
Enterotoxigenic *Escherichia coli*	1-3 d	Watery diarrhea, abdominal cramps, some vomiting	3->7 d	Water or food contaminated with human feces	Stool culture. ETEC requires special laboratory techniques for identification. If suspected, must request specific testing	Supportive care. Antibiotics are rarely needed except in severe cases. Recommended antibiotics include TMP/SMX and quinolones
Listeria monocytogenes	9-48 h for gastrointestinal symptoms; 2-6 wk for invasive disease	Fever, muscle aches, and nausea or diarrhea. Pregnant women may have mild flulike illness, and the infection can lead to premature delivery or stillbirth. Elderly or immunocompromised patients may have bacteremia or meningitis. Infant infected from mother at risk for sepsis or meningitis	Variable / At birth and infancy	Fresh soft cheeses, unpasteurized milk, inadequately pasteurized milk, ready-to-eat deli meats, hot dogs	Blood or cerebrospinal fluid cultures. Asymptomatic fecal carriage occurs; therefore, stool culture usually not helpful. Antibody to listeriolysin O may be helpful to identify outbreak retrospectively	Supportive care and antibiotics. Intravenous ampicillin, penicillin, or TMP/SMX are recommended for invasive disease
Salmonella spp.	1-3 d	Diarrhea, fever, abdominal cramps, vomiting. *S typhi* and *S paratyphi* produce typhoid with insidious onset characterized by fever, headache, constipation, malaise, chills, and myalgia; diarrhea is uncommon, and vomiting is not usually severe	4-7 d	Contaminated eggs, poultry; unpasteurized milk, juice, or cheese; contaminated raw fruits and vegetables (eg, alfalfa sprouts, melons). *S typhi* epidemics are often related to fecal contamination of water supplies or street-vended foods	Routine stool cultures	Supportive care. Other than for *S typhi* and *S paratyphi*, antibiotics are not indicated unless there is extraintestinal spread or the risk of extraintestinal spread. Consider ampicillin, gentamicin, TMP/SMX, or quinolones if indicated. A vaccine exists for *S typhi*
Shigella spp.	24-48 h	Abdominal cramps, fever, and diarrhea. Stools may contain blood and mucus	4-7 d	Food or water contaminated with human fecal material. Usually person-to-person spread, fecal-oral transmission. Ready-to-eat foods (eg, raw vegetables, salads, sandwiches) touched by infected food workers	Routine stool cultures	Supportive care. TMP/SMX recommended in the United States if organism is susceptible; nalidixic acid or other quinolones may be indicated if organism is resistant, especially in developing countries

Table 1 (continued) Foodborne Illnesses Caused by Bacteria and Viruses

Etiologic Factor	Incubation Period	Signs and Symptoms	Duration of Illness	Associated Foods	Laboratory Testing	Treatment
Staphylococcus aureus (preformed enterotoxin)	1-6 h	Sudden onset of severe nausea and vomiting. Abdominal cramps. Diarrhea and fever may be present	24-48 h	Unrefrigerated or improperly refrigerated meats, potato and egg salads, cream pastries	Normally a clinical diagnosis. Stool, vomitus, and food can be tested for toxin and cultured if indicated	Supportive care
Vibrio cholerae (toxin)	24-72 h	Profuse watery diarrhea and vomiting, which can lead to severe dehydration and death within hours	3-7 d; causes life-threatening dehydration	Contaminated water, fish, and shellfish; street-vended food typically from Latin America or Asia	Stool culture; *V cholerae* requires special media to grow. If *V cholerae* is suspected, must request specific testing	Supportive care with aggressive oral and intravenous rehydration. In cases of confirmed cholera, tetracycline or doxycycline is recommended for adults and TMP/SMX for children (age, <8 y)
Vibrio parahaemolyticus	2-48 h	Watery diarrhea, abdominal cramps, nausea, vomiting	2-5 d	Undercooked or raw seafood, such as fish, shellfish	Stool cultures. *V parahaemolyticus* requires special media to grow. If *V parahaemolyticus* is suspected, request specific testing	Supportive care. Antibiotics are recommended in severe cases: tetracycline, doxycycline, gentamicin, and cefotaxime
Vibrio vulnificus	1-7 d	Vomiting, diarrhea, abdominal pain, bacteremia, and wound infections. More common in immunocompromised persons or in patients with chronic liver disease (presenting with bullous skin lesions). May be fatal in patients with liver disease and in immunocompromised persons	2-8 d	Undercooked or raw shellfish, especially oysters; other contaminated seafood; and open wounds exposed to sea water	Stool, wound, or blood cultures. *V vulnificus* requires special media to grow. If *V vulnificus* is suspected, must request specific testing	Supportive care and antibiotics. Tetracycline, doxycycline, and ceftazidime are recommended
Yersinia enterocolitica and Yersinia pseudotuberculosis	24-48 h	Appendicitislike symptoms (diarrhea, vomiting, fever and abdominal pain) occur primarily in older children and young adults. May have a scarlatiniform rash with *Y pseudotuberculosis*	1-3 wk, usually self-limiting	Undercooked pork, unpasteurized milk or tofu; contaminated water. Infection has occurred in infants whose caregivers handled chitterlings	Stool, vomitus, or blood culture. *Yersinia* requires special media to grow. If suspected, must request specific testing. Serologic testing is available in research and reference laboratories	Supportive care. If septicemia or other invasive disease occurs, antibiotic therapy with gentamicin or cefotaxime (doxycycline and ciprofloxacin are also effective)

Agent	Incubation period	Duration	Signs and symptoms	Vehicle/source	Laboratory testing	Prevention/treatment
Hepatitis A	28 d average (range, 15-50 d)	Variable, 2 wk-3 mo	Diarrhea, dark urine, jaundice, and flulike symptoms (ie, fever, headache, nausea, and abdominal pain)	Shellfish harvested from contaminated waters, raw produce, contaminated drinking water, uncooked foods, and cooked foods that are not reheated after contact with infected food handler	Increase in ALT and bilirubin. Positive IgM and antihepatitis A antibodies	Supportive care. Prevention with immunization
Noroviruses (and other caliciviruses)	12-48 h	12-60 h	Nausea, vomiting, abdominal cramping, diarrhea, fever, myalgia, and some headache. Diarrhea is more prevalent in adults and vomiting is more prevalent in children	Shellfish, fecally contaminated foods, ready-to-eat foods (eg, salads, sandwiches, ice, cookies, fruit) touched by infected food workers	Routine RT-PCR and electromicroscopy on fresh, unpreserved stool samples. Clinical diagnosis, negative bacterial cultures. Stool is negative for WBCs	Supportive care, such as rehydration. Good hygiene
Rotavirus	1-3 d	4-8 d	Vomiting, watery diarrhea, low-grade fever. Temporary lactose intolerance may occur. Infants and children, the elderly, and immunocompromised persons are especially vulnerable	Fecally contaminated foods. Reacy-to-eat foods (eg, salads, fruits) touched by infected food workers	Identification of virus in stool with immunoassay	Supportive care. Severe diarrhea may require fluid and electrolyte replacement
Other viral agents (astroviruses, adenoviruses, parvoviruses)	10-70 h	2-9 d	Nausea, vomiting, diarrhea, malaise, abdominal pain, headache, fever	Fecally contaminated foods. Ready-to-eat foods touched by infected food workers. Some shellfish	Identification of the virus in early acute stool samples. Serologic testing. Commercial ELISA kits are now available for adenoviruses and astroviruses	Supportive care. Condition is usually mild and self-limiting. Good hygiene

Abbreviations: ALT, alanine aminotransferase; ELISA, enzyme-linked immunosorbent assay; ETEC, enterotoxigenic *Escherichia coli*; IgM, immunoglobulin M; RT-PCR, reverse transcription–polymerase chain reaction; TMP/SMX, trimethoprim-sulfamethoxazole; WBC, white blood cell.
Adapted from: Centers for Disease Control and Prevention. Diagnosis and management of foodborne illnesses: a primer for physicians and other health care professionals. MMWR. 2004;53(RR-4).

the bacteria (71°C [160°F]). Other food sources may be inoculated by animal feces (present in fields where fruit falls to the ground or near farm workers who handle fruits and vegetables); food subsequently is not sufficiently washed or pasteurized to eliminate bacterial contamination.

E coli O157:H7 and related bacteria produce Shiga toxin, which is implicated in many outbreaks; symptoms include severe stomach cramps, diarrhea (often bloody), and vomiting. Shiga toxin may cause fever, although the fever temperature usually is not very high (<38.5°C [<101°F]). The average length of illness is 5 to 7 days. Some infections are mild, but others are severe or even life threatening.

Of persons infected with *E coli* O157:H7, 5% to 10% may have **hemolytic uremic syndrome** (HUS). HUS is a potentially life-threatening complication, and its symptoms include fatigue, pallor, and decreased frequency of urination. Persons with HUS should be hospitalized because of the risk of kidney failure, among other serious problems. Most persons with HUS recover within a few weeks, but some have permanent organ damage or die of the syndrome.

Infection With *Campylobacter*

Campylobacter is both the most common cause of bacterial gastroenteritis in the world and the most commonly identified pathogen for diarrhea in industrialized nations. Although serious outcomes are not as prevalent with this bacterium as with salmonella, it still is the cause of serious outcomes, being the most common event preceding Guillain-Barré syndrome.

Clinical manifestations typically involve an average of 3 days of incubation (range, 1-7 d), which is most commonly followed by abdominal pain and diarrhea. In one-third of cases, individuals may have fever and malaise with no gastrointestinal disease. The fever may last for a day or more before the diarrhea occurs, and the infection may cause rigors, diffuse body aches, dizziness, and delirium.

The diarrhea stage lasts 7 days on average, often with blood present in the diarrhea by the second or third day. Abdominal pain and cramping can be severe and may mimic other conditions, such as appendicitis. Other acute complications of *Campylobacter* infections include cholecystitis, pancreatitis, hepatitis, peritonitis, hemorrhage, HUS, rashes, strangulation of ileostomy stoma, pericarditis, myocarditis, and cellulitis. Secondary, late complications of *Campylobacter* include Guillain-Barré syndrome and reactive arthritis.

For most cases of this illness, treatment involves supportive hydration and maintenance of electrolyte levels. Occasionally, infections may require hospitalization and antibiotic treatment. Typically, hospitalization is reserved only for patients who are at increased risk or have severe disease. These patients include individuals who are severely ill, elderly, pregnant, or immunocompromised and those with bloody stools, a high fever, extraintestinal infection, worsening or relapsing symptoms, or symptoms lasting longer than 1 week.

Listerial Infection

Listeria monocytogenes is the cause of listeriosis, a rare but deadly foodborne disease with a mortality rate of approximately 20%. Listeriosis is most likely to occur in immunocompromised persons, the elderly, and women who are pregnant. Febrile gastroenteritis due to listerial infection usually occurs after a large inoculum of bacteria from contaminated food. Ingestion of delicatessen meat, raw hot dogs, and unpasteurized soft cheese are risk factors for listeriosis.

The incubation period may be as long as 6 weeks in these populations with increased risk, but it can be as short as 6 to 10 hours during outbreaks in previously healthy adults. Symptoms of gastroenteritis due to *Listeria* include fever, watery diarrhea, nausea, vomiting, headache, and pains in joints and muscles. Symptoms typically last 2 days or less, and most patients recover completely. Invasive infections are rare, but they are most likely to occur in persons at high risk. They may lead to sepsis, meningoencephalitis (especially in neonates), cerebritis (sometimes leading to brain abscess), and rhombencephalitis (brainstem encephalitis). Listerial gastroenteritis is diagnosed with stool cultures, and secondary outcomes are detected through blood and cerebrospinal fluid cultures.

Fortunately, *Listeria* tends to be susceptible to most antibiotics, and recommended treatment generally favors ampicillin or penicillin G. In most patients with limited gastroenteritis, the illness has already resolved by the time a definite diagnosis is made, and thus no further treatment is needed.

Infection With *Salmonella*

Nontyphoidal salmonella gastroenteritis is generally indistinguishable from other forms of bacterial gastroenteritis and continues to be a common cause of diarrhea. Symptoms include nausea, vomiting, fever, and cramping, which typically occur at 8 to 72 hours after exposure. Contaminated food or water is the source of exposure. Symptom severity corresponds with the amount of bacteria present in the source.

As with the other causes of gastroenteritis mentioned herein, medical treatment is supportive care, and antibiotic treatment is primarily reserved for severe or extended infections and for persons with a history of immune deficiency. Antibiotics recommended for treatment of persons with preserved renal function include fluoroquinolones, trimethoprim-sulfamethoxazole, amoxicillin, and, if intravenous administration is needed, a third-generation cephalosporin.

Persons who have had resolution of diarrhea commonly continue to shed bacteria for up to 5 weeks. Follow-up cultures are not recommended after the original diagnosis has been made. **Ongoing treatment is not necessary or advised except in carriers** who had a positive culture 1 month after acute illness, followed by a confirmed positive culture 1 year later. Even so, treatment should only be considered for persons who may have other reasons for eradication treatment, such as those working in day care, food handlers, and those with family members who have immunodeficiency (Table 1).

Phytotoxins

Phytotoxins originate from phytoplankton, a group that includes algae and single-celled organisms, such as diatoms and dinoflagellates. Amnesiac shellfish poisoning, neurotoxic shellfish poisoning, paralytic shellfish poisoning, diarrheic shellfish poisoning, and ciguatera fish poisoning are foodborne illnesses resulting from ingestion of fish or shellfish that have had exposure to phytoplankton with accumulation of toxins from these sources. The first 4 of these conditions occur when individuals eat shellfish that have a bioaccumulation of toxins originally produced by biotoxic algae and plankton that are food sources for the shellfish. **Ciguatera fish poisoning** is caused by herbivorous fish grazing on algae that produce ciguatera toxin precursors. Large carnivorous fish associated with coral reefs, such as barracuda, snapper, grouper, and jacks, then consume the herbivorous fish. The ciguatera toxins accumulate in the predator fish and can cause poisoning when consumed by humans.

Mycotoxins

Many molds are associated with disease, as well as being sources of beneficial agents for medical uses. Beneficial agents include such antibiotics as penicillin and such immune suppressants as cyclosporine, as well as medications for control of postpartum hemorrhage and migraine headaches, such as ergot alkaloids. Exposure to mycotoxins may occur through ingestion, inhalation, and dermal exposure.

Bovine Spongiform Encephalopathy

Bovine spongiform encephalopathy (BSE) is a neurodegenerative disease of cattle associated with consumption of contaminated feed and is thought to be a **prion-transmitted disease**. The largest outbreak of this disease has occurred in the United Kingdom and a lesser outbreak occurred in the European Union. Experts believe that cattle acquire the disease by being given processed bovine offal as a component of feed. The infectious agent for this disease is most likely a prion, a protein that transmits disease.

Evidence suggests that the prion for BSE can lay dormant in the soil and remain infectious for an extended time, thus infected cattle and other cervids that have died and are decomposing may release prions into the environment for cattle to later acquire.

Interest in BSE began to increase when the disease was associated with **variant Creutzfeldt-Jakob disease** (vCJD) in humans. The largest number of cases parallel countries with the highest incidence of BSE. vCJD has been associated with a diet high in beef and beef products, as well as chicken. The latency for developing symptoms is thought to be years. Progressive mental deterioration and myoclonus are the hallmark features of vCJD.

Symptoms of vCJD differ from those of Creutzfeldt-Jakob disease in that they occur less rapidly, tend to affect a younger cohort, and often present with psychiatric symptoms (depression, anxiety, and psychosis) before development of myoclonic symptoms, such as gait disorders, involuntary movements, and slurred speech. Moderate to severe cognitive decline is eventually an end result in almost all persons infected with this agent. Death is uniformly the result and occurs within an average of 14 months, rather than the 5 months for Creutzfeldt-Jakob disease.

Prevention of vCJD focuses primarily on eliminating its sources in the food supply through various regulations. Eliminating cattle older than 3 years and "downer" cows (those that cannot stand), as well as stopping the practice of using processed animal parts in cattle feed, has been the primary method to remove the infectious material from the food supply.

- Foodborne diseases are common, affecting an estimated 76 million people annually, and differ in results that range from a rapid onset of gastrointestinal symptoms to death.
- Many causes of foodborne illness are bacteria and viruses, and some causes require special laboratory tests that need to be requested at sample submission.
- Persons most susceptible to the effects of foodborne illness are elderly individuals, persons with immunosuppression, and women who are pregnant.

Physical Stressors

Heat Stress

The potential for heat stress occurs in environments that cause increased internal body temperature. Factors that contribute to heat stress include the metabolic cost of work, environmental factors (air temperature, humidity, air movement, and radiant heat exchange), and clothing requirements. The American Conference on Governmental Industrial Hygienists (ACGIH) provides tools designed to prevent most workers from experiencing a core body temperature greater than 38°C (100.4°F). Activities that have the potential to induce a high degree of heat stress include those that involve high indoor or outdoor temperatures, radiant heat sources, high humidity levels, direct physical contact with hot objects, strenuous physical activity, or use of personal protective equipment that shields the body from hazardous biological, chemical, or radiologic agents but in doing so limits the removal of excess body heat and perspiration. Mild or moderate heat stress may cause discomfort and affect performance and safety but is not harmful to health. Severe heat stress may cause heat-related disorders. Usually a minor problem for healthy individuals, heat stress is often difficult to predict because individual susceptibility varies. It may become serious for people with heart or respiratory problems or those who are exposed to prolonged high temperatures. In acute cases of severe heat stress, symptoms can occur in as little as 15 minutes. Table 2 provides additional information on heat stress disorders.

Cold Stress

Injury from frostbite and hypothermia occurs at low temperatures and can be extreme when the windchill factor is very low. Fatal exposure to cold temperatures is usually the result of accidental exposure from failure to escape low air temperatures or from immersion in low-temperature water. For the case of a single, occasional exposure to cold temperature, the ACGIH recommends that **core body temperature should not be allowed to drop lower than 35°C (95°F)** and that all parts of the body be protected, including hands, feet, and head. Clinical signs and symptoms of cold stress are described in Table 3.

Sun Exposure

Solar radiation is a form of nonionizing radiation that can have negative health effects and primarily involves exposure to UV radiation, of which the sun is the major source. UV radiation involves wavelengths from 160 nm to 400 nm and is often categorized as near UV or UV-A, middle UV or UV-B, far UV or UV-C, and vacuum.

The health effects of UV radiation typically are divided into acute and long-term effects. Acute effects typically affect the skin and eyes. Immediate changes occur with sun exposure and are directly related to the intensity and duration of the exposure, as well as individual susceptibility. Persons with more melanin have greater protection because melanin absorbs radiation from the whole spectrum of UV light.

Acute exposure to UV radiation may also cause ocular damage. UV radiation is absorbed mostly by the cornea, and excessive exposure can damage vision. Caution is especially important when working with occupational exposure to strong UV sources, such as lasers, where irreversible

Table 2 Heat Stress Disorders

Heat stroke	Medical emergency. Temperature regulation fails; body temperature rises to critical levels (rectal temperature, 41°C [105.8°F]). Patient confused with irrational behavior; loss of consciousness; convulsions, lack of sweating; hot, dry skin. While waiting for medical assistance, place worker in shade and remove outer clothing; wet skin and increase air movement around patient to improve evaporative cooling. Provide fluids.
Heat exhaustion	Causes headache, nausea, vertigo, weakness, thirst, and giddiness, all of which respond to the patient's removal from the hot environment, fluid replacement, and rest.
Heat cramps	Due to electrolyte imbalance (lack of water replenishment) caused by hard physical labor in a hot environment (sweating). Water should be taken every 15-20 min in a hot environment. Working 6-8 h in heavy protective gear may result in loss of sodium. Drinking carbohydrate-electrolyte replacement liquids minimizes physiologic disturbances during recovery.
Heat collapse	Heat collapse (fainting) occurs when the brain does not receive adequate oxygen because of blood pooling in the extremities. Onset can be rapid and unpredictable. Heat collapse can be prevented by gradually becoming acclimatized to the hot environment.
Heat rash	Rash (prickly heat) consists of red papules and often appears in areas persistently wetted by sweat or where clothing is restrictive. Sweating causes prickling sensation. Papules can become infected if left untreated. Rash is the most common problem in a hot work environment and often disappears when patient returns to cool environment.
Heat fatigue	Impaired performance of skilled sensorimotor, mental, or vigilance jobs, usually caused by lack of acclimatization. Treatment consists of removing the patient from the hot environment. Heat fatigue can be prevented though acclimatization.

damage, including photokeratitis and conjunctivitis, can occur.

Prolonged exposure of the skin to the sun over many years results in elastosis (loss of elasticity), and the skin takes on a wrinkled, leathery look. Elastosis leads to premature aging and is most often evident in workers who spend long hours outdoors.

Some agents and medications can interact with sunlight to cause more severe results. Hence, it is especially important for clinicians to inform patients of the photosensitizing potential of these medications and antibiotics.

Another long-term effect of UV radiation is increased risk of skin cancer, which has been recognized for more

Table 3 Progressive Clinical Signs of Hypothermia

Core Temperature, °C	Clinical Signs
37	Normal oral temperature
36	Metabolic rate increases in attempt to compensate for heat loss
35	Maximum shivering
34	Patient conscious and responsive, blood pressure normal, shivering continues
33	Severe hypothermia below this temperature
32	Consciousness clouded, low blood pressure, pupils dilated but reactive to light, shivering ceases
30	Progressive loss of consciousness, muscle rigidity, readings of pulse and blood pressure difficult to obtain, decreasing respiratory rate
28	Ventricular fibrillation possible
27	Voluntary motion ceases, pupils nonreactive to light, deep tendon and superficial reflexes absent
26	Patient seldom conscious
25	Pulmonary edema
22	Maximum risk of ventricular fibrillation
20	Cardiac arrest

than a century. White persons are at higher risk for skin cancer than persons with darker skin, especially if they spend more time outdoors or live close to the equator. Lifestyle choices, such as getting a suntan, may be responsible for increased incidence of skin cancers. Worldwide, rates of squamous cell carcinoma have risen considerably over the last 25 years. Educating patients to avoid sun exposure from 10 AM to 2 PM—when the sun's rays are strongest—and to use topical lotions with sun-blocking protection is likely to help reduce the rate of future skin cancers.

Some controversy exists around the role of UV radiation in the development of malignant melanomas. There is no good animal model for malignant melanoma, and data on the relation between UV radiation and melanomas come from epidemiologic studies. Several studies have found that the frequency of severe sunburns in childhood is predictive of malignant melanoma risk, but this association does not hold true for adult exposures.

Prevention of UV exposure includes limiting total time in the sun, timing the exposure to when the sun's rays are less strong, wearing appropriate clothing, and wearing sunscreen during every exposure. Prevention of ocular problems includes the use of UV-protective eyeglasses, goggles, and plastic shields, especially in industrial settings.

The benefits of UV radiation primarily involve the synthesis of vitamin D, which plays an important role in calcium absorption. Vitamin D can be obtained through supplements and fortified diets, but when these are not available, sun exposure is the best way for humans to have adequate levels of vitamin D.

Ozone

Global concentrations of ozone precursors, including volatile organic compounds and nitrogen oxides, have steadily increased in the ambient atmosphere, due to increasing combustion of petroleum-based fuels used in automobiles and other motorized equipment. Ozone is a highly reactive oxidizing compound, reacting with intracellular lipid-based molecules to form free radicals, aldehydes, hydrogen peroxide, and various other toxic by-products. It has been shown to have direct cytotoxic effects, but experts also believe that ozone injures tissues through inflammatory response pathways.

Several controlled studies have identified that the inhalation of ozone by healthy human subjects reduces expiratory airflow that is sequentially associated with increased concentration of the gas, respiratory rate, and duration of exposure. This reduction in airflow seems to be associated with an involuntary inhibition of inspiratory effort through neurally mediated stimulation of airway C fibers. Certain populations, such as persons with asthma or chronic respiratory disease, have been shown in epidemiologic studies to have increased emergency department visit rates and hospitalizations on days with measured high ambient ozone levels. The measured forced expiratory volume in the first second of expiration does not necessarily fall acutely with acute exposure to ozone, likely because the proposed mechanism involving reduction in inspiratory capacity—rather than bronchoconstriction—causes acute obstructive airflow physiologic response. Patients with the tendency to have bronchoconstriction from any etiologic factor are generally cautioned to avoid outdoor exposure during times of elevated ambient ozone levels.

The ozone layer absorbs radiation of less than 290 nm (ie, vacuum and UV-C waves) and prevents exposure of the Earth to these wavelengths. Considerable discussion in the past few decades has focused on the decreasing coverage of the ozone layer, with some estimates of a 2% loss during the past 2 decades. Discussion has focused primarily on the impact of chlorofluorocarbons (CFCs), which are currently used as a component in the manufacture of refrigerator and air conditioner coolants in the United States. CFC use has been banned as a propellant for spray cans. However, production of CFCs is growing at a worldwide rate of 5% per year despite efforts to limit their use. **CFCs catalyze the destruction of ozone**, and CFCs used currently take up to a century to degrade.

Ionizing Radiation

The use of various sources of ionizing radiation in developed countries is highly regulated, and thus, serious bioeffects from occupational radiation exposure are rare. The recommended maximum permissible occupational radiation doses in the United States are 50 mSv as the effective whole-body dose, 150 mSv to the lens of the eye, and 500 mSv to the skin, hands, or feet. Worker doses rarely approach or exceed these limits.

Biologic effects of ionizing radiation are grouped into 2 general categories: deterministic and stochastic. A **deterministic effect** is defined as a somatic effect that occurs above a threshold dose and increases in severity with increasing dose above the threshold. Examples are skin damage and lens opacities. Skin damage is most likely to occur in patients during high-dose fluoroscopic procedures, such as complicated angioplasty cases. The threshold for skin damage (erythema followed by blistering and necrosis at extremely high doses) is about 3 Gy to 6 Gy for x-rays in the diagnostic energy range (for diagnostic x-rays, a Gy is equivalent to 1,000 mSv). Thus, skin effects are not observed in workers unless they are involved in an accidental exposure to radiation doses far in excess of the regulatory limit of 500 mSv.

Cataract development requires acute doses in excess of 1 Gy or a lifetime dose of about 10 Gy (1,000 rem) to the lens of the eye. During a 40-year career, a worker would need to receive about 250 mSv per year to the eye to have radiation-induced cataracts. Cardiologists and interventional radiologists who have the potential to receive the 150-mSv annual limit to the lens of the eye wear protective lenses, such as goggles with leaded glass, to keep the lens dose well under the limit. Thus, radiation-induced cataracts are not likely to be observed in workers.

A third clinically significant deterministic effect of radiation is structural anomalies for abnormal development or growth of the embryo and fetus. However, the maximum permissible radiation dose to the fetus is 0.5 mSv and the threshold for deterministic effects in the fetus is 1,000 mSv or more. Thus, the risk of fetal anomalies from occupational radiation exposure is negligible.

A stochastic effect is defined as an **all-or-none response** in which the probability of the effect increases with radiation dose while the severity is independent of dose (eg, occurrence of cancer). Also, solid tumors have a latent period of approximately 20 years, so they may not express themselves within the lifetime of the worker. The risk of cancer is low or negligible for workers whose occupational radiation exposure is less than the 50-mSv annual limit. However, since theoretically there is no threshold for this risk, radiation protection programs are expected to include procedures to keep occupational doses as far below the occupational dose limit as reasonably achievable. The National Research Council of the National Academy of Sciences provides estimates of cancer risk in its report from the Committee to Assess Health Risks From Exposure to Low Levels of Ionizing Radiation. Risk is dependent on the radiation dose, the organ exposed, and the age and sex of the exposed individual. The overall risk of death from solid cancer, regardless of age and sex, is approximately 500 deaths per 100,000 persons exposed to 100 mGy (ie, 100 mSv for medical x-rays and most radionuclides that emit gamma rays).

Nonionizing Radiation

Biologic effects of nonionizing radiation have been recognized and reasonably understood for some time. Few workplaces produce field strengths of concern. Nonionizing radiation includes static magnetic and subradiofrequency fields, radiofrequency and microwave radiation, and light, infrared, and ultraviolet radiation. The ACGIH has established **threshold limit values** (TLVs) to protect workers from excess exposure to these fields. A TLV is the **maximum unprotected workplace field strength or radiation field** under which nearly all workers (except the most sensitive workers) may be exposed repeatedly without adverse health effects. Various hazards have been shown in laboratory studies of nonionizing radiation above these levels, including startle reactions from spark discharges, contact currents from ungrounded conductors within the field, and ignition of flammable materials. The TLV may not protect against electromagnetic interference with pacemaker function. There is no convincing evidence of adverse health effects below these limits.

Noise

Although noise levels are not excessive in most work environments, nuisance levels of noise exist in some work areas and can contribute to stress or to some loss of hearing. These levels of noise may startle, annoy, or distract workers and, when excessive, may cause pain or physical damage to the ear and even temporary or permanent hearing loss. Noise may be an immediate safety concern when it interferes with speech communication by preventing individuals from warning others of safety hazards or immediate danger. The TLV for noise refers to sound pressure levels and durations of exposure that represent conditions under which nearly all workers may be exposed repeatedly without adverse effects on hearing. Workers should not be exposed to more than 85 dBA for an 8-hour period. Greater TLVs of noise may be permitted for shorter periods (eg, 88 dBA for up to 4 hours, 91 dBA for up to 2 hours, 94 dBA for up to 1 hour, and 97 dBA for up to 30 minutes). A hearing conservation program that includes audiometric testing is necessary when workers are exposed to noise levels at or above the TLVs.

- Heat stress, defined for workers as the effect of a core body temperature greater than 38°C (100.4°F), is often difficult to predict because individual susceptibility varies.

- Injury from frostbite and hypothermia can be extreme, even fatal, and prevention involves avoiding a decline in inner core temperature to 35°C (95°F).
- UV radiation from sun exposure can cause acute (skin and eyes) and long-term (skin) effects that may result in an increased risk of skin cancer, yet a benefit of UV radiation is vitamin D synthesis.
- Ozone, which protects the Earth from low-wavelength radiation, is also an oxidizing compound that reacts with intracellular lipid-based molecules and may effect an involuntary inhibition of inspiratory effort.
- Biologic effects of ionizing radiation are grouped into deterministic (eg, eyes, skin), which increase as the dose increases above a threshold level, and stochastic, which have an all-or-none response and for which the probability of the effect increases with radiation dose while the severity is independent of dose (eg, cancer).
- Nonionizing radiation includes static magnetic and subradiofrequency fields, radiofrequency and microwave radiation, and light, infrared, and ultraviolet radiation, yet few workplaces produce field strengths of a concern to health.
- Noise levels are not excessive in most work environments, but some have nuisance levels of noise that can contribute to stress and hearing loss.

Solid-Waste Management

Community Systems

Until the past few decades, many communities considered household garbage, yard waste, cans, bottles, newspapers, ashes, discarded building materials, electronic products, and other common trash as solid or municipal waste. They were not considered hazardous and were usually transported to the town dump, where this municipal waste was periodically burned and sometimes buried. Today, communities require collection and transport of household waste to a government-permitted landfill or incinerator, and many require recycling of such materials as newspapers, aluminum and other metal cans, and glass and plastic bottles. The goals of most community solid-waste programs include encouragement of environmentally sound solid-waste management practices, maximization of reuse or recycling of recoverable resources, and fostering of resource conservation. The most environmentally sound management of solid waste is achieved when communities implement practices in accordance with the EPA's preferred order: source reduction first, recycling and composting second, and disposal in landfills or waste combustors last.

Individual Sewage Disposal Systems

Domestic activities, such as cooking, cleaning, laundry, or bathing, create wastewater that, through ingestion or bodily contact, can result in disease, severe illness, and, in some instances, death due to bacteria, viruses, and parasites contained in the waste. Therefore, proper treatment of the wastewater is important. For homes and vacation properties not connected to a municipal sewer, a properly designed, constructed, and maintained individual sewage disposal system (ie, septic system) provides long-term, effective treatment of household wastewater. However, a malfunctioning system can contaminate groundwater that might be a source of drinking water.

A **septic system** has 4 main components: a pipe from the home, a septic tank, a drain field, and soil. Household wastewater is delivered through the pipe to the septic tank, a buried, watertight container made of concrete, fiberglass, or polyethylene. Solids settle out from the wastewater in the tank (forming sludge) and oil and grease floats to the surface (creating scum). The solid materials undergo partial decomposition at the bottom of the tank; the sludge and scum are pumped periodically to prevent buildup and the floating of solid material into the drain field. Wastewater enters the drain field and is pushed into the soil whenever new wastewater enters the septic tank. Microbes in the soil digest or remove nutrients, other microbes, and most contaminants from wastewater before it eventually reaches groundwater.

Septic systems need to be monitored and maintained to prevent their failing. Failure of the septic system could result in harmful microbes and hazardous materials entering the groundwater and, eventually, a drinking water supply. Typical pollutants that may escape an improperly maintained septic system include nitrogen compounds, phosphorous, and disease-causing bacteria and viruses. One-fourth of US homes use septic systems, resulting in the daily release of more than 4 billion gallons of wastewater into the soil. Inadequately treated sewage from septic systems poses a considerable threat to human health because it can contaminate drinking water wells. It can also contaminate nearby surface waters, thereby increasing the chance of swimmers contracting various infectious diseases that range from eye and ear infections to acute gastrointestinal illness and such diseases as hepatitis.

- The most environmentally sound solid-waste management is achieved by communities when their practices are in accordance with the EPA's preferred sequential order: source reduction, recycling and composting, and disposal in landfills or waste combustors.
- Households not connected to municipal sewer should have a properly designed and well-maintained septic system, incorporating a wastewater pipe from the

house to a buried septic tank, which then sends separated waste to a drain field where it percolates through soil.

Management of Hazardous Materials

Many communities have established policies and procedures to identify and separate hazardous waste from the solid-waste stream and offer various options for safely disposing of hazardous household waste. Such a waste treatment program requires definition and identification of hazardous waste, regulation of generators and transporters, and regulation of operators of facilities that treat, store, or dispose of hazardous waste.

Materials often banned from disposal in municipal solid-waste landfills include common household items such as paints, cleaners and chemicals, motor oil and oil filters, batteries, electronic products, and pesticides. Improper disposal of household hazardous wastes includes pouring them down the drain, on the ground, into storm sewers, or, in some cases, putting them out with the trash. The dangers of such disposal methods might not be immediately obvious, but improper disposal can pollute the environment and pose a threat to human health.

In addition to household hazardous waste, considerable volumes of hazardous waste are generated by business and industry, including chemical manufacturers, the construction industry, hospitals and healthcare organizations, dental offices, industrial and research laboratories, and the paper and printing industry. The wastes from these sources include strong acids and bases, spent solvents, reactive wastes, heavy-metal solutions, and cyanide wastes. The EPA and US states individually regulate disposal of these hazardous wastes through implementation of the **Resource Conservation and Recovery Act** (RCRA), which created a system for the management, treatment, storage, and disposal of hazardous waste.

Under RCRA, the EPA ensures that hazardous waste is managed safely from the moment it is generated, while it is transported, treated, or stored, and until it is finally disposed of. This process is called the "cradle to grave" management system that defines requirements for hazardous-waste identification; generators, transporters, treatment, storage, and disposal facilities; recycling; and universal wastes, land disposal restrictions, combustion, and permitting. Also, specific regulations govern the requirements and procedures for the EPA to authorize states to administer the RCRA program. Anyone or any facility that generates, transports, treats, stores, or disposes of hazardous waste and any entity that produces, burns, distributes, or markets any waste-derived fuels must notify the EPA of its activities and comply with

the RCRA. The EPA may issue an administrative order or impose a civil penalty to any person who violates the RCRA. It also may bring a civil action against anyone who fails to comply with such an administrative order.

- The dangers of improper disposal methods of hazardous waste from households and industry, such as pouring them down the drain or into storm sewers, may not be obvious immediately, but such disposal can pollute the environment and threaten human health.

Land Use Planning

Land use planning is the systematic assessment of land and water potential for selecting and adopting the best land use options. Planning also provides guidance in cases of conflict between rural land use and urban or industrial expansion, indicating which areas of land are most valuable. Communities decide to embark on land use planning for various reasons that preserve and enhance quality of life and maintain and protect public health, safety, and well-being. Planning may help the community qualify for grant and loan programs, provide consistency among its ordinances, and provide a healthy landscape that includes trails for walking and biking. Various tools are used to help the community address land use issues consistently, prioritize projects, and obtain public input. Problems addressed by land use planning include the development of zoning ordinances and public transportation and the establishment of transportation corridors.

Land use planning also involves anticipation of the need for change, as well as the public's reactions to it. In some cases, an existing situation cannot continue because the land is being degraded. Examples of unwise land use are the clearance of forest on steep land or on poor soil for which sustainable systems of farming have not been developed; overgrazing of pastures; and industrial, agricultural, and urban activities that produce pollution.

Planning can help communities identify the best use for land. For any particular use, certain areas are better suited than others. Planning can help match potential land use with the areas that will yield the greatest benefits at the least cost. Land use also must be socially acceptable.

- The systematic assessment of land and water potential for selecting and adopting the best land use options, land use planning addresses the development of zoning ordinances and public transportation and the establishment of transportation corridors as a community changes.

Environmental Disasters

Many environmental disasters that likely are familiar to the reader have received considerable attention by the press. Those disasters that were manmade were subsequently the subject of legal action. Many environmental disasters originated in nature and caused widespread loss of life and economic devastation. We highlight perhaps the most well-known episodes (Box).

Of manmade disasters, there may be some debate as to the significance, the number of deaths, and the illness attributed to each episode. Although these episodes are rated 1 through 10 in the Box, they are not in an important ordinal ranking because of the difficulty in making a direct comparison of their outcomes. Key historical anthropogenic environmental disasters are summarized in Table 4.

Natural disasters also have caused heavy tolls on humanity, and their effects in antiquity are difficult to quantify. These types of disasters caused many deaths and substantial disease and disability. Secondary effects often added further damage to populations, with problems such as the loss of emergency services, transportation, communication, and safety.

Box Major Natural Disasters of Recent History

1. Global epidemics—the plague (1348-1350), the Spanish flu (1918), and AIDS (1981 to present)
2. Bangladesh arsenic crisis (1994 to present)
3. Asian earthquake and tsunami of 2004
4. Hurricane Katrina (2005) and Hurricane Mitch (1998)
5. Earthquakes of Izmit, Turkey, in 1999
6. Dutch flood disaster of 1953
7. Roraima wildfires of Brazil in 1998
8. Mount Pinatubo volcanic eruption in the Philippines (1991)
9. The Ellington, Missouri, tornado of 1925
10. Dust storms of Beijing, China, and Queensland, Australia (recurring)

- The outcomes of environmental disasters, whether of nature or manmade, have consisted of widespread loss of life, substantial disease and disability, and economic devastation. Their full effects are difficult to quantify.

Table 4 Anthropogenic Environmental Disasters

Location/Population	Year	Chemical	Cause	Effects
Bhopal, India Union Carbide Corp plant	1984	Methyl isocyanate	Human error, disabled safety mechanisms	4,000 estimated acute deaths, 50,000 persons with chronic health effects, including respiratory effects and blindness
Chernobyl, Ukraine Nuclear power plant	1986	Radioactive material (^{137}Cs and ^{131}I) from core breach and fire	Errors in reactor design, errors in judgment	31 immediate deaths, death from chronic effects estimated at 30,000-300,000; numerous evacuees and an economic impact
London, England	1952	Coal combustion products and vehicle emissions	Cold winter temperatures, weather inversion, and normal practice for residential and commercial heating	12,000 estimated deaths from acute effects on vulnerable infants, children, and elderly persons with underlying respiratory and cardiovascular disease
Seveso, Italy Chemical manufacturer	1976	TCDD	Human error, uncontrolled thermal reaction	3,300 acute animal deaths, 80,000 feed animals sacrificed to prevent TCDD entering food chain, 447 persons with skin reactions (chloracne)
Major oil spills	1978-current	Crude oil 2,000-260,000 tons	Numerous, primarily errors in judgment	Numerous effects on and deaths of aquatic life and water fowl, major economic impacts to fishing and tourism industries in some locations

Abbreviation: TCDD, tetrachlorodibenzo-*p*-dioxin.

Climate Change

Climate is related to physical features of the Earth and its atmosphere, as well as energy from the sun. Depletion of the ozone layer and accumulation of greenhouse gases are global concerns that are implicated in the gradual warming of the Earth. The melting of polar ice caps and the melt-off of mountainous glaciers will reflect less incoming solar radiation and allow additional elevations in temperature. Marked deviation in the normal fluctuations of temperature may lead to changes in land use, precipitation patterns, and desertification. These effects in turn will likely lead to changes in migration, population distribution, and food production and to overpopulation.

- Depletion of the ozone layer and accumulation of greenhouse gases are global concerns that are implicated in the gradual warming of the Earth.

Global Issues and Threats

Nuclear Warfare

The threat of potential nuclear warfare and nuclear terrorism is of great concern in the current geopolitical environment. In addition to the escalating number of nations acquiring advanced technology to use in nuclear weapons, tensions are escalating between some nations, increasing the possibility of their use. In addition to this threat, the breakup of the former Soviet Union has raised concerns of weapon-grade plutonium being diverted to subversive groups for use in terrorist activities (eg, "dirty bombs").

This potentially disastrous use of nuclear material has been a consideration in disaster planning for nations that are potential targets, including the United States. The CDC has substantial resources for health professionals on instruction and communication of emergency response to these threats (http://emergency.cdc.gov/planning/responseguide.asp).

Biological Warfare and Bioterrorism

The CDC classifies biological agents that could be used as weapons into 3 categories. Category A agents have the characteristics of organisms that pose a risk to national security because they can be easily disseminated or transmitted from person to person; result in high mortality rates and have the potential for major public health impact; might cause public panic and social disruption; and require special action for public health preparedness. **Category A agents** include anthrax, botulism, plague, smallpox, tularemia, and viral hemorrhagic fevers, such as infections with Ebola, Marburg, and Lassa. A summary of category A agents including symptom manifestations, diagnosis, and treatment are summarized in Table 5.

Category B agents are less virulent but still are capable of use as weapons and can be a threat to public health. They are moderately easy to disseminate; result in moderate morbidity rates and low mortality rates; and require specific enhancements of CDC's diagnostic capacity and enhanced disease surveillance. Category B agents include brucellosis, clostridium toxin, food safety threats such as *E coli* O157:H7, ricin toxin, typhus fever, viral encephalitis such as western equine encephalitis, and water safety threats such as *Vibrio cholerae* and *Cryptosporidium parvum*.

Category C agents are defined as emerging pathogens that have the capability of being used as potential threats because of their availability; ease of production and dissemination; and potential for high morbidity and mortality rates and major health impact. Examples of category C agents are Nipah virus and Hantavirus.

Chemical Warfare and Terrorism

Chemical warfare is the use of chemicals to produce an irritant, disabling effect that in many instances will cause death. These agents can be categorized by the type of chemical or the effects (Table 6).

- The threat of nuclear warfare has been escalating as more countries have the nuclear technology for the creation of nuclear weapons and as tensions among countries flare.
- Agents of biological warfare are divided into categories A, B, and C in accordance with their ease of dissemination, their availability, and their potential deleterious effect on large numbers of people.
- Chemical warfare and terrorism is the use of chemicals to produce an irritant, disabling effect that in many instances will cause death.

Table 5 Summary of Category A Bioterrorism Agents

Disease (Causatory Organisms)	Presentation	Transmission	Diagnostic Test	Isolation[a]	Postexposure Prophylaxis	Treatment
Anthrax (*Bacillus anthracis*)						
Inhalation	Fever with chills, malaise, nonproductive cough, nausea, and/or vomiting. May progress rapidly to respiratory failure	Inhalation of anthrax spores	Sputum, blood, and/or cerebrospinal fluid culture; PCR	Standard	Duration, 60 d *or* 100 d plus anthrax vaccine; ciprofloxacin, 500 mg orally every 12 h *or* doxycycline, 100 mg orally every 12 h *or* amoxicillin, 500 mg orally every 8 h if strain is susceptible	Ciprofloxacin, 400 mg IV every 12 h *or* doxycycline, 200-mg IV load followed by 100 mg IV every 12 h *and* 1 or 2 additional antimicrobials[b,c]
Gastrointestinal	Fever, abdominal pain, anorexia, nausea, and vomiting. May have hematemesis and bloody diarrhea	Eating undercooked, contaminated meat	Blood and/or stool cultures	Standard	As above	As above
Cutaneous	Pruritic macule or papule that progresses to vesicular lesions, which develop into a black eschar with surrounding edema	Direct contact with spores or with infected skin lesions	Vesicular fluid, exudate, and/or eschar culture; biopsy of cutaneous lesion	Standard	As above	Ciprofloxacin, 500 mg orally every 12 h *or* doxycycline, 100 mg orally every 12 h; both for a total of 60 d in the setting of a bioterrorism event
Smallpox (variola virus)	High fever, myalgia, headache, and maculopapular rash with centripetal evolution and synchronous onset. Vesicular at first and then pustular	Respiratory droplets, direct contact with skin lesions or secretions	Pharyngeal swab and/or scab material EM; ELISA, RFLP analysis, PCR virus characterization	Airborne and contact	Vaccinia immune globulin (best within 24 h of exposure)	Supportive care; cidofovir (proven effectiveness in vitro)
Tularemia (*Francisella tularensis*)	Most common syndromes Ulceroglandular: cutaneous papule that becomes pustular and eventually ulcerates; lymphadenopathy Typhoidal: fever, abdominal pain, diarrhea, vomiting Other syndromes include oculoglandular and oropharyngeal tularemia and tularemia pneumonia	Inoculation of infected body fluids of animals, bites of infected deerflies, ticks, or mosquitoes	Blood, sputum, serum culture; EM of tissue PCR, immunoblotting, pulsed-field gel electrophoresis	Standard	Doxycycline, 100 mg orally every 12 h for 14 d *or* ciprofloxacin, 500 mg orally every 12 h for 14 d	Streptomycin, 1 g IM every 12 h for 10 d *or* gentamicin, 5 mg/kg daily IM or IV for 10 d

Table 5 (continued) Summary of Category A Bioterrorism Agents

Disease (Causatory Organisms)	Presentation	Transmission	Diagnostic Test	Isolation[a]	Postexposure Prophylaxis	Treatment
Botulism (Clostridium botulinum)	Acute, afebrile, descending flaccid paralysis usually accompanied by ptosis, blurred vision, dysarthria, dysphonia, and dysphagia	Respiratory droplets, food or wound contamination	Serum, stool, gastric aspirate, vomitus for detection of toxin and culture; Ag-ELISA; bioassay using mice for toxin analysis	Standard	Pentavalent toxoid	Antitoxins, supportive care, ventilatory care if needed
Pneumonic plague (Yersinia pestis)	High fever, cough, hemoptysis, nausea, vomiting, and headache; may rapidly progress to respiratory failure	Flea vectors from rodents, respiratory droplets	Blood, sputum, lymph node aspirate Gram or Wright-Giemsa stain; Ag-ELISA in urine, serology for IgM and IgG, IFA	Droplet	Doxycycline, 200 mg orally every 12 h for 10 d or ciprofloxacin, 500 mg orally every 12 h for 10 d	Streptomycin, 1 g IM every 12 h for 10 d or gentamicin, 5 mg/kg per day IM or IV for 10 d or gentamicin, 2 mg/kg loading dose followed by 1.7 mg/kg IM or IV every 8 h for 10 d
Viral hemorrhagic fever (varies)	Varies with virus origin CCHF: hemorrhagic complications and DIC Marburg, Ebola: DIC, maculopapular rash RVF: hepatitis, retinitis Bunyaviridae, Flaviviridae: acute febrile illness, signs of vascular permeability	Differs with each viral syndrome. Commonly transmitted through contact with infected animal reservoirs or arthropod vectors	Serum, blood virus isolation; Ag-ELISA, RT-PCR, Ab-ELISA	Airborne and contact	Isolation precautions	Supportive therapy CCHF/ arenavirus: ribavirin, 30 mg/kg IV initial dose, followed by 15 mg/kg IV every 6 h for 4 d and 7.5 mg/kg IV every 8 h for 6 d; convalescent plasma may be useful for AHF, Lassa fever, and CCHF

Abbreviations: Ab, antibody; Ag, antigen; AHF, argentine hemorrhagic fever; CCHF, Congo-Crimean hemorrhagic fever; DIC, disseminated intravascular coagulation; ELISA, enzyme-linked immunosorbent assay; EM, electron microscopy; IFA, immunofluorescent assay; IgG, immunoglobulin G; IgM, immunoglobulin M; IM, intramuscular; IV, intravenous; PCR, polymerase chain reaction; RFLP, restriction fragment length polymorphism; RT-PCR, reverse transcriptase PCR; RVF, Rift Valley fever.

[a] Data from Miller JM. Agents of bioterrorism: preparing for bioterrorism at the community health care level. Infect Dis Clin North Am. 2001;15:1127-56 and Centers for Disease Control and Prevention [Internet]. Guideline for isolation precautions: preventing transmission of infectious agents in healthcare settings 2007. [cited 26 Sep 2009]. Atlanta (GA): CDC. Available from: http://www.cdc.gov/ncidod/dhqp/gl_isolation.html.

[b] Including rifampin, imipenem, vancomycin, chloramphenicol, clindamycin, clarithromycin, or IV penicillin.

[c] Antimicrobial therapy may be switched to ciprofloxacin, 500 mg orally every 12 h, or doxycycline, 100 mg orally every 12 h, once clinically appropriate and continued for 60 days.

Table 6 Common Agents Used for Chemical Terrorism

Category	Examples	Major Organ System Affected	Treatment
Biotoxins	Ricin, digitalis, saxitoxin	Various systems depending on individual agent	Varies depending on specific agent
Blister agents and vesicants	2-Chloroethenyldichloroarsine (lewisite), mustard gas, phosgene oxime	Eyes, skin, respiratory tract	Supportive care
Blood agents	Arsine, cyanide	Oxygen transport, cellular respiration	Supportive care, no antidote for arsine; amyl nitrite perles and intravenous infusions of sodium nitrite and sodium thiosulfate for cyanide
Caustic acids	Hydrofluoric acid	Skin, skeletal, respiratory and gastrointestinal tracts	Supportive care, calcium gluconate for respiratory tract
Choking and pulmonary agents	Ammonia, phosgene	Respiratory tract and mucous membranes	Supportive care, particularly for airway
Incapacitating agents	BZ, fentanyl	CNS	Supportive care (airway, breathing, cardiac system)
Long-acting anticoagulants	Brodifacoum (superwarfarin)	Circulatory	Supportive care, no established regimen
Metals	Arsenic, thallium	Gastrointestinal tract, cardiac, and CNS initially, then multisystem failure	Chelation treatment early in course
Nerve agents	Sarin, VX	Anticholinesterase inhibitors, particularly affect nervous system but lead to multisystem failure	Atropine, decontamination, supportive
Organic solvents	Carbon tetrachloride	Respiratory and skin irritant; at high doses, CNS depressant and cause of cardiac arrhythmias	Supportive care, irrigation and decontamination
Riot control agents/ tear gas	Mace, pepper spray	Ocular, respiratory tract, skin and mucous membranes	Supportive care
Toxic alcohols	Ethylene glycol	Gastrointestinal tract; metabolites toxic to CNS, cardiac, and kidneys	Prompt administration of ethanol or 4-methylpyrazole
Vomiting agents	Diphenylamine chlorarsine (adamsite)	Ocular; respiratory and gastrointestinal tracts	Supportive care; a nonlethal agent group

Abbreviations: BZ, quinuclidin-3-yl-hydroxy(diphenyl) acetate; CNS, central nervous system; VX, various methylphosphonothioate agents.

SUGGESTED READING

American Conference of Governmental Industrial Hygienists. Threshold limit values for chemical substances and physical agents and biological exposure indices. Cincinnati (OH): ACGIH. c2009.

Brooks SM, Gochfeld M, Herzstein J, Jackson JJ, Schenker MB. Environmental medicine. St. Louis (MO): Mosby. c1995.

Centers for Disease Control and Prevention. Diagnosis and management of foodborne illnesses: a primer for physicians and other health care professionals. MMWR. 2004;53(RR-4).

Environmental Protection Agency [Internet]. RCRA statute, regulations & enforcement. [cited 12 Oct 2008]. Washington (DC): EPA. Available from: http://pubweb.epa.gov/enforcement/civil/rcra/rcraenfstatreq.html.

Environmental Protection Agency [Internet]. Standards and practices for all appropriate inquiries. [cited 13 Oct 2008]. Available from: http://www.epa.gov/wastes/nonhaz/municipal/index.htm.

Environmental Protection Agency [Internet]. Wastes, non-hazardous waste, municipal solid waste. [cited 12 Oct 2008]. Washington (DC): EPA. Available from: http://pubweb.epa.gov/wastes/nonhaz/municipal/index.htm.

Etzel RA. Mycotoxins. JAMA. 2002 Jan 23-30;287(4): 425-7.

Koren H, Biesi M. Handbook of environmental health and safety: principles and practices. 3rd ed. Vol 2. Boca Raton (FL): Lewis Publishers. c1996.

National Council on Radiation Protection and Measurements. Limitations on exposure to ionizing radiation. NCRP Report No. 116. Bethesda (MD): NCRP. 1993.

Sara MN. Site assessment and remediation handbook. 2nd ed. Boca Raton (FL): Lewis Publishers. c2003.

Questions and Answers

Questions

1. Members of a 25-person work unit contacted the Occupational Medicine Department with concerns that a new computed tomography (CT) scanner installed 1 year earlier in an adjacent room was the cause of 5 cancer deaths in the past year. Shielding had been installed in the walls of the CT room at construction. The Radiation Safety Office monitored the radiation dose in the work unit and found a dose rate of 0.2 mSv per year attributable to the CT installation. On the basis of the National Academy of Science estimates for radiation-induced solid cancers, what is the likelihood that the 5 cancer deaths were caused by the radiation exposure from the CT scanner?
   a. 1 chance in 100,000
   b. 5 chances in 100,000
   c. 25 chances in 100,000
   d. 0, because 0.2 mSv is below the threshold for cancer induction
   e. Negligible, because the latent period for solid tumors is approximately 20 years

2. Acoustical measurements by the in-house industrial hygiene department show that workers in the printing unit are exposed to high levels of noise for 4 hours during the workday and approximately 60 dBA during the other 4 hours. At what sound level should the employees be placed on a hearing conservation program?
   a. ≥85 dBA
   b. ≥88 dBA
   c. ≥100 dBA
   d. Protection against noise-induced hearing loss is not necessary since the duration of high level noise is less than 8 hours
   e. A hearing conservation program is not necessary when the average noise level ([4 hours at 60 dBA + 4 hours at ___dBA]/2), is less than 85 dBA for 8 hours.

3. A 6-year-old girl is brought to her physician's office by her parents after the onset of nausea, vomiting, and bloody diarrhea. She is dehydrated, and her physician admits her to the hospital service for hydration. During her stay, she is found to have severely elevated levels of blood urea nitrogen and creatinine, with insufficient urine output. Stool cultures are pending. The child has seafood and dairy allergies. She has not eaten foods in those categories. She attended a state fair with her parents 5 days ago and ate hamburgers, hot dogs, and French fries. The most likely causative organism is which of the following?
   a. *Vibrio vulnificus*
   b. Hepatitis A
   c. *Escherichia coli* O157:H7
   d. *Listeria*

4. Postal workers at a processing center noted that a poorly sealed envelope was leaking a white powder. Authorities closed the facility and the powder was evaluated. If workers had skin lesions and rapid onset of pneumonia with acute respiratory distress syndrome, the most likely causative agent is which of the following?
   a. Botulinum toxin
   b. Digitalis
   c. Anthrax
   d. Ricin

5. An organism that has *not* been associated with carcinogenic properties is which of the following?
   a. *Fusarium moniliforme* (fumonisins)
   b. Hepatitis B virus
   c. *Aspergillus flavus* (aflatoxins)
   d. *Claviceps purpura* (ergot alkaloids)

6. During a health risk assessment, a patient volunteered that he used short-term tests to determine radon levels in several rooms of his home. All results on the main and second floors, including bedrooms, were 3 to 3.5 pCi/L, but the level in a finished basement bedroom where his teenaged son spent approximately 10 hours per day was 12 pCi/L. Since the average level was under 4 pCi/L and since the basement bedroom is finished and the radon in this room would be hard to mitigate, what advice would you offer?

7. Which of the following examples does *not* describe a point source of pollution?
   a. Noise from a jet engine
   b. Bright light from a football stadium
   c. Discolored water from an oil refinery discharge outlet
   d. Seismic vibration from a passing locomotive
   e. Elevated nitrate levels in groundwater near agricultural fields

8. Of the following compounds, which is associated as much with indoor air pollution as with contamination of the ambient environment?
   a. Particulate matter
   b. Sulfur dioxide
   c. Carbon monoxide
   d. Nitrogen dioxide
   e. Ozone

9. Which of the following parameters would be considered *least* reliable in assessing the prognosis of a 57-year-old man who was found obtunded in his home after the discovery that his propane-fueled furnace had malfunctioned?
   a. Oxygen saturation
   b. Sequential carboxyhemoglobin levels
   c. Persistent mental confusion on mental status examination
   d. Arterial blood gas analyses
   e. Low hematocrit levels

Answers

1. Answer e.

Regulations require that the annual radiation exposure rate in areas adjacent to the CT scanner not exceed 1 mSv. The measured exposure rate of 0.2 mSv is well within this limit. The lifetime risk of fatal cancer from radiation exposure, 0.05 per Sv (0.00005 per mSv), multiplied by an annual dose rate of 0.2 mSv equals 1 chance in 100,000. This low level of risk is negligible considering that the lifetime risk of sporadic fatal cancer is approximately 25%. In addition, since the latent period for solid tumors is about 20 years after radiation exposure, it is unlikely that any of these cancers were caused by exposure to radiation from the CT scanner.

2. Answer b.

Workers exposed to noise level at or above the threshold limit value (TLV) must be placed on a hearing conservation program that includes follow-up monitoring, annual audiometric testing, and hearing protection. The TLV for an 8-hour work period is 85 dBA. Higher noise levels are permitted for shorter periods (eg, 88, 91, or 94 dBA for 4, 2, or 1 hour per day, respectively).

3. Answer c.

All of the organisms listed could cause a diarrheal disease. *Vibrio* is most associated with ingestion of raw seafood, such as oysters. *Listeria* is most often associated with ingestion of soft cheeses. Since the child has allergies to these foods, they are less likely a cause of her symptoms. Hepatitis A and *E coli* O157:H7 infection both can cause diarrhea, but *E coli* is most often associated with hamburger that is not fully cooked. It is associated with hemolytic uremic syndrome, which can lead to renal insufficiency and renal failure, which is consistent with this child's decline in renal function.

4. Answer c.

All of the listed agents could be implicated in the use of biological agents as weapons. Botulinum toxin is associated with paralysis and weakness of muscles; ricin is associated with diarrhea, inhibition of protein synthesis, and shock. Early symptoms of digitalis ingestion include nausea, vomiting, anorexia, diarrhea, abdominal pain, wild hallucinations, delirium, and severe headache. Depending on the severity of the toxicosis, the person may later have irregular and slow pulse, tremors, various cerebral disturbances (especially of a visual nature [eg, unusual color visions with objects appearing yellowish to green, blue halos around lights]), convulsions, and deadly disturbances of the heart. Anthrax is the only agent listed that causes boillike changes or black eschars. Pulmonary symptoms include cold or flulike symptoms for several days, followed by severe respiratory collapse, acute respiratory distress syndrome, and death.

5. Answer d.

Claviceps purpura is a source of ergot alkaloids, and no carcinogenic properties have been reported as having association with exposure. *Fusarium* toxins have been linked with esophageal cancer, hepatitis B (and hepatitis C) is associated with liver cancer, and *Aspergillus* produces aflatoxins and is also associated with liver cancer.

6. Answer.

Although the risk from 12 pCi/L is probably not high, there are 2 issues of concern. First is the age of the individual who is most highly exposed. The tissues of young people are more susceptible to the potentially damaging effects of radiation, including the free radicals produced when radiation interacts with the body. Thus, it is concerning that the person exposed to this high level of radon is young and has many more years of potential exposure to radon and other sources of radiation in his lifetime. Second is the duration of daily exposure. Since people spend a greater fraction of the day in their bedroom (eg, 8 hours sleeping plus additional time reading or doing homework), the radon level in the bedroom is probably more consequential than the radon level in any other room of the house. The Environmental Protection Agency (EPA) recommends that the maximum exposure to radon not exceed 4 pCi/L. Therefore, this homeowner should conduct another short-term test or, preferably, a long-term test, to verify that the radon levels exceed 4 pCi/L. The test should include rooms adjacent to the basement bedroom and the utility room if it is located nearby. If results confirm that the radon level exceeds 4 pCi/L, remedial action should be taken to decrease the radon concentration. It is possible that successful mitigation can be accomplished without expensive alterations to the house, depending on the house construction. For example, if the utility room includes a sump pump, the pump could be covered and sealed and connected with a 4-in polyvinyl chloride pipe to an exhaust fan that vents to the outdoors. It also is possible that one of the drain lines to the sump lay under the bedroom in question and that venting the sump will create enough negative pressure under the floor to decrease the radon concentration to less than 4 pCi/L. Other inexpensive actions may also help. For the do-it-yourself homeowner, general guidance provided by EPA may be adequate. For others, a radon professional may be able to suggest an inexpensive fix. After remedial action, a subsequent short-term test should be conducted to confirm that the action was adequate.

7. Answer e.

Each of the incorrect responses describes an example of point-source pollution of varying types. A point source of pollution is a single identifiable *localized* source of air, water, thermal, noise, or light pollution. Nonpoint-source pollution, unlike pollution from industrial and sewage treatment plants, comes from many diffuse sources. Nonpoint-source pollution is caused by rainfall or snowmelt moving over and through the ground. As the runoff moves, it picks up and carries away natural and manmade pollutants, finally depositing them into lakes, rivers, wetlands, coastal waters, and even underground sources of drinking water.

8. Answer d.

Oxides of nitrogen, which are predominantly nitrogen dioxide, are produced from the burning of fossil fuels in motor vehicles. Unlike the other compounds listed, nitrogen dioxide is also a common indoor air contaminant whose sources include gas cooking stoves, gas furnaces, and kerosene space heaters. The emission from these devices results in indoor nitrogen dioxide levels that frequently exceed levels found in the ambient air outdoors.

9. Answer a.

Oxygen saturation measurements rely on a machine-calculated difference in light wave absorbance of each of the 2 wavelengths. On the basis of the ratio of changing absorbance of the red and infrared light caused by the difference in color between oxygen-bound (bright red) and oxygen-unbound (dark red or, in severe cases, blue) blood hemoglobin, a measure of oxygenation (the percentage of hemoglobin molecules bound with oxygen molecules) can be made. In the case of carbon monoxide poisoning (as suggested in this case of an obtunded individual in a residence with a malfunctioning furnace), bound carboxyhemoglobin often causes a falsely elevated oxygen saturation level and cannot be used reliably to predict clinical outcome or efficacy of treatment. Carboxyhemoglobin levels greater than 10% suggest acute carbon monoxide exposure, and levels may be followed over time to assess overall status. By comparison, persistent mental confusion portends a poor clinical prognosis. Arterial blood gas analysis, although lacking some precision, may be used to assess respiratory status and oxygenation of peripheral tissues. Anemia is associated with worse clinical prognosis since more of the available erythrocytes may be bound with carbon monoxide during acute toxic exposures.

14

OCCUPATIONAL MEDICINE

Robert R. Orford, MD, MS, MPH; and Hamid Rehman, MD, MPH

Occupational medicine is the medical specialty devoted to 1) prevention and management of occupational injury, illness, and disability, and 2) promotion of health and productivity of workers, their families, and communities. Historically, occupational medicine was termed industrial medicine when heavy industry (eg, lumbering, automobile manufacturing, mining, railroads, steel manufacturing) employed physicians to provide acute medical and surgical care for workers. However, by 1945, medical programs had spread to business organizations that predominantly were staffed with clerical and service employees (eg, banks, insurance companies, mercantile establishments). The broader designation of occupational medicine then came into common use. Occupational medicine was recognized as a specialty by the American Board of Preventive Medicine in 1955.

Occupational Health Services

The International Labour Organization established general principles for the provision of occupational health services during the 1985 Occupational Health Services Convention. They defined occupational health services as:

> . . .services entrusted with essentially preventive functions and responsible for advising the employer, the workers and their representatives in the undertaking on (i) the requirements for establishing and maintaining a safe and healthy working environment which will facilitate optimal physical

and mental health in relation to work; (ii) the adaptation of work to the capabilities of workers in the light of their state of physical and mental health.

> (International Labour Organization. Convention concerning occupational health services. C161. ILO, Geneva, 1985.)

Occupational health services are defined using this international standard (Box 1). The occupational physician provides leadership and consultation services.

Workplace Health and Surveillance

The National Institute for Occupational Safety and Health (NIOSH) defines occupational health surveillance as the "tracking [of] occupational injuries, illnesses, hazards, and exposures." They further note that "Occupational surveillance data are used to guide efforts to improve worker safety and health, and to monitor trends and progress over time." To achieve these goals, **risks from health hazards in the workplace must first be identified and assessed**. Every occupational health service should have its own workplace health surveillance program, designed specifically for the needs of the workplace(s) for which it is responsible.

In the United States, work-related injury and illness data are collected using the Occupational Safety and Health Administration (OSHA) forms (Form 300 Log [http://www.osha.gov/recordkeeping/new-osha300form1-1-04.pdf]). These records must be maintained for 5 years after the year to which they pertain. Recordable cases include any death, nonfatal illness, or nonfatal injury that results in loss of

Box 1 Functions of Occupational Health Services.

1. Identification and assessment of the risks from health hazards in the workplace

2. Surveillance of the factors in the working environment and working practices that may affect worker health, including sanitary installations, canteens, and housing, when these facilities are provided by the employer

3. Advice on planning and organization of work, including the design of workplaces; on the choice, maintenance, and condition of machinery and other equipment; and on substances used in work

4. Participation in the development of programs for the improvement of working practices, as well as testing and evaluation of health aspects of new equipment

5. Advice on occupational health, safety, and hygiene and on ergonomics in individual and collective protective equipment

6. Surveillance of workers' health in relation to work

7. Promoting the adaptation of work to the worker

8. Contribution to measures of vocational rehabilitation

9. Collaboration in providing information, training, and education in the fields of occupational health, hygiene, and ergonomics

10. Organizing first aid and emergency treatment

11. Participation in analysis of occupational accidents and occupational diseases

Adapted from the International Labour Organization [Internet]. Geneva: The Organization; Occupational Health Services Convention, 1985, No. 161; [cited 4 Mar 2009]. Available from: http://webfusion.ilo.org/public/db/standards/normes/appl/appl-displayConv.cfm?conv=C161&hdroff=1&lang=EN. Used with permission.

consciousness, restriction of work or motion, transfer to another job, medical treatment (other than first aid), or any combination of these outcomes.

Health risk assessments may be elective or may be mandated by state or federal regulations. Assessments include appropriate laboratory tests to facilitate earlier identification of health problems and permit interventions. Depending on exposure levels and other factors, medical examinations may be required for workers exposed to asbestos, cadmium, lead, and noise and for workers who use respirators or are involved with hazardous waste operations and emergency response. US government agencies (eg, Department of Defense, Department of Energy, Federal Aviation Administration) require medical examinations for their employees and those subject to agency oversight.

Hazard Recognition, Evaluation, and Control

Occupational hazards may be broadly categorized as physical (traumatic or nontraumatic [eg, noise, radiation]), chemical, biological, or psychological. Hazards such as fire or high noise levels are easy to recognize, but others require knowledge of the workplace (eg, to identify noxious gases, microbial agents) and special training (eg, to evaluate and control hazards). The OSHA Hazard Communication Standard (29 CFR 1919.1200) requires employers to make employees aware of possible occupational hazards by using safety labels, providing **material safety data sheets** (MSDSs), and creating training programs and a written hazard communication program. Proper emergency procedures must be developed and effective safety equipment made available.

MSDSs should be readily available (print copy or online) at the work site and from the occupational health service. MSDSs are designed to inform workers, supervisors, occupational health staff, and emergency personnel about handling or working with chemical substances. They include information about physical characteristics (eg, melting point, boiling point, flash point), reactivity, toxic and health effects, first aid procedures, storage, disposal, protective equipment, and how to handle a spill, leak, or other accident. Proprietary, publicly available databases and poison control centers also may be helpful in obtaining information regarding chemical exposures.

Because employee knowledge of hazards and safe work habits is essential to prevent occupational illness, each institution should establish policies that ensure that workers are familiar with potential hazards and encouraged to follow safe work practices. Employees should be trained to access and use available hazard information (read and interpret labels and MSDSs). They also should be trained to identify characteristics of work site hazards. All should be familiar with the **employee protection plan**, which details use of personal protective equipment, safe work practices, and engineering controls. Employees should be trained to detect the presence of hazardous materials (ie, use basic senses such as vision, smell). Proper glove and respirator selection should be stressed. If respirators (OSHA standard) are required, the occupational health service should ensure that workers are properly fitted and trained to use them.

- The goal of occupational health services is to provide a safe and healthy working environment. The occupational physician provides leadership and consultation services.
- Risks from health hazards in the workplace must be identified and assessed. Control and preventive measures are then taken.
- Each institution should establish policies that ensure employees are familiar with potential hazards and use safe work practices.
- Material safety data sheets (MSDSs) are designed to inform workers, supervisors, occupational health staff, and emergency personnel about handling or working with chemical substances.

Clinical, Occupational, and Environmental Medicine and Toxicology

An **occupational health program** will perform preplacement and periodic health examinations to assess fitness to work and fitness to use personal protective equipment. If necessary, restrictions will be placed. Medical conditions and immunizations are documented and preventive health behaviors are encouraged. Education is part of the occupational health program (eg, how to use respirators and other personal protective equipment, infection control procedures), as is care of employees with work-related exposures, injuries, or illnesses. The occupational health program also monitors exposure to chemical and biological hazards and maintains employee health records.

It is important to identify the cause of likely workplace-related symptoms. Doing so helps to treat affected workers, may stop progression of an occupational disease (by eliminating or reducing the exposures of concern), and helps prevent occupational disease among as yet unaffected workers. Determining the cause of an occupational illness will also reduce the costs of medical care, indemnity, and permanent disability that may result from the condition. Box 2 describes the key criteria for the diagnosis of an occupational or environmental disease. These criteria for diagnosing illness due to toxic chemical exposures are relatively easy to apply when a **threshold limit value** (TLV) has been established; exposures below the TLV are unlikely to have adverse health effects. Table 1 lists examples of common chemical exposures, routes of absorption, and clinical effects.

The approach described in Box 2 is difficult to use when the exposures involve carcinogens and allergens. Carcinogens do not appear to have a definitive threshold under which they are completely safe; the probability of cancer increases with the intensity and duration of exposure. With allergens, a considerable exposure is required for sensitization, but after sensitization has occurred, a

very low level of exposure can trigger a reaction or symptoms (this pattern is commonly observed after exposure to epoxies or toluene diisocyanate).

In developed countries, legislation and managerial controls have reduced the frequency of occupational and environmental diseases due to toxic chemical exposure. However, occupational and environmental diseases continue to be a huge burden in developing countries.

- Knowing the cause of an occupational illness helps to treat affected workers, may stop progression of disease, and helps prevent new cases of illness.
- Carcinogens do not have a definitive safe threshold; the probability of cancer increases with the intensity and duration of exposure.
- Considerable exposure to an allergen is required for sensitization; however, after sensitization has occurred, a very low level of exposure can trigger a reaction or symptoms.

Occupational Diseases

Skin Disease

Work-related skin diseases are fairly common but often are underreported because of failure to recognize the workplace association. Skin diseases typically affect workers in manufacturing, material production, food production, machining, health care, forestry, electroplating, printing, and leather industries. Contact dermatitis, both irritant and allergic forms, accounts for 90% of cases of occupational skin disease (Table 2).

Irritant contact dermatitis is a nonimmunologic reaction that occurs after prolonged exposure to a relatively weak skin irritant such as soap, water, or a solvent. Stronger skin irritants (eg, alkalis, acids) are more likely to cause burns than dermatitis. Thin skin, such as that on the dorsal surfaces of the hands or eyelids, is affected more frequently than other areas. Irritant contact dermatitis is generally associated with the following principles: 1) a higher concentration of the chemical is required to cause the rash; 2) it affects most workers doing similar activities; 3) the rash affects exposed parts of the body; and 4) removal of offending agents results in quick improvement. However, differentiating between allergic and irritant contact dermatitis is often difficult.

Allergic contact dermatitis is an immunologic reaction to an antigen; it may occur after a very low level of exposure. It affects relatively few people, and it takes some time for sensitization to develop. Once present, it continues to worsen with continued exposure. The rash affects exposed parts of the body but may be unilateral or asymmetric. It may affect skin on the face or waistline when the offending agent is transferred by the hands or clothing. Pruritus is

Box 2 Diagnosis of an Occupational or Environmental Disease

1. The symptoms and signs, including the laboratory data, fit with known health effects of a chemical. One example is the well-known causal association between asbestos exposure and mesothelioma.

2. Objective data confirm a sufficient level of exposure to the hazardous agent.

3. The interval between the suspected exposure and clinical symptoms fits with the known pathophysiology of the disease. This information can be obtained by occupational history and employment records.

4. If a preexisting, nonoccupational disease has similar symptoms, consider the possibility of disease causation or exacerbation by an occupational exposure.

Table 1 Routes and Effects of Exposure to Toxins Often in the Workplace

Toxin	Routes and Effects of Exposure
Metals[a]	
Arsenic	May enter via the lungs, skin, or gastrointestinal tract. Arsenic compounds are used as insecticides and weed killers. Causes respiratory and gastrointestinal symptoms and, in high doses, death. Can cause lung cancer.
Beryllium	Usually enters via the lungs. Causes granulomas in the lungs; lesions appear similar to those of sarcoidosis.
Cadmium	Usually enters via the lungs. Displaces zinc in enzyme systems, often damaging the renal tubules. Causes metal fume fever (disorder also can be caused by other metal fumes).
Lead	Usually enters via the gastrointestinal tract or lungs. Displaces calcium in chemical reactions. Inorganic form of lead causes gastrointestinal (including abdominal pain) and neurologic (neuropathy) symptoms. Organic compounds of lead cause diffuse neurologic symptoms. Other effects include glomerulonephritis and hypertension.
Mercury	May enter via the lungs, skin, or gastrointestinal tract. Used in the past by milliners to make felt for hats. Chronic exposure damages the central nervous system, with the elemental form of mercury tending to cause tremors ("hatter's shakes") and the organic forms tending to cause psychiatric symptoms ("mad as a hatter") and even dementia. Mercury also damages the kidneys.
Zinc	Usually enters via the lungs. Inhaling zinc oxide causes metal fume fever.
Insecticides, herbicides, and fungicides	
Organophosphates	Usually enter via the skin from handling but can enter via the lungs. Blocks acetylcholinesterase activity and produces central nervous system and peripheral nerve damage.
Pentachlorophenol	Usually enters via the skin. Used as a wood preservative. Interferes with cellular respiration. Causes anorexia and respiratory symptoms and, in high doses, coma and death.
Polychlorinated biphenyls	Enter via the skin or lungs. Are teratogens and possibly also carcinogens.
Hydrocarbon solvents[b]	
Benzene	Absorbed through the lungs and skin. Is a lipid-soluble aromatic solvent that is used widely in industry. Chronic exposure can result in suppression of bone marrow, subsequent aplastic anemia is possible.
Carbon tetrachloride	Absorbed readily through the lungs. Is a lipid-soluble chlorinated hydrocarbon not widely used in industry because of extreme toxicity to kidneys and liver, but it is the prototype of this chemical class. Damage to either the kidneys or liver can predominate. Renal tubular necrosis may follow acute exposure, and hepatic centrilobular necrosis tends to predominate after chronic exposure, especially in the presence of ethanol or after hepatic damage by ethanol.
Toluene	Usually inhaled. Is a lipid-soluble aromatic solvent in products such as glue. Primarily causes central nervous system effects, including hallucinations (which is why glue is sometimes sniffed).
Asphyxiants[c]	
Carbon dioxide	Enters the body via the lungs and stimulates the respiratory center. Is a nonreactive asphyxiant. Begins to produce symptoms of rapid breathing when concentration reaches about 3% in the air. In high concentrations, causes coma and death.
Carbon monoxide	Enters the body via the lungs. Is a chemical asphyxiant that is ubiquitous in urban society (a product of automobile exhaust and sometimes of poorly ventilated space heaters). Combines with hemoglobin to form carboxyhemoglobin; when 50% or more of the hemoglobin is in the form of carboxyhemoglobin, fainting and death are likely. Some carbon monoxide may be inhaled during cigarette smoking.

Table 1 (continued) Routes and Effects of Exposure to Toxins Often in the Workplace

Toxin	Routes and Effects of Exposure
Asphyxiants, continued[c]	
Hydrogen cyanide	Enters the body via the lungs or gastrointestinal tract. Is a chemical asphyxiant. Toxicity is retained in cyanide salts because it is the reactive cyanide moiety that interferes with cytochrome oxidase. Causes headaches, rapid breathing, and, frequently, death.
Hydrogen sulfide	Absorbed through the lungs. Is a chemical asphyxiant that is as dangerous as hydrogen cyanide, but its odor usually warns of its presence before hazardous levels develop. Causes symptoms and effects similar to those of hydrogen cyanide.
Methane	Enters the body via the lungs. Is a nonreactive asphyxiant that is mainly a problem in mines, causing severe respiratory symptoms. The greater danger is from explosion.
Nitrogen	Enters the body via the lungs. Is a nonreactive asphyxiant that used to be a problem in mines but now presents a hazard primarily to deep sea divers. Divers accumulate nitrogen in the fatty tissues during dives at high pressure. As divers approach the surface, nitrogen reenters the blood, and if the pressure is reduced too rapidly, it forms small bubbles in the blood that interfere with circulation, especially to the brain. This process causes "the bends."
Miscellaneous organic compounds	
Resins	Usually enter via the skin, although may enter via the lungs. Produces asthma, irritation and allergic sensitization of the skin, and irritation of the eyes.
Vinyl chloride	Absorbed through the lungs and skin. Is ubiquitous in industry because it is used to make plastics. Can cause sclerodermatous skin lesions, Raynaud phenomenon, bone lesions in the hand, and liver damage. The monomer form causes hemangiosarcoma of the liver in a small proportion of persons who are exposed.

[a] Metals often cause toxicity by interfering with enzyme reactions that have a metal cofactor.
[b] Lipid-soluble hydrocarbon solvents build up in tissues with high levels of lipids (eg, the central nervous system); all have narcotic effects. Central nervous system effects are exacerbated by alcohol. Exposure to more than one solvent may result in complex interactions.
[c] Asphyxiants can be divided into 2 groups. The first group consists of gases that have no direct toxic effect but can reduce the partial pressure of oxygen in the lungs to dangerous levels; these gases are often called simple or nonreactive asphyxiants. The second group consists of gases that interfere with respiration at the cellular level; these are called chemical or reactive asphyxiants.
Adapted from Jekel JF, Katz DL, Elmore JG. Epidemiology, biostatistics and preventive medicine. 2nd ed. Philadelphia (PA): Saunders; c2001; p. 297. Used with permission.

Table 2 Common Causes and Occupations Associated With Irritant and Allergic Contact Dermatitis

Cause of Dermatitis	Occupation
Irritant dermatitis	
Fiberglass	Construction
Oil	Machining
Solvent	Painting, cleaning
Detergent	Housekeeping, cosmetology
Cement	Construction
Allergic dermatitis	
Latex or rubber	Laboratory and health care work (gloves)
Nickel	Electroplating
Colophony	Electronics
Formaldehyde	Laboratory and health care work
Hair dye	Cosmetology
Epoxy resin	Painting

commonly associated with rash. In photoallergic contact dermatitis, the sensitization reaction to an antigen is initiated after exposure to ultraviolet light. Diagnosis of allergic contact dermatitis is made on the basis of history and clinical findings. It is further confirmed by laboratory tests (eg, patch tests). When the cause is unknown, patch testing with multiple antigens is performed. For photoallergic reactions, photopatch testing with ultraviolet light is performed. Alternatively, radioallergosorbent testing may be used to measure blood levels of specific antibodies against a sensitizing substance (eg, latex IgE for latex allergy). Allergic contact dermatitis improves with removal of the sensitizing agent.

Oil acne and folliculitis are relatively less common skin conditions that may occur after exposure to solvents and lubricants. Preventive and treatment strategies are mainly geared toward avoiding direct contact with unprotected skin.

Skin tumors can occur after occupational exposure to polycyclic hydrocarbons, arsenic, inorganic metals, ultraviolet light, and radiation. They may also occur after burns or recurrent trauma. It may be difficult to establish a relationship between occupational exposure and skin cancers because of changing job responsibilities.

It is important to identify workers with conditions that may predispose them to skin disease. Educating workers at risk is a key preventive measure. For example, fair-skinned workers who are occupationally exposed to sun for extended periods should take sun protection measures. Health care workers with preexisting hand eczema are more likely to have an exacerbation if they wash their hands frequently. For people with irritant dermatitis from latex gloves, preventive measures such as provision of vinyl or neoprene gloves may be helpful.

Lung Disease

Lung disease is the most common occupational illness in the United States. It usually is caused by prolonged exposure to a toxic or irritant chemical but also may be triggered by one high-level exposure. Smoking may synergistically increase the severity of an occupational illness. Occupational lung disease is preventable but not always curable. The most common occupational lung diseases are asthma, lung cancer, and interstitial lung disease (others are listed in Table 3).

Occupational Asthma

Occupational asthma is a chronic inflammatory disease of the airway lining. Hypersensitivity to a chemical, dust,

Table 3 Select Occupational Lung Diseases

Disease	Exposure	Occupation
Asthma	Isocyanates	Plastic industry
	Wood dust	Wood work
	Wheat flour	Flour mill
	Animal dander	Poultry, laboratory work
	Cutting oils	Machining
Hypersensitivity pneumonitis	Moldy hay	Farming
	Cutting oil	Machining
Silicosis	Silica	Mining, foundry work
Pneumoconiosis	Coal	Mining
Asbestosis	Asbestos	Mining, construction, maintenance
Lung cancer	Asbestos	Construction, maintenance
	Coal tar	Steel work
	Chromium	Metal plating
	Radon	Mining
	Arsenic	Pesticide-related work

vapor, gas, or fume present in the workplace leads to airway inflammation, local tissue swelling, and excess mucus production; symptoms are similar to those of nonoccupational asthma. The consequent airway narrowing causes breathing difficulty. Even a very low level of exposure to an offending agent can trigger symptoms such as wheezing, chest tightness, cough, and shortness of breath. Symptoms usually occur when a worker is actively exposed to an irritant or allergen, but they may occur several hours or sometimes several days after the work shift. After the airway becomes hyperreactive, other substances such as cigarette smoke, cold air, or house dust may precipitate symptoms. Exposed workers with a personal or family history of allergies or asthma have greater risk of occupational asthma. However, disease can also develop among those with no history of allergies.

The diagnosis of occupational asthma is made by obtaining a detailed medical and employment history and determining the chemicals to which a worker is potentially exposed. MSDSs can be quite helpful because they describe the chemical nature of a substance, health effects, and recommended protective measures while handling the particular substance. Similarly, it is important to review information about work conditions, including control measures and protective equipment used, and whether any coworkers have similar symptoms. A thorough physical examination, with consideration of other possible causes of symptoms, is mandatory. Special tests such as pulmonary function tests (eg, serial spirometry before and after the work shift or at the start and end of the work week) may help identify an association between symptoms and the work environment. **Challenge testing** with the offending substance may be needed for the definitive diagnosis; such a test must be conducted in a specialized laboratory in a pulmonary medicine facility.

Bronchodilators may be effective for relieving symptoms, but the main treatment is **avoiding exposure** to the offending agent. Respirators and masks are unlikely to completely eliminate the exposure and associated symptoms. Transfer to a different area of the same workplace may be helpful. A job change should be recommended only after serious consideration of the diagnosis, causative factors, and treatment, and only when deemed medically necessary. Occupational asthma usually is reversible if exposure can be stopped early; however, it can be permanent if the exposure continues in the presence of symptoms.

Occupational Lung Cancer

Occupational exposure accounts for 5% to 27% of lung cancers. Most commonly implicated carcinogens include asbestos, radon, and cigarette smoke (passive exposure). The latency period between exposure and lung cancer occurrence can be long. Nonoccupational factors, including exposure through the home environment and hobbies, must also be explored. Manifestations of asbestos exposure range from benign pleural plaques to interstitial lung disease (termed **asbestosis**), lung cancer, and pleural cancer (termed **malignant mesothelioma**). Lung cancer is also associated with radon. OSHA requires periodic medical evaluation for workers exposed to asbestos, arsenic, acrylonitrile, vinyl chloride, bis(chloromethyl) ether, cadmium, coke oven emissions, and silica.

Occupational Interstitial Lung Disease

Inflammation of the lung parenchyma may be caused by various environmental and occupational exposures that lead to lung destruction and fibrosis. Commonly implicated agents include asbestos, silica, and organic and inorganic dust. However, interstitial lung disease can be observed without occupational or environmental exposure—alternative diagnoses can include sarcoidosis, idiopathic pulmonary fibrosis, and various collagen vascular syndromes.

Diseases of the Organs of Metabolism and Excretion

The liver is one of the primary organs involved in metabolizing absorbed chemicals. Hence, it may be the principal organ affected by toxicants. Chemicals such as nitroaromatics, ethanol, resins, halogenated aromatics, chlorinated hydrocarbons, and vinyl chloride can cause acute liver injury, hepatic failure, or chronic liver disease with fibrosis.

The kidney also may be affected by toxic occupational and environmental exposures. High-level exposure may cause acute renal failure, and low-level exposure may cause chronic renal failure. Agents that commonly affect the kidneys include mercury, cadmium, chromium, arsine, and halogenated hydrocarbons.

Hearing Loss and Eye Injury

Occupational noise exposure leads to high-frequency hearing loss (3,000-4,000 Hz), usually after many years of exposure. Later, it affects lower-frequency tones (500-2,000 Hz), resulting in functional hearing–related disability. The OSHA **permissible exposure limit** (PEL) for occupational noise exposure is 90 dB for 8 hours.

Workers exposed to noise levels of 85 dB or higher must be enrolled in a **hearing conservation program**, which requires use of appropriate hearing-protection devices and periodic hearing evaluations to document any change in hearing thresholds. The program itself must be evaluated periodically to ensure noise control and hearing protection of exposed workers. Occupational ototoxic agents also exist, these include certain solvents, heavy metals, and carbon monoxide.

Occupational eye damage may result from chemical spills, mechanical trauma such as contusions and lacerations, and radiation exposure. Proper eye protection can help reduce injury risk.

Musculoskeletal Disorders

Work-related musculoskeletal disorders are common concerns in clinical practice; they often include neck and low back pain, shoulder pain due to rotator cuff tendinopathy, medial and lateral epicondylitis, de Quervain tenosynovitis, and forearm tendinitis. The incidence of musculoskeletal disorders is increasing, and these are the most common concerns among the workers. Certain risk factors predispose workers to musculoskeletal injuries, including awkward and static postures, excessive force, psychosocial stresses, vibration, mechanical stresses, and cold temperatures. Industries with higher rates of work-related musculoskeletal injuries include construction, food preparation, manufacturing, health care, and meat packing.

The general criteria described in Box 2 for diagnosing occupational diseases can also be applied to work-related musculoskeletal conditions. Furthermore, they can be used to identify treatment and prevention options. Timely identification of areas with higher incidence rates of work-related musculoskeletal disorders facilitates identification and correction of ergonomic and psychosocial factors. These factors can be controlled through engineering and administrative means.

- Contact dermatitis, both irritant and allergic forms, accounts for 90% of cases of occupational skin disease.
- Occupational lung disease usually is caused by prolonged exposure to a toxic or irritant chemical but also may be triggered by one high-level exposure.
- Occupational asthma usually is reversible if exposure can be stopped early; treatment usually is avoidance of the offending agent.
- Malignant mesothelioma is associated with asbestos exposure, and lung cancer is associated with radon exposure.
- Because the liver metabolizes many absorbed chemicals, it may be the principal organ affected by toxicants. However, the kidneys also may be affected by toxic occupational and environmental exposures.
- Occupational noise exposure can cause high- and low-frequency hearing loss with time, resulting in functional hearing–related disability.
- Work-related musculoskeletal disorders are common concerns. Factors that influence development of musculoskeletal disorders may be controlled through engineering and administrative means.

Industrial Hygiene

Industrial hygiene, also termed occupational hygiene, is the discipline of anticipating, recognizing, evaluating, and controlling health hazards in the work environment. The objectives of industrial hygiene are to protect the health and well-being of workers and to safeguard the community at large. Occupational health physicians should work closely with occupational or industrial hygienists when evaluating workplace hazards and when designing and implementing control measures.

TLVs have been established for physical and chemical agents; these define the level of daily exposure considered acceptable (safe) for workers. They are meant to protect all workers from adverse health effects caused by chronic exposure to harmful agents. Levels are selected on the basis of human experience and findings from animal studies. The American Conference of Governmental Industrial Hygienists (ACGIH) has been the principal organization involved in the development of TLVs; their TLVs have been accepted internationally and are updated annually.

PELs are regulatory occupational exposure limits set or adopted by OSHA. In 1970, OSHA adopted the 1968 ACGIH TLVs (29 CFR 1910.1000). In 1989, OSHA published revisions for approximately 376 substances, with changes mostly derived directly from ACGIH TLVs. However, in 1989, the 11th Circuit Court overturned the 1970 rulemaking in response to legal action by employers and organized labor. Note that PELs and TLVs are not absolute safe limits; rather, they are widely acknowledged as a compromise between scientific knowledge and political expediency. Since 1989, OSHA has issued only a few specific standards, mostly for toxic chemicals (cadmium [1992], methylenedianiline [1992], formaldehyde [1992], lead in construction [1993], asbestos [1994], 3-butadiene [1996], methylene chloride [1998], and hexavalent chromium [2006]) and for some aspects of protection and monitoring. Most exposure limits are defined as 8-hour, time-weighted averages. In addition, upper limits were established; these are not to be exceeded during an 8-hour shift. Short-term exposure limits are used in emergency and rescue situations; these are defined using exposure times no longer than 15 minutes.

Exposure is quantified by industrial hygienists, who analyze the process and dispersion of a contaminant through the environment and estimate the effects of protective equipment. Depending on the chemical or physical agent, different methods are used to assess exposure. A direct reading instrument may be used, or a wipe sample can be submitted for physical, chemical, or biological analysis. Exposure also may be quantified by analyzing urine, exhaled air, or blood samples from workers. Biological exposure indices also are published by the ACGIH; these describe biological levels of a chemical or its metabolites after any route of exposure. For example, the blood lead level in a worker is a measure of the dose of lead absorbed by inhalation, by ingestion, or through the skin.

After assessment has been completed, various control measures are used to keep exposures within recommended limits. The best measures are **engineering controls**, which include ventilation, process modification, enclosure, substitution with safer chemicals, and hygienic work practices. **Administrative controls** include reducing the number of workers exposed to a hazardous process or changing the number or duration of shift breaks and rest periods. **Personal protection measures** are the least desirable because of the need for compliance by individual workers and the possibility of equipment failure or misuse. Personal protective equipment should be implemented only after engineering and administrative control measures have been executed to the best possible level. Personal protective equipment includes gloves, safety glasses, nonpermeable clothing, and respirators. Workers must be properly fitted and trained to use protective equipment.

Occupational Hazards

A hazard is defined as an environmental factor that can cause worker illness, injury, or discomfort. Exposure to hazards can cause immediate or delayed responses. Hazards can be chemical, physical, and biological.

Chemical hazards include airborne gases, vapors, and particulates (dusts or fumes). Exposure most commonly occurs through inhalation or skin contact. The hazard level is determined by the inherent toxicity of the agent (ie, the capacity of the agent to cause harm or injury) and the probability of exposure (ie, the conditions of its use). The severity of a hazard is affected by a number of factors, including work patterns, how the chemical is used, specific job activities, duration of exposure, temperature, ventilation and airflow pattern, use of safety equipment, and general housekeeping.

Physical hazards may be traumatic, ergonomic, or nontraumatic. Traumatic hazards include crushing injuries or falls. Ergonomic hazards include awkward postures or improper work procedures (eg, poor lifting practices, repetitive motions, poorly designed tools). Nontraumatic physical hazards include noise, vibration, temperature, pressure, and ionizing radiation. These categories have some overlap. Health effects of physical hazards may be immediate and cumulative. Noise exposure may cause psychological effects, result in poor job performance, or cause hearing loss that affects communication and safety (eg, inability to hear an alarm). The effects of noise exposure can be influenced by individual susceptibility, sound energy, duration of exposure, and duration of employment.

Biological hazards include living organisms and their products. For example, blood and body fluid exposures are biological hazards for health care and laboratory workers.

Environmental Management

Occupational and environmental risks, particularly physical hazards, may be obvious to the casual observer. However, subtle threats to health and safety are common.

For example, gases such as radon can be detected only by instrumentation. A structural weakness in a building or airframe may not be readily apparent, but it can fail and result in catastrophic human injury or death. **Risk management** refers to the recognition, evaluation, and control of environmental factors that can cause injury or illness in individuals or populations. Further details on risk management are provided in the chapter on environmental health (Chapter 13).

- The objectives of industrial (occupational) hygiene are to protect the health and well-being of workers and to safeguard the community at large by anticipating, recognizing, evaluating, and controlling health hazards in the work environment.
- Threshold limit values (TLVs) and permissible exposure limits (PELs) define the level of acceptable exposure to harmful agents but are not absolute safe limits.
- Engineering and administrative controls are the best measures to keep exposures within recommended limits. Personal protection is the least desirable control measure because of the need for compliance by individual workers and the possibility of equipment failure or misuse.
- Environmental factors that can cause worker illness, injury, or discomfort include chemical, physical, and biological hazards. In risk management, these hazards must be recognized, evaluated, and controlled to prevent injury or illness in individuals or populations.

Workers' Compensation

Workers' compensation programs were introduced in Europe at the end of the 19th century and in the United States and Canada early in the 20th century. These programs are required by law and provide no-fault insurance to workers who are injured during the course of their employment. Workers' compensation insurance is sold to employers by private companies in most states, although 12 states and all Canadian provinces operate a state or provincial fund (the largest is the State Compensation Insurance Fund of California). In many states, employers may also be self-insured. The government has workers' compensation funds established for federal employees.

Programs vary by state or province, but they generally provide payment for the injured worker's medical care (no personal expenses), indemnification for short-term wage loss due to inability to work, and long-term financial support or a lump-sum monetary payout if a permanent impairment occurs (ie, loss or impairment of a body part or sensory function). Medical fees and salary indemnification schedules vary considerably because they are set by each state or province.

In most cases, a worker's only legal remedy for a job-related accident or illness is through the workers' compensation system. The employer avoids legal action from employees for injuries that occur on company property, but the medical, indemnification, and administrative costs are high, particularly for employers with multistate operations. Some multistate employers have negotiated agreements with labor unions that identify a single state that will have jurisdiction, regardless of the geographic location of the accident. Some states require medical services to be provided in accordance with occupational medical treatment guidelines; this helps ensure that employees receive evidence-based treatment and also reduces claim costs.

Management and administration of workers' compensation by state governments and employers should assure fairness, encourage appropriate medical management and early recovery, and minimize financial losses for the worker and employer. When a work-related injury occurs, the worker must promptly notify the supervisor, and 1 or more reports must be filed by the worker, the employer, or the physician or health care provider. The insurer determines the compensability of the claim, and payment for medical services and salary replacement is made. To qualify for benefits, the injured person must be employed by the organization when the injury occurs, the injury must be work-related or work must have made a substantial contribution to occurrence of the injury, and the worker must be covered by workers' compensation legislation. Employees may not claim benefits fraudulently, and the employer or insurer may sometimes investigate the legitimacy of a claim.

When considering permanent loss of a body part or sensory function, the medical definition of permanent impairment in many states is largely based on the most recent edition of the American Medical Association's *Guides to the Evaluation of Permanent Impairment*. When injuries to multiple body parts have occurred, or when injuries are not readily definable, a government regulatory body or an administrative law judge may adjudicate payment of the claim. Many factors are involved in these decisions, including physical limitations, education, and work experience.

An alternative-duty (light-duty) program is provided by many employers for workers who are not able to perform their original duties because of a work-related injury. Either the physician caring for the worker or an occupational health physician who has examined the worker should set limitations on physical activity (eg, lifting, pushing, pulling).

Record Keeping

Occupational injuries and illnesses should be recorded for legal, medical, and epidemiological purposes. In the United States, the OSHA 300 Log is used for this purpose, but a form designed by the occupational health service of the employer also may be required. A key point is that no reporting mechanism should include the employee's diagnostic information.

The reported data may be used by employers to direct resources toward improving workplace safety; in aggregate, data should be used by governments to identify interventions that address industries, employers, and processes with the greatest risks. With sufficient time, the logs can help evaluate the effectiveness of interventions, provided that the data are valid and the log reliably maintained.

- Workers' compensation programs generally pay for the injured worker's medical care and cover short-term wage loss. Long-term financial support may be provided if a permanent impairment occurs.
- To qualify for benefits, the injured person must be employed by the organization when the injury occurs, the injury must be work-related, and the worker must be covered by workers' compensation legislation.
- An alternative-duty (light-duty) program is provided by many employers for workers who are not able to return to their original duties.
- Occupational injury data should be recorded for legal, medical, and epidemiological purposes. These data may be used by employers to improve workplace safety and by governments to identify interventions that address industries, employers, and processes with the greatest risks.

Occupational Health and Safety Law

Expert Testimony

Occupational physicians may be called upon to provide expert assistance in legal, administrative, and legislative proceedings and to testify in hearings or trials as expert witnesses. The expert witness should have no direct personal or pecuniary interest in the outcome of the case. The medical expert witness assists the court in understanding complex medical or scientific issues, and the witness's testimony should be founded on a thorough and critical review of pertinent medical and scientific facts, available data, and relevant literature. Experts should specify whether their opinions are based on personal experience, specific studies in the peer-reviewed literature, or "professional opinions" generally accepted by specialists in the field. Transcripts of depositions and courtroom testimony are public records, subject to independent peer review by colleagues and professional organizations, and testimony in some states may be subject to the jurisdiction and review of appropriate licensing or disciplinary boards.

In the 1993 Daubert vs Merrell Dow Pharmaceuticals decision, the US Supreme Court determined that scientific evidence presented in court must be both relevant and reliable. They suggested 4 questions to ask when determining whether scientific evidence was admissible:

1) Is the evidence based on a testable theory or technique?
2) Has the theory or technique been peer reviewed?
3) In the case of a particular technique, does it have a known error rate and standards controlling the technique's operation?
4) Is the underlying science generally accepted?

The "Daubert criteria" now are applied to federal and to some state jurisdictions. Unfortunately, what started as a well-intentioned attempt to ensure reliable and relevant evidence has been exploited by some to protect polluters and manufacturers of dangerous products from product liability and personal injury lawsuits.

Government Organizations

In 1970, the US Congress passed the Occupational Safety and Health Act to enforce health and safety standards in workplaces. The Occupational Safety and Health Act of 1971 created OSHA and NIOSH.

OSHA is the primary regulatory agency for occupational safety and health. OSHA is managed by an Assistant Secretary of the Department of Labor. **OSHA field offices are responsible for enforcing regulatory standards**, which apply to workplaces throughout the United States. Officers may inspect workplaces at any time and may be requested to do so by an employer, labor representative, or worker. If a serious occupational health or safety violation is found, the worksite can be closed or a fine may be levied. States may elect to have their own OSHA programs, and half have done so. Any state program must, at minimum, meet all regulations and requirements established by the federal OSHA.

NIOSH is part of the Department of Health and Human Services and administratively is considered part of the Centers for Disease Control and Prevention. Like OSHA, NIOSH has the authority to conduct inspections, to question employees and employers, and to even use warrants to acquire information about workplace conditions. However, **NIOSH is not a regulatory agency** and cannot levy penalties; thus, it can also serve as a consultative body. NIOSH further serves the occupational and environmental health community as an educational resource, providing educational materials and financial support for programs such as residencies in occupational medicine. NIOSH also provides funding for research in occupational and environmental medicine.

Employment Law

Employment law mediates the relationship between employers and employees (or labor unions, when applicable).

It addresses the fundamental inequality between employers and employees and establishes conditions for issues such as employment, termination of employment, minimum wage, and hours of work. Two laws of particular importance to physicians in the United States are the Americans with Disabilities Act and the Family and Medical Leave Act.

The **Americans with Disabilities Act** prohibits discrimination against disabled persons. Title 1 of the act applies to employment, specifically to employers with 15 or more employees, and is enforced by the Equal Employment Opportunities Commission. The legislation affects management decision-making at the time of hiring, during employment, and at termination for qualified individuals. A qualified individual is defined as someone with a physical or mental impairment that substantially limits one or more major life activities; this person must have a record of such impairment or must be regarded as having such impairment. A qualified individual must meet job-related requirements (eg, education, work experience, training skills, licensing, certification) and must be able to perform the essential functions of the job. Outcomes of background checks, drug tests, and agility tests must be acceptable before employment. Exclusions include current drug users, persons with non-heterosexual orientation, and persons with certain behavior disorders (eg, kleptomania, pyromania).

The **Family and Medical Leave Act** provides eligible employees with up to 12 weeks of unpaid, job-protected leave per year. To be eligible, an employee must have worked for at least 12 months and for 1,250 hours during the previous 12 months. This legislation was designed to help employees balance their work and family responsibilities by allowing them to take reasonable, unpaid leave for qualifying family and medical reasons. Qualifying conditions include a serious health condition of the employee; a serious health condition of a spouse, parent, or child (specifically, a minor or disabled child); birth, adoption, or placement of a child or foster child; care of a family member injured during active duty; and time needed to cover qualifying exigencies related to active duty. Certification of the qualifying condition by a medical provider is required. The absence may run concurrently with short-term disability or workers' compensation leave.

- The Daubert criteria are used in federal (and some state) courts to determine admissibility of scientific evidence from expert witnesses.
- The Occupational Safety and Health Administration (OSHA) is the primary regulatory agency that enforces standards for occupational safety and health in the workplace.
- The National Institute for Occupational Safety and Health (NIOSH) can conduct worksite inspections but is not a regulatory agency.
- The Americans with Disabilities Act prohibits employment discrimination against qualified individuals.

- The Family and Medical Leave Act provides eligible employees with up to 12 weeks of unpaid, job-protected leave per year for qualified conditions.

SUGGESTED READING

Andersson GBJ, Cocchiarella L. Guides to the evaluation of permanent impairment. 5th ed. Chicago (IL): American Medical Association; c2001.

Bowler RM, Cone JE. Occupational medicine secrets. Philadelphia (PA): Hanley & Belfus; c1999.

LaDou J. Current occupational & environmental medicine. 3rd ed. New York: Lange Medical Books, McGraw-Hill; c2004.

Levy BS, Wegman DH, Baron SL, Sokas RK. Occupational and environmental health: recognizing and preventing disease and injury. 5th ed. Philadelphia (PA): Lippincott Williams & Wilkins; c2006.

McCunney RJ. A practical approach to occupational and environmental medicine. 3rd ed. Philadelphia (PA): Lippincott Williams & Wilkins; c2003.

Plog BA, Quinlan PJ. Fundamentals of industrial hygiene. 5th ed. Itasca (IL): National Safety Council; c2002.

Rosenstock L, Cullen M, Brodkin C, Redlich C. Textbook of clinical occupational and environmental medicine. 2nd ed. Philadelphia (PA): Elsevier; c2005.

Questions and Answers

Questions

1. A middle-aged man presents with a chronic cough. Which of the following is most helpful in establishing the diagnosis?
   a. Tobacco use
   b. Detailed occupational history
   c. Pulmonary function tests
   d. Chest radiograph
   e. All of the above
2. Asbestos is associated with which of the following diseases?
   a. Mesothelioma
   b. Lung cancer
   c. Asbestosis
   d. Pleural plaques
   e. All of the above
3. A young clinical assistant comes to you with hand dermatitis. She has been working at her current job for 3 months. You determine that she has allergic contact dermatitis from wearing latex gloves. What is the best treatment for her condition?
   a. Limit hand washing
   b. Apply topical corticosteroids
   c. Use hand moisturizer
   d. Wear nonlatex gloves
   e. Change the job
4. Which of the following federal agencies are part of the Department of Health and Human Services?
   a. Equal Employment Opportunity Commission
   b. National Institute for Occupational Safety and Health
   c. Occupational Health and Safety Administration
   d. Federal Aviation Administration
   e. American Conference of Governmental Industrial Hygienists
5. Medical investigation of an occupational health problem may involve which of the following?
   a. Determining whether a hazardous substance is present
   b. Measuring environmental and/or biological levels of the hazardous substance

c. Determining whether deleterious health effects are observed in the exposed population

d. a and b

e. a, b, and c

6. Clinical features of lead toxicity include all *except*:

a. Radial neuropathy

b. Acute abdominal pain

c. Chronic glomerulonephritis

d. Polycythemia

e. Hypertension

7. Which of the following accurately describes occupational asthma?

a. It occurs in all workers who use toluene diisocyanate above the threshold limit value.

b. It is characterized by symptoms that are different from nonoccupational asthma.

c. It responds to removal of the triggering agent but does not respond to bronchodilators.

d. It may make airways hyperreactive to smoke, cold air, or house dust.

e. It occurs only among those with no history of allergies.

Answers

1. **Answer e.**

   Chronic cough may be attributable to many occupational and nonoccupational causes. To help determine the diagnosis, it is important to take a detailed history, including inquiring about hobbies and occupational activities. Pulmonary function tests will aid in identifying the specific disease and evaluating its severity.

2. **Answer e.**

   Asbestos is known to cause mesothelioma, lung cancer, and asbestosis. All can occur in the same exposed person. The route of exposure is mainly through inhalation.

3. **Answer d.**

   Ultimately, the best therapeutic and preventive action for allergic contact dermatitis is to eliminate the exposure of concern (in this case, latex gloves). However, active disease can be controlled by reducing exposure to irritants, by frequent hand washing, and by using topical corticosteroids and hand moisturizer.

4. **Answer c.**

   The Occupational Safety and Health Administration is part of the Department of Labor. It was established in 1971 by the Occupational Safety and Health Act.

5. **Answer e.**

   To investigate an occupational health problem, the occupational health professional should determine that the hazardous substance is present, determine worker exposure to the substance, and determine whether observed health effects are known to be associated with the exposure.

6. **Answer d.**

   Lead exposure does not cause polycythemia. It is associated with neuropathy (with a tendency to affect the radial nerve), acute abdominal pain, chronic glomerulonephritis, hypertension, and anemia.

7. **Answer d.**

   Occupational asthma is a chronic inflammatory disease of the airway lining; symptoms are the same as those of nonoccupational asthma and include wheezing, chest tightness, cough, and shortness of breath. It usually responds to bronchodilators and usually is reversible if exposure can be stopped early. It does not affect all exposed workers but may develop among those with no history of allergies. It may make the airways hyperreactive to substances such as cigarette smoke, cold air, or house dust.

15

AEROSPACE MEDICINE

Lawrence Steinkraus, MD, MPH; and Jan Stepanek, MD, MPH

Portions of this chapter were presented at the Western Occupational Health Conference, Scottsdale, Arizona, September 12, 2009, copyrighted and used with permission of Mayo Foundation for Medical Education and Research.

Aerospace medicine focuses on the clinical care, research, and operational support of the health, safety, and performance of crewmembers and passengers of air and space vehicles, together with the support personnel who assist operation of such vehicles. This population often works and lives in remote, isolated, extreme, or enclosed environments under conditions of physical and psychological stress. Practitioners strive for an optimal human-machine match in occupational settings rich with environmental hazards and engineering countermeasures.

American Board of Preventive Medicine

Atmosphere and Gas Laws

Earth exists within a gaseous envelope from sea level to nearly 300 to 400 mi (480-640 km) out into space. The atmosphere is an oxidizing environment consisting of multiple gases and water vapor—99% is nitrogen and oxygen, and the rest is mostly inert gases and carbon dioxide. The atmosphere is classified into zones on the basis of temperature:

1) **Troposphere**: most weather is here; varying moisture content, turbulent air, constant rate of decrease in temperature with altitude.
2) **Stratosphere**: almost complete absence of moisture; nearly uniform temperature of −55°C, varying with latitude more than altitude; most ozone exists at the stratopause level.
3) **Mesosphere**: steady drop in temperature; where most meteors disappear.
4) **Thermosphere**: gradual increase in temperature; no upper limit; domain of auroras.

An exception to the rule on classification on the basis of temperature, the ionosphere starts roughly 50 mi (80 km) up and ends at about 600 mi (965 km). Gases here are ionized as a result of photochemical and photoelectric reactions with solar ultraviolet irradiation. The ionosphere acts as a reflector for long-wavelength electromagnetic radiation, allowing radio communications beyond line of sight. Solar disturbances (flares and sunspots) initiate changes in the ionosphere that can at times disrupt radiofrequency-based communications.

Atmospheric Pressure Zones

The atmosphere may also be characterized by pressure zones:

1) **Physiologic**: surface to 10,000 ft (3,050 m).
2) **Physiologic deficient**: 10,000-50,000 ft (3,050-15,240 m); oxygen required.
3) **Space equivalent**: 50,000 ft to 120 mi (15,240 m to 193 km); pressure decreases to 1 mm Hg; full-pressure suit or pressurized cabin required.
4) **Space**: above 120 mi (193 km).

Gas Laws

Understanding of the 5 basic gas laws aids understanding of aeromedical health impacts:

1) **Law of Boyle-Mariotte**: volume varies inversely with pressure; $V_1/V_2 = P_2/P_1$
   a) At 18,000 ft (5,500 m), a gas bubble is twice its sea-level size.
   b) Wet gas occupies more volume than dry; gases in the body are saturated.
   c) Volume changes lead to more health problems than any other physiologic consequence of flight, other than hypoxia.
2) **Law of Dalton**: pressure of mixed gases; total pressure = sum of each of the individual gas pressures; explains partial pressures and why less oxygen is available per volume at altitude.
3) **Henry's Law**: quantity of gas dissolved in a liquid is proportional to the partial pressure of the gas in contact with the liquid; the law responsible for decompression illness and decompression sickness (DCS).
4) **Charles-Gay-Lussac's Law**: with constant pressure, volume is proportional to temperature; $V_1/V_2 = T_1/T_2$
5) **General gas law**: $P_1V_1/T_1 = P_2V_2/T_2$ (combines laws of Charles-Gay-Lussac and Boyle-Mariotte)

- Understanding of the 5 basic gas laws aids understanding of aeromedically significant effects, specifically hypoxia, volume changes at higher altitudes, and decompression illness.

Respiratory Physiology and Decompressive Stress

As we ascend to altitude, whether on the ground scaling a mountain or in an aircraft, the environment is one of changing pressure due to the Law of Dalton, changing volume due to the Law of Boyle-Mariotte, and finally also changing dissolved inert gas loads in the body due to the Law of Henry (Table 1). The main difference is the time during which this change occurs.

Respiration

Respiration allows the body to take up oxygen and rid itself of carbon dioxide. This process consists of ventilation, pulmonary diffusion, transportation of gases to tissues, diffusion, and finally, cellular use. The alveolar oxygen tension, determined by barometric pressure, ventilation, and inspired gas oxygen content, is by far the most important determinant of arterial oxygen tension and resulting hemoglobin saturation.

Table 1 Effects of Altitude Exposure

Ascent	Illness	Relevant Gas Law
Gradual (terrestrial)[a]	Altitude illness (acute or chronic)	Dalton
Rapid (aerospace)[b]	Decompression sickness	Henry
		Boyle-Mariotte
	Dysbaric symptoms	Dalton
	Hypoxia	

[a] Problems with oxygen.
[b] Problems with nitrogen, oxygen, pressure, and volume.

The **oxygen-hemoglobin dissociation curve** (Figure 1) allows one to estimate a person's oxygenation status with a noninvasive measurement of oxygen saturation of the hemoglobin molecule with an oximeter. Useful numbers to remember on the curve include 40 mm Hg, where oxygen saturation is 75% (normal venous partial pressure of oxygen [PO_2]). At 60 mm Hg, the curve falls steeply, and a small change in saturation is equivalent to a large change in PO_2. The normal range for PO_2 is 80 to 100 mm Hg (95%-97% saturation).

Hyperventilation will ensue below an alveolar PO_2 of 55 to 60 mm Hg, resulting in a decrease in the partial pressure of carbon dioxide and **respiratory alkalosis,** which in turn decreases P_{50}, resulting in decreased tissue oxygenation and increased nerve irritability.

Hypoxia

Hypoxia is defined as the lack of sufficient oxygen supply to the body cells or body tissues; it is caused by an inadequate supply of oxygen, inadequate transportation of oxygen, or inability of the body tissues to use oxygen. We distinguish 4 general types of hypoxia:

1) **Hypoxic hypoxia**: the most hazardous physiologic threat to flight crew at increasing altitude; is caused by

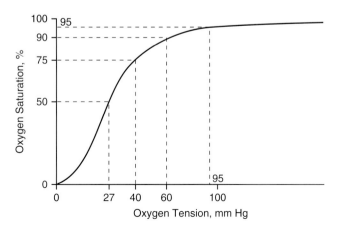

Figure 1 Oxygen-Hemoglobin Dissociation Curve.

decreased partial pressure of oxygen in the ambient atmosphere. Supplemental oxygen will combat hypoxic hypoxia successfully if crewmembers recognize hypoxic signs and symptoms. In the event of a depressurization or failure of an oxygen system, descent to lower altitudes, typically below 10,000 ft (3,000 m), is a way to increase oxygen in the ambient air.

2) **Stagnant hypoxia**: is caused by decreased tissue profusion or circulation of blood flow to the tissues. It can occur with sustained acceleration (G forces) and, in case of circulatory failure, with the heart being unable to successfully pump blood and sustain blood pressure.

3) **Histotoxic hypoxia**: the inability of the body to use oxygen at the cell and tissue level because of toxins that impair those functions. A classic mechanism for this to occur is cyanide poisoning.

4) **Anemic or hypemic hypoxia**: the decreased ability of the blood to carry oxygen to the body tissues. This can be due to a lack of red blood cells as the carriers of oxygen or to contamination of the red blood cells and the hemoglobin with a substance such as carbon monoxide, which impairs the ability of the blood to transport oxygen. Smokers, by virtue of having carbon monoxide in their bloodstream from their cigarette smoking, are at an increased-altitude equivalent while at sea level because of hypemic hypoxia.

Duration of Consciousness Without Supplemental Oxygen

The **effective performance time** or **time of useful consciousness** is defined by the Federal Aviation Administration (FAA) as "the amount of time in which a person is able to effectively or adequately perform flight duties with an insufficient supply of oxygen." Effective performance time decreases with increasing altitude and eventually coincides with circulation time for blood to go from the lungs to the brain at altitudes in excess of 43,000 ft (13,100 m). It is useful to remember that effective performance time at 18,000 ft (5,500 m) is 20 to 30 minutes; at 35,000 ft (10,500 m), it is 30 to 60 seconds; and at 43,000 ft (13,100 m), it is less than 10 seconds. These values will be divided in half if experienced in the context of a rapid decompression.

Treatment of Hypoxia

Hypoxic incapacitation is treated by applying oxygen. Use of oxygen masks by crew and passengers is a practical and efficient way to accomplish this task. At altitudes greater than 50,000 ft (15,240 m), a full-pressure suit or a closed cabin is needed because pressure breathing alone will not sufficiently combat the physiology of low environmental pressure and the resultant low oxygen content and insufficient oxygen

tension to allow for body tissue oxygenation and gas exchange.

Cabin pressurization, which allows passengers to fly comfortably at cabin pressure altitudes of 6,000 to 8,000 ft (1,800-2,400 m), helps combat hypoxia. Aircraft engines produce bleed (bypass) air that is then air conditioned, filtered, and distributed in the aircraft cabin via airflow systems above the passengers, with airflow down to the floor. Commercial aircraft have aft outflow valves that, combined with the bleed air setting from the engines, determine cabin pressure. Recirculation of the aircraft cabin air allows for additional moisture to be retained inside the cabin for the purposes of passenger comfort.

- A person's oxygenation status can be estimated with a noninvasive, transcutaneous oximeter measurement and an oxygen-hemoglobin dissociation curve.
- Commercial aircraft are pressurized to the equivalent of 6,000 to 8,000 ft (1,800-2,400 m) altitude. The airflow pattern and air filtration help reduce risk of infectious disease transmission.

Trapped Gases and Change of Gas Volumes

Changes of gas volumes are governed by the Law of Boyle-Mariotte, which states that with constant temperature, the product of a pressure and the volume of a gas stay constant. Thus, with decreasing pressure, **gas volume will increase when going to altitude**, and the inverse will be true when going to depth.

It is important to remember the changes in volume that can be expected when flying to altitude. At sea level, the volume of a given unit will double at 18,000 ft (5,500 m), triple at 28,000 ft (8,500 m), and quintuple at 39,000 ft (12,000 m). This has profound ramifications for airspaces such as the middle ear, the sinuses, and sometimes, carious teeth. On ascent, expansion of gases is first experienced, and pressure equilibrium through connecting ducts is usually accomplished; but upon descent, significant discomfort can be felt if there is no ability to equilibrate the pressures within these airspaces and gas becomes trapped.

In a normal middle ear, there is equal pressure between the eardrum and the external ear because the eustachian tube allows pressure from the mouth and nose to equilibrate with the middle ear. With a cold, swelling of the eustachian tube may occur, and it is not possible for the air to equilibrate between the middle ear and ambient pressure. With descent from altitude, ambient pressure will increase, thus creating a relative vacuum in the middle ear, resulting in pain and possibly vertigo (alternobaric vertigo). The analogous mechanism may occur with sinuses.

Physical Phenomena of Decompression and its Consequences

Flight at high altitude in a pressurized aircraft always carries a small risk of loss of cabin pressurization. In civilian operations, about 40 to 50 decompression events are reported every year, which equals about 1 decompression for every 50,000 flying hours. Loss of cabin pressurization results in a sequence of physical phenomena that may have significant physiologic consequences.

Decompression Rate

The decompression rate in an aircraft at altitude depends on the size of the breach of the hull of the aircraft; loss of a door will result in a very rapid decompression, whereas a gradual leak will result in a slow and possibly dangerously imperceptible decompression. Any decompression that occurs in less than 0.5 seconds is considered to be explosive in nature.

Phenomena of Decompression

Phenomena that can be encountered with rapid or explosive decompression are a loud noise, strong wind blast, fogging, and rapid onset of hypoxia. Time of useful consciousness is cut in half by a rapid decompression. There is a distinct possibility of DCS if decompression occurs above 18,000 ft (5,500 m).

Gas Bubble Formation

As we live at the bottom of the atmosphere (at sea level), our bodies are saturated with inert gases, mainly nitrogen. If we rapidly decrease the ambient pressure surrounding our bodies—like the rapid opening of a carbonated beverage container—we may experience a set of signs and symptoms that may be due to free gas bubbles developing and evolving within our body tissues.

The principle behind these phenomena is based on the Law of Henry. Decreases in ambient pressure (ascent to altitude or ascent to sea level from a dive) may result in DCS. Haldane noted that DCS could be prevented by avoiding pressure ratios exceeding a 2:1 in pressure changes. With rapid ascent to high altitude without prebreathing oxygen or when flying at high altitude, a rapid decompression may result in development of nitrogen bubbles in tissues. This is known as **aviator bends** or **altitude DCS**.

Decompression Illness

The term "decompression illness" is often used interchangeably with DCS. By definition, decompression illness encompasses the entity of DCS and arterial gas embolization. Arterial gas embolization occurs with introduction of significant gas loads into the circulation, usually because of pulmonary or iatrogenic injury. The transported air results in injury in critical vascular territories such as the brain, heart, and other tissues.

In this context, it also is important to mention that flying after diving is riskier because of increases in inert gases being dissolved in our bodies. The recommended waiting period before going to flight altitudes of 8,000 ft (2,400 m) is at least 12 hours after non–decompression-stop diving and 24 to 48 hours after decompression-stop diving. If flight will be in a nonpressurized aircraft above 8,000 ft (2,400 m), the recommended waiting time is at least 24 hours after any scuba diving.

Manifestations of DCS

The evolved gas in altitude DCS typically manifests with pain in and around joints. More serious is the affliction of heart and lungs, which is termed the **chokes** (chest pain and burning sensation underneath the chest that, if not corrected, could cause collapse and unconsciousness). Neurologic signs of DCS may involve a sense of tingling, itching, or rash on the body (cutis marmorata), problems with vision, temporary paralysis, and seizures. Should any such symptoms occur in the context of a decompression at altitude, treatment with 100% high-flow oxygen via a tight-sealing mask and immediate medical attention for possible treatment in a hyperbaric chamber should be instituted.

- Changes in volume should be expected when flying to altitude. These volume changes may elicit signs and symptoms in trapped airspaces such as the middle ear, the sinuses, and sometimes, carious teeth.
- Preventive measures include breathing pure oxygen in advance to flush nitrogen from the body before planned ascents.
- Signs and symptoms of decompression illness may include pain in and around joints. More serious is the affliction of heart and lungs or neurologic problems. Transported air can injure critical vascular territories such as the brain, heart, and other tissues.
- Treatment of neurologic symptoms involves 100% high-flow oxygen and recompression in a hyperbaric chamber as soon as practical under the guidance of a physician experienced in treating decompression illness.

Acceleration Physics and Physiology

Aircraft Design

Aircraft design has evolved with the growing understanding of physics affecting objects moving in airstreams at varied speeds. Important elements include aircraft function (passenger transport, cargo transport, air-to-air combat, stealth capability, agility in harsh environments), economics, and environment. Striking a balance between speed and utility, for instance, in the commercial industry, has been a constant challenge. Although it seems reasonable to have high speed, economic factors may dictate more carrying capacity and slower speeds; thus the Concorde Supersonic Transport, which delivered fewer passengers faster, never became a profitable operation compared with the Boeing 747 or Airbus 380. Design also influences medically relevant effects, including hypobaria and resulting degree of hypoxia, acceleration tolerance, exposure to toxins or disease vectors, and even legroom.

Application of Forces

As humans fly, vehicles and bodies are influenced by various application of forces. Depending on how these forces are applied, they can be useful, tolerated, or deleterious. Understanding these forces help protect flyers and prevent injury. Force may be penetrating if the applied area is small and/or if the impacted surface is fragile (eg, bullets), or it may be blunt if it affects a larger area of the body (eg, more typical for restrained occupants). The concepts of stress and strain are used in understanding how aircraft materials respond to forces and how biological tissues such as bones respond; this is critical when designing protection systems such as helmets. Applied stress causes strains in materials or tissues; stress is independent of the material, but material and tissue characteristics dictate what will happen with imposed stress.

Restraint Systems

To prevent injuries, restraint systems have been developed. The goal of restraint systems is to isolate the human from the vehicle during short-term (transient) events by minimizing applied acceleration forces to the body and redistributing velocity changes over a longer period. There are numerous forms of restraint, from lap belts to air bags. Restraint system effectiveness depends on multiple factors: how well restraint configurations transmit loads; ability of restraints to control motion; restraint contact pressure (eg, tight seat belt); load-carrying capability of the restrained anatomic segments (eg, biologic limits); avoiding secondary impacts (eg, head on steering wheel); avoiding acceleration amplification (eg, bottoming); and maximizing time to accomplish required velocity changes.

Five factors influence passenger survival in crashes, described by the acronym **CREEP**:

1) **C**rashworthiness (aircraft structures and design)
2) **R**estraint (described above)
3) **E**nvironment (surrounding area that body may strike)

4) **E**nergy absorption
5) **P**ostcrash factors (fire, emergency medical response)

In designing safety systems, human impact tolerances must be considered.

Egress or Escape

An alternative to remaining inside aircraft with restraints is to egress or escape. Parachute use has been well known for centuries, but with the higher speeds of aircraft, better systems were needed to allow crew to initially escape the aircraft before parachute use. Strong wind blasts and excessive G forces have prevented crews from escaping aircraft, and ejection seats were developed to counter this problem. (On the surface of the Earth, bodies are subjected to an acceleration force of 32 ft/sec^2 [9.81 m/sec^2], giving us "weight"; this acceleration is termed 1 G.) Rocket propulsion technologies have produced the higher trajectories necessary to clear aircraft structures for high-speed escape, as well as for escape during low-speed and zero-zero (zero-velocity and zero-altitude) ejections.

- Aircraft design considers aircraft function and economic and environmental factors. Design also influences medically relevant effects, including hypobaria and resulting degree of hypoxia, acceleration tolerance, exposure to toxins or disease vectors, and even legroom.
- Understanding penetrating and blunt forces help protect flyers and prevent injury. The concepts of stress and strain are used in understanding how aircraft materials respond to forces and how biological tissues such as bones respond.
- The goal of restraint systems is to isolate the human from the vehicle during short-term (transient) events by minimizing applied acceleration forces to the body and redistributing velocity changes over a longer period.
- Five factors influence passenger survival in crashes: crashworthiness, restraint, environment, energy absorption, and postcrash factors (acronym CREEP).
- An alternative to remaining inside aircraft with restraints is to egress or escape with ejection seats and parachutes.

Spatial Orientation

The primary source of the information we use to orient ourselves in the 3-dimensional aerospace environment is visual (90%). The rest comes from vestibular and kinesthetic sources. Orientation is a complex process involving **orientational perception** (upright vs upside down), which helps us in understanding where we are relative to other physical objects in space and **locational (geographic)**

perception, which places us in, as opposed to above, the plane of the Earth's surface (the map). Orientational clues can be primary and dependent on clues from the natural environment such as proprioceptive, vestibular, and visual preconscious signals that evolved over millennia of nonaerial survival. Although these signals may be appropriate on the ground or in low arboreal settings, they subject us to certain **spatial disorientation illusions** in specific aerospace operational settings. Further, secondary or conscious processing reconstructed from focal visual, verbal, or other symbolic data (eg, flight instruments) helps us in orienting ourselves, but it is subject to certain information processing errors that may lead to disorientation. As roughly 14% of all civilian fatal aircraft accidents are attributed to spatial disorientation, and when a crash occurs where spatial disorientation is the leading contributing factor, it has 90% fatality rate, it is important to understand some of the basics in this area. Figure 2 outlines the various elements involved in spatial orientation.

Motion Sickness

A common result of movement in the aerospace environment is motion sickness. The specific symptoms that occur in response to motion tend to be typical and predictable and include lethargy, apathy, and stomach awareness, followed by nausea, pallor, and cold perspiration, then retching, vomiting, and collapse. **Airsickness**, **space motion sickness**, **and flight simulator sickness** are the 3 primary aerospace forms of motion sickness. Cited incidence rates of aviation trainee airsickness range from 10% to 40%. Most modern air forces have a fairly consistent loss of 1% to 2% of pilot trainees for persistent motion sickness. Flight simulator sickness is relatively new and more widely reported, with increasing use of more advanced simulators. The cause of simulator sickness is the mismatch between the presented visual image of the simulation and the expected but absent kinesthetic cues such as proprioceptive and matching neurovestibular cues. Sufferers tend to be more experienced crews performing in wide field-of-view or dome-type simulators. No treatment is 100% successful. Basic treatments include reassurance that this is normal and not a true medical illness and that most flyers adapt given time, exposure, and appropriate habits (avoiding self-induced stressors); anxiety only accelerates and worsens the chain of events.

- The primary source of the information we use to orient ourselves in the 3-dimensional aerospace environment is visual (90%). The rest comes from vestibular and kinesthetic sources.
- Orientation clues from the natural environment such as proprioceptive, vestibular, and visual preconscious signals subject us to certain spatial disorientation illusions in specific aerospace operational settings, which may contribute to aircraft accidents.
- A common result of movement in the aerospace environment is motion sickness. Most flyers adapt given time, exposure, and appropriate habits.

Space Medicine

Brief History of Human Space Flight

The Russian cosmonaut Yuri Gagarin became the first human to go into space on April 12, 1961, aboard Vostok 1. Extensive animal testing preceded the first human space

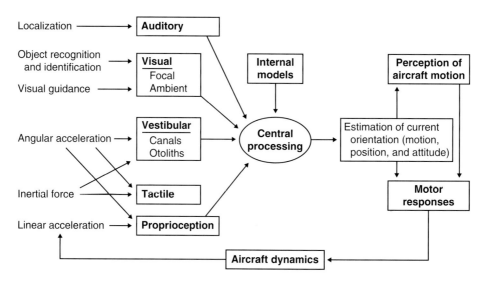

Figure 2 Mechanisms of Spatial Orientation in Flight. (Adapted from Previc FH, Ercoline WR. Spatial disorientation in aviation. Reston [VA]: American Institute of Aeronautics and Astronautics, Inc. c2004. Used with permission.)

flight. Sputnik 2 flew a biomedically instrumented dog ("Laika") into orbit, and the spacecraft supported the animal for 6 days; the results from these experiments revealed that heart rate, respiratory rate, blood pressure, as well as overall performance, appeared to be maintained in microgravity. At the end of the Gemini program in 1966, spaceflight was recognized as being associated with decreased red cell mass, postflight orthostatic intolerance, loss of body calcium, and diminished postflight exercise capacity. The exploration of the biomedical aspects of longer-duration sojourns in space prompted the creation of manned orbital laboratories to study some of the effects of a microgravity environment on humans during extended spaceflight. The Russian Salyut and US Skylab programs fulfilled this very mission, and the biomedical results from these flights still form a relevant foundation in space medicine today. It was concluded as a result of these flights that humans were able to operate effectively in space for periods up to 3 months and, given effective countermeasures, possibly longer. The International Space Station has seen continuous crew presence since 2000 and is the current platform for life sciences research and countermeasure validation and testing. The current mean flight duration is 28 days, and a mere 40 individuals have spent more than 6 months in space.

Relevant Biomedical Aspects of Human Spaceflight

As humans enter space, physiologic adaptive changes ensue, primarily from the altered gravitational environment and the resulting absence of hydrostatic pressure gradients.

Space Motion Sickness

When astronauts experience microgravity at low-earth orbit, there is a period of adaptation of the neurovestibular system due to absent gravitational force vectors, absent proprioceptive gravitational inputs, and the new visual environment, with the challenge of defining "up" and "down." Space motion sickness can occur within the first 72 hours and affect upward of 66% of astronauts; when experienced during a first flight, there is a 77% chance of getting it on the next flight as well. Current countermeasures include use of promethazine, preflight adaptation training (results in 19%-54% reduction in space motion sickness severity), and autogenic training. Selection of motion sickness–resistant individuals is not effective. Astronauts avoid provocative head movements and avoid mission-critical tasks (eg, extravehicular activity) in the first 72 hours as additional risk-mitigation strategies.

Fluid Shifts

Removal of hydrostatic pressure gradients in microgravity results in fluid shifts to the central circulation, which in turn results in a compensatory, adaptive redistribution of plasma over time. These shifts occur within the first 6 to 10 hours in orbit. The relative venous congestion of the central vascular compartment leads to distention of veins and vascular plexi of the head, resulting in perceived stuffiness akin to sinus congestion. The lower extremities experience a relative loss of fluids, which leads to the apt term "chicken leg syndrome" to describe the appearance of markedly thinner legs in microgravity. Fluid shifts also tend to suppress thirst when first arriving in orbit and sometimes are worsened by space motion sickness.

Cardiovascular Changes

In the Apollo program, cardiac rhythm changes were seen during extravehicular activity and during lunar excursions and were thought to be due to low levels of potassium in the face of large workloads for the astronauts. A 14-beat run of ventricular tachycardia was registered during an extravehicular activity on Mir-2 in 1987, resulting in an abbreviated mission. Russian medical operations have recorded 75 abnormal electrocardiograms over 10 years of work on Mir. Echocardiography data show a short-term change (during the first 17 days of flight) of increased stroke volume by 46%, followed by a decrease by 10% to 16% at 1, 3, and 5 months in space. Consistent with these changes is the initial short-term increase in cardiac output of 22% to 29%, followed by a decrease in cardiac output by 17% to 20% at 1, 3, and 5 months.

Postflight Orthostatic Intolerance

Postflight orthostatic intolerance occurs in 20% to 67% of crew. The perception of astronauts postflight is that the 1 G_z environment feels more like 4 G_z, and postural instability is associated with walking and orthostatic intolerance with standing. Countermeasures include use of G-suits and fluid loading before reentry, and studies have shown body cooling increases total peripheral resistance. Maintenance of cardiovascular fitness with use of aerobic and strength training in orbit, as well as use of lower body, negative-pressure devices in orbit, is a consideration.

Pulmonary Function Changes

The functioning of the lungs and gas exchange overall has not been found to be a clinical concern that warrants specific countermeasures. Long-term effects of altered pulmonary pressures and airflow distribution in the lungs are not known.

Anthropometric Changes

The absence of gravitational axial loading on the body results in increased hydration of the intervertebral discs, with resultant elongation of the spine and thus a rather swift change in height of the astronaut of 5 to 6 cm. The neutral body position also changes as a result of absent gravity vectors, and the body assumes a position with arms slightly angled in front of the chest and legs slightly bent at the knee and hip level.

Changes in the Musculoskeletal System

Due to the lack of need for muscular compensation for gravitational loading muscles, especially extensor muscles, atrophy may reach 10% to 20% on short-term missions, while it may be higher on long-duration missions. Muscle atrophy contributes to postflight postural control and locomotor changes. Countermeasures include consistent resistance and aerobic exercises while in orbit.

Bone loss occurs during spaceflight at a rate of about 1% to 2% per month; the areas that lose the most bone are the weight-bearing bones in the legs and lower spine. Crews on 6-month missions have lost up to 20% of lower extremity bone mass. Fracture risk becomes an important concern, especially if extravehicular activity is planned after a long-duration mission (Mars).

Unfortunately, it is not possible to prevent bone and muscle loss based on regular exercise alone. A combination of prudent diet, exercise, and potentially pharmacologic measures is needed as a multifaceted countermeasure to this problem.

Psychosocial Aspects of Spaceflight

The spaceflight environment is unique in that it frequently places a crew together that consists of members with different cultural, sexual, and ethnic backgrounds. This diverse environment is a potential source for a multitude of factors that influence crew culture, from different communication styles to different attitudes and approaches to problem solving.

The goal in the selection process is to remove significant psychopathology (schizophrenia, depression, bipolar disorder, etc); this is achieved by standardized neuropsychometric testing, including the MMPI (Minnesota Multiphasic Personality Inventory Scale) and MCMI (Million Clinical Multiaxial Inventory). Key is the assessment of whether the individual being screened is a potential risk to flying safety. The answer can be found by combining psychometric tests with psychiatric interviews.

Long-Duration Missions

The rigor and duration of the exposure that a crew will undergo on a mission to Mars is significant. With current technology, a mission is anticipated to be of 30 months' duration, with outbound and inbound flights being 4 to 6 months long, on-site duration is scheduled to be 18 months, with G transitions being on the order of 4 G_x/G_z.

Risks include radiation exposure, medical events, and the obvious challenges (eg, bone loss, muscular atrophy, cardiovascular deconditioning, and neurovestibular adaptations) that are brought on by microgravity. The most serious threat for long-duration space missions is the threat of radiation exposure, which can be markedly accentuated with solar flare activity. Shielding of the crew from radiation is a required life-support function of the space vehicle. Aggressive risk mitigation of any preventable disease processes is one of the key factors of long-duration mission operations because treatment options may be limited, given the relative lack of medical resources.

- When astronauts experience microgravity at low-Earth orbit, there is a period of adaptation of the neurovestibular system due to absent gravitational force vectors, absent proprioceptive gravitational inputs, and the new visual environment.
- Removal of hydrostatic pressure gradients in microgravity results in fluid shifts to the central circulation, which in turn results in a compensatory, adaptive redistribution of plasma over time.
- Echocardiography data show a short-term change in stroke volume and cardiac output when in space.
- Postflight orthostatic intolerance and postural instability can affect some individuals. Countermeasures include use of G-suits, fluid loading before reentry, and body cooling. Maintenance of cardiovascular fitness and performing strength training in orbit are considerations.
- The absence of gravitational axial loading on the body results in elongation of the spine. Due to the lack of need for muscular compensation for gravitational loading muscles, atrophy may reach 10% to 20% on short-term missions.
- Bone loss occurs during spaceflight at a rate of about 1% to 2% per month; the areas that lose the most bone are the weight-bearing bones in the legs and lower spine, making fracture risk an important concern. It is not possible to prevent bone and muscle loss based on regular exercise alone.
- The diversity of spaceflight crew members may affect the culture of the working environment. The goal in the crew selection process is to remove significant psychopathology (schizophrenia, depression, bipolar disorder, etc).
- The most serious threat for long-duration space missions is the threat of radiation exposure, which can be markedly accentuated with solar flare activity. Other risks include medical events and the physical challenges of weightlessness.

Aeromedical Transport

More than 4 billion people travel each year by air, with 2.5 billion by commercial aircraft. As more people fly, it is expected that more will have potential medical issues, either in-flight or before flight. Data are scarce on medical emergencies in flight. One medical group, consulting for a major US airline, noted that for roughly 4 million flights over 6 years, there were 2,000 in-flight medical incidents requiring medical consultation.

With increased numbers of travelers of all ages and medical conditions, the number requiring and requesting medical assistance for transport has been increasing. Costs tend to be high and coordination complex. Travelers are advised to contact their physicians for pretravel advice, to address preventable issues (immunizations, appropriate medications, precoordination of medical requirements), and to educate themselves on potential hazards.

Stressors of Flight

Inherent in flight are a number of physiologic stressors that can have impacts ranging from annoying to fatal.

1) **Decreased partial pressure of oxygen or hypoxia**: most commercial aircraft have cabin pressure altitudes up to a maximum of 8,000 ft (2,400 m), at which the partial pressure of oxygen is the equivalent of 15.5% at sea level. FAA requirements for flight limit cabin pressure altitude to a maximum of 8,000 ft (2,400 m), except during emergencies. In nominal flight operations, the maximum cabin pressure altitude is rarely reached; in most operations, the cabin pressure altitude is around 6,000 ft (1,800 m). Although most healthy passengers will tolerate decreases in oxygen availability, passengers with cardiac and pulmonary conditions often need extra attention. The Aerospace Medical Association has published guidelines that can assist physicians in advising travelers.

2) **Acceleration and G forces**: generally not a concern for standard civilian passenger flight; utility or sport flyers may be exposed to significant acceleration forces; military crews are certainly expected to operate in physiologically challenging environments.

3) **Vibration**: the body has specific natural frequencies, depending on its density and make-up; the vulnerable range is 0.1 to 40 Hz. Effects range from discomfort to disruption of physiologic processes. Impacts can be direct, as with increased pain for patients with fractures, to indirect, as when communication is interrupted or degraded.

4) **Noise**: inherent to aeromedical operations; impacts can include fatigue, blood pressure elevation, and hearing loss (acute and chronic); operational effects include difficulty hearing alarms, listening with stethoscopes, or communicating.

5) **Humidity**: cabin air in aircraft tends to be very dry (3%-15% relative humidity), resulting in dry nasal and respiratory passages, skin irritation, and other effects.

6) **Barometric pressure changes and hypobaria**: the primary effect of lowered cabin pressures (Law of Boyle-Mariotte) relates to gas expansion of trapped gas in pulmonary, gastrointestinal, and ear-nose-throat body systems. Effects can be problematic in medical equipment such as tracheal cuff tubes, pneumatic splints, and vacuum devices. Hypobaria may rarely cause spontaneous pneumothorax in trauma patients with significant respiratory compromise. Gastrointestinal tract gas expansion may cause diaphragmatic crowding, leading to lower tidal volumes.

7) **Jet lag**: as long-duration international flights have become more common, the problem of **desynchronosis**, or jet lag, has arisen. West-to-East travel is the most upsetting for biorhythms; typically 1 day is required for each time zone crossed for full adjustment; appropriate planning and sleep management (crew rest) can alleviate many of the problems; military and civilian crews are expected to meet minimum crew rest requirements to address some of these problems. Pharmacological solutions, including sleep-inducing agents such as temazepam, can help passengers adjust to transmeridian travel; as yet, only the military allows activating agents such as dextroamphetamines and modafinil for maintaining crew wakefulness in certain mission contexts; persons with diabetes mellitus and others who rely on natural body cycles for medication administration may encounter problems.

8) **Thermal stress**: heat increases body temperature and cold produces muscle shivering, increasing the metabolic rate and oxygen demand on the body. This is particularly true in ventilator-dependent patients and patients with decreased peripheral perfusion in shock; although civilian passenger aircraft generally are air conditioned, military and some civilian utility category operations (eg, firefighting, crop dusting) subject crews and passengers to wide ranges of thermal stress, from arctic to jungle levels.

9) **Toxins**: tobacco is no longer an issue, as use in flight has been generally banned in civilian and military settings. Concerns about residual insecticide after disinsection, fuel combustion byproducts with use of bleed air for pressurization, and off-gassing from aircraft surfaces are areas of controversy, particularly for aircrew who have longer exposures to aircraft environments.

10) **Exposure to infection**: while current modern jet design allows for high air exchange rates and high-efficiency particulate air filters, there remains some risk to on-board passengers and crews when transporting passengers with some infectious diseases. Tuberculosis, influenza, severe acute respiratory syndrome, and other respiratory illnesses may be transmitted to fellow passengers; typically, the risk increases with proximity and longer exposure time. Airflow in aircraft is a mixture of outside and inside air. Most modern aircraft have laminar flow systems wherein air is introduced at the ceiling level and removed at the floor level. Exchange rates of cabin air (10-20 volumes per hour) typically are much higher than standard offices and households. Thus, in the case of respiratory infections, it is unlikely for passengers to acquire these infections under normal operational circumstances. Risk factors include prolonged ground times when circulation rates are reduced or when the air conditioning is shut off, and proximity to infected passengers (usually 1 to 2 rows or seats, maximal distance). Of course, the usual contact risks remain for door handles and other common objects, and these are more likely related to transmission of common colds and gastrointestinal tract infections. In aircraft with front-to-back flow designs, **placement of patients with infectious disease in the rear of the aircraft** is reasonable, along with use of appropriate personal protective equipment and infection control schema. When risk for contagion exists and air travel is required, it is critical to know aircraft specific airflow systems because not all are the same.

11) **Restricted mobility**: seated immobility in any context of transportation carries the risk of deep venous thrombosis, and travel by air is no exception; to date, data have not shown conclusively that excess risk is associated with the hypobaric environment. That said, any at-risk passengers should be cautioned to take appropriate preventive measures such as stretching, walking, and maintaining hydration.

12) **Airsickness**: most commercial passengers do not experience this problem because typical flight profiles avoid excess turbulence and accelerative forces. Incidence increases with turbulence (nearly 100% in hurricane penetration aircraft) and preexisting illnesses (sinusitis, otitis, gastroenteritis, etc).

Medical Oxygen

Some airlines provide medical oxygen to passengers in flight. The airline should be contacted 48 to 72 hours before the flight, and a medical statement regarding the necessary flow-rates provided to enable the airline to determine the volume of oxygen needed for the patient. The airline provides continuous-flow oxygen with a face mask or nasal cannula, with flow rates of up to 4 L/min. Airlines do not provide oxygen for passengers before or after a flight. Separate arrangements with local oxygen providers must be made accordingly. The use of oxygen in flight is covered under Medicare Part B for Medicare beneficiaries with a certificate of medical necessity. The FAA recently (2005) authorized use of oxygen concentrators in flight for patients.

- Travelers are advised to contact their physicians for pretravel advice, to address preventable issues (immunizations, appropriate medications, precoordination of medical requirements), and to educate themselves on potential hazards.
- Physiologic stressors of commercial flight can include decreased partial pressure of oxygen, vibration, noise, humidity, expansion of trapped gases (trauma patients may have spontaneous pneumothorax), and thermal stress.
- Jet lag (desynchronosis) has become more common with increasing international travel. Typically, 1 day is required for each time zone crossed for full adjustment. Persons with insulin-treated diabetes mellitus may encounter problems.
- A cabin pressure altitude of 8,000 ft (2,400 m) is the maximum altitude recommended by the Federal Aviation Administration (FAA) in civilian air transport of passengers. Gas expansion is expected but can affect the body (eg, barotrauma to the middle ear).
- Modern jet designs have laminar air flow systems and high air-exchange rates; thus, extensive and free transmission of respiratory infection is unlikely.
- Seated immobility carries the risk of deep venous thrombosis. Any at-risk passengers should be cautioned to take appropriate preventive measures such as stretching, walking, and maintaining hydration.
- With sufficient advance notice, airlines can provide continuous-flow oxygen with a face mask or nasal cannula to patients, with flow rates of up to 4 L/min. The use of oxygen in flight is covered under Medicare Part B for Medicare beneficiaries if the patient has a certificate of medical necessity.

Relevant Passenger Medical Conditions

Passenger medical conditions commonly needing preflight evaluations (in passengers travelling without medical escort team) are listed below.

1) **Cardiovascular disease**: contraindications to flight are listed in Table 2. Some patients will require oxygen

Table 2 Cardiac Conditions Contraindicating Flight in Unaccompanied Passengers

Uncomplicated myocardial infarction within 2-3 wk

Complicated myocardial infarction within 6 wk

Unstable angina

Congestive heart failure, severe, decompensated

Uncontrolled hypertension

Coronary artery bypass graft within 10-14 d

Cerebrovascular accident within 2 wk

Uncontrolled ventricular or supraventricular tachycardia

Eisenmenger syndrome

Severe symptomatic valvular heart disease

and may need medication adjustments to optimize their cardiac status.

2) **Deep venous thrombosis**: passengers at high risk for thrombosis should be taking appropriate anticlotting agents and be advised on hydration, regular exercise, and stretching, use of compression stockings, and signs and symptoms of deep venous thrombosis.

3) **Chronic pulmonary disease**: patients should have further testing if ground-level oximetry is below 95%. The single most helpful test is the arterial blood gas. Alveoloar partial pressure of oxygen (PaO_2) at ground level is the best predictor of altitude PaO_2. A PaO_2 exceeding 70 mm Hg is in most cases adequate for travel without in-flight medical oxygen. A hypoxic challenge test at 15% inspired oxygen may assist in the decision to prescribe in-flight oxygen, sometimes in conjunction with a walking test. Oxygen requirements exceeding 4 L/min are a contraindication to standard commercial travel. Hypercapnia on arterial blood gas is a sign of poor pulmonary reserve and possibly increased risk at altitude. Patients with severe, poorly controlled asthma should consider ground transportation. Patients with mild or well-controlled asthma should always carry their medications on board.

4) **Seizure disorders**: lower cabin oxygen levels, fatigue, jet lag, alcohol use, and other stressors may trigger seizures. Medications need to be dosed properly and passengers should be cautioned on precautions. Air travel is not recommended for those with frequent, uncontrolled seizures.

5) **Stroke**: recent stroke or transient ischemic events warrant caution for potential passengers and consideration for delay in travel until fully stable.

6) **Conditions affecting the ear, nose, and throat**: the middle ear and the different sinuses constitute potential areas for trapped gas to develop with resultant complications. Use of topical and oral decongestants, nasal saline, and frequent clearing maneuvers (eg, Toynbee, swallowing, and Valsalva) may be needed. Ideally, passengers should not fly with colds.

7) **Diabetes mellitus**: especially for patients with type 1 disease and when crossing multiple time zones or traveling to less developed destinations, insulin dosage and administration times may be problematic.

8) **Pregnancy and infants**: contraindications to air travel for pregnant passengers include current bleeding, pain, history of premature deliveries, cervical incompetence, and being past the 36th week of gestation. The healthy newborn may safely fly 1 week postpartum.

9) **Air travel after surgery**: travel should be avoided after surgery of the central nervous system, abdomen, chest, and hollow viscus for at least 3 to 4 days to allow for postoperative absorption of gas.

Individuals with any contagious disease that could be transmitted to other passengers should postpone air travel until they are no longer contagious. Of particular concern is tuberculosis. Prospective passengers who have tuberculosis should have had adequate therapy and be noninfectious before flight. The World Health Organization has published guidelines on air travel with tuberculosis.

If the physician has fully reviewed the prospective traveler's condition and there is any question regarding the suitability to fly or any special requests for assistance, airlines should be contacted. Some airlines require a medical certificate from the health care provider stating that the passenger is currently stable and fit for air travel. For contagious diseases, the certificate should also state that the passenger is not currently infectious. Physicians may be asked to assist in other ways such as facilitating seat upgrades (allowing more room and reclining options) and ticket refunds (when illness precludes travel) and provision of advice on special equipment like supplemental oxygen.

Aeromedical Transportation Issues (for Patients With Medical Escort Teams)

Some medical conditions of importance for aeromedical transportation are listed below. Appropriate equipment, staffing, and logistical issues are noted for each condition.

1) **Cardiovascular**: cardiopulmonary resuscitation on board before flight (defibrillator); oxygen available and adjusted for cabin pressure and preflight requirements; caution on electrical devices such as external pacemakers; use medical teams with advanced cardiac resuscitation skills and equipment if intensive care unit–level care might be needed; hemoglobin below 8.5 g/dL can be a problem for oxygen delivery for patients, especially in the context of concurrent diseases and acute status (trauma).

2) **Pulmonary**: untreated pneumothorax is an absolute contraindication to movement by air unless cabin altitude can be maintained at destination level; do not remove chest tubes preflight unless the patient can be observed for more than 24 hours; saline should be used for endotracheal cuffs; careful tailoring of oxygen requirements for those with chronic obstructive pulmonary disease.

3) **Gastrointestinal**: postsurgery patients may have air pockets; nasogastric tubes recommended for possible ileus to decompress the stomach; colostomy patients will have greater output volume (need more bags); caution on recent surgical anastomoses as possibility for gas expansion.

4) **Surgical**: for orthopedic patients, avoid casts unless bivalved for tissue expansion; no swinging weights for traction, use springs only (acceleration effects); do not use pneumatic splints; have window casts over wounds for rapid reassessment, if needed; for trauma patients, caution on compartment syndromes, use of drains.

5) **Neuropsychiatry**: patients with elevated intracranial pressures need appropriate oxygen support and cabin pressure restrictions, use caution if intracerebral air is present; need to position appropriately (usually head first) to avoid acceleration injuries; psychiatric patients need preflight coordination for appropriate medical attendant support, and decisions are required on chemical and physical restraints because suicidal, homicidal, and psychotic patients can pose grave risk to passengers and crew if not controlled.

6) **Special populations**: women with high-risk pregnancies need oxygen support, cabin pressure restriction to avoid gas distension, proper medical team support for potential labor; physician needs to accompany patient; neonates need an appropriate, controlled-environment life support system and trained support team, including physician.

7) **Decompression illness**: patients need 100% oxygen and cabin-altitude control; sea-level cabin pressure best, next best is origination airport altitude; use a helicopter only as last resort.

Cabin Environment in High-Altitude Operations

Cabin Air Quality

Numerous factors contribute to good cabin air quality, including pressurization, oxygen content, carbon dioxide content, temperature, ozone content, humidity, bioaerosols, and tobacco smoke. The single most important factor that significantly improved cabin air quality was the introduction of smoking bans onboard aircraft. The air in aircraft is completely exchanged every 3 to 4 minutes, as opposed to every 12 minutes in a residential home. Up to 30% to 50% of the air is recirculated. All air is filtered via high-efficiency particulate air filters that capture particles the size of 0.3 micrometers or larger. Carbon dioxide levels are usually maintained at levels of 0.5% (equivalent to sea level). Laminar airflow (ceiling to floor) reduces risks for infectious disease transmission.

In-Flight Medical Support to Passengers

All commercial airlines have some capability to provide in-flight emergency medical care. Medical kits and flight crews with medical training vary in type and quality, depending on country and airline. International and longer-distance flights tend to have more expanded kits. In 2004, automated defibrillators became required on US aircraft carrying at least 7,500 pounds of payload and one (or more) flight attendants.

Although flight attendants are typically trained to recognize common symptoms of distress and respond to medical emergencies with basic resuscitation techniques, they may ask for assistance from passengers with medical credentials. When there is no onboard assistance, or more help is needed, many airlines use air-to-ground communications to coordinate with in-house or contracted medical services. Airlines with their own medical departments frequently take emergency calls from their aircraft or have a designated emergency call routing system. In some cases, diversion to the nearest airport is required; the senior pilot makes this decision. Cardiac complaints are the primary cause for flight diversions, but second in number are neurologic complaints (dizziness, seizure, severe headaches, etc), which are the most common in-flight medical issues.

FAA regulations (14CFR121.803 Appendix A) now require enhanced medical kits onboard commercial aircraft. Required elements include a blood pressure kit, stethoscope, airways, syringes, needles, 50% dextrose, epinephrine 1:1000, diphenhydramine injectable, nitroglycerin tablets, and instructions for use of the kit components. The International Civil Aviation Organization (ICAO) regulations have similar requirements. When a physician is called upon to assist, he/she is covered by Good Samaritan immunity, part of the 1998 Aviation Medical Assistance Act. Internationally, most countries follow this example.

- Flight is not contraindicated for numerous medical conditions, but patients traveling without a medical escort team should seek preflight evaluation and counseling from their physicians.
- Some airlines require a medical certificate from the health care provider stating that the passenger is currently stable or noninfectious and fit for air travel.
- Aeromedical transportation of patients with more serious medical conditions requires appropriate equipment, staffing, and coordination of logistical issues.
- The air in aircraft is completely exchanged every 3 to 4 minutes. All air is filtered via high-efficiency particulate air filters that capture particles the size of 0.3 micrometers or larger. The single most important

factor that significantly improved cabin air quality was the introduction of smoking bans on aircraft.

- During cases of in-flight medical emergencies, many airlines use air-to-ground communications to coordinate with in-house or contracted medical services. If a physician passenger is called upon to assist, his or her actions are covered legally by Good Samaritan immunity.

Medical Standards, Clinical Aviation, and Civil Aviation

Civil Aviation Regulations

The Civil Aviation Agency (precursor to the FAA) was created in 1925 through the Air Commerce Act. In 1944, the International Civil Aviation Conference met in Chicago and agreed upon the Convention on International Civil Aviation, known as the Chicago Convention. Reaffirming the principle of national sovereignty in airspace, it laid the groundwork for a global organization for civil aviation and created machinery to ensure uniform standards and practices for flight safety and operations. The ICAO, part of the United Nations, was the result of this convention. Its goal is to promote the safe, orderly, and efficient growth of international civil aviation. In 1958, the FAA replaced the Civil Aviation Agency under the Department of Transportation.

The Federal Air Surgeon heads the Office of Aerospace Medicine. This office is the principal FAA staff element overseeing physical fitness of airmen and other persons associated with safety in flight, medical certification, the designated Aviation Medical Examiner system, occupational health programs, aviation medical research, medical factors in civil accident investigation, aeromedical education, and biostatistical data for use in human factors evaluations.

International Civil Aviation

More than half of air traffic is international. Air routes are the highways for world commerce and have brought with them international challenges from coordination of techniques and laws to dissemination of technical and economic information. Safety through consistency requires standardized airport construction, navigational aids, and weather-reporting systems. Errors caused by misunderstanding or inexperience could be catastrophic, underlining the importance of standardization of operational practices. ICAO, the principle non-US aviation oversight organization, is based in Montreal and is the primary international agency outside the FAA addressing these issues. ICAO studies problems, applies new technology, and provides technical assistance through the United Nations development program. ICAO's aviation medicine section maintains current and valid specifications of a medical nature within ICAO regulations and guidance. ICAO's standards are the minimum standards required of contracting states, unless the states elect not to comply, in which case ICAO publishes the differences, with possible negative impacts on the noncompliant states (eg, restrictions on flights to and from those states).

Civil Aviation Operations

Commercial air carriers (airlines) in the United States have crews including pilots, first officers, flight engineers, and flight attendants. The first 3 groups require **FAA certification** to fly legally. Part of this certification is medical, and airline transport pilot certification requires a first-class medical certificate, the most stringent under FAA rules. The flight engineer and first officer require second-class medical certificates. Mandatory retirement for airline transport pilots is now age 65.

Pilots (other than those above) being paid to fly and not flying more than 9 passengers in turbine-powered aircraft require a commercial pilot certificate and second-class medical certificate. Included here are air taxi and air commuter operations, corporate pilots, and utility aircraft operators. There is no upper age limit for these pilots. Private pilots, not flying for pay, require at least a third-class FAA medical certificate, and there is no upper age limit.

Sport pilot certification is a relatively new designation by the FAA; this is needed to operate low-speed aircraft. The sport pilot certificate does not entail a medical examination; rather, a valid US driver's license is a surrogate for medical safety and eligibility to fly. Some aircraft, such as ultralights, do not require pilots to be certified. For US glider and balloon operations, only a self-proclamation of health status is necessary.

Flight attendants do not require FAA medical certification. Occupational exposures include cabin air, nutrition, circadian rhythm shifts with travel, temperature fluctuation, infectious disease exposure, exposure to violence, and humidity. The upper limit for age is 70 years, and they can fly with well-controlled diabetes mellitus and with a history of epilepsy, if controlled by medication. Periodic examinations are determined by individual airlines.

There are over 25,000 air traffic controllers in the United States. Their primary jobs are to maintain safe separation of aircraft on airfields and within larger, geographically defined zones and to expedite efficient and safe aircraft movement in flight and on the ground. The FAA oversees their certification, and they require regular medical examinations to maintain their certification, similar to pilots. Conditions affecting controllers include shift work and fatigue, variable stress levels, and ergonomic issues.

Aircraft Certification

FAA requires design, performance, and operational safety information from the manufacturer to certify aircraft for use.

Categories of airworthiness include fixed-wing airline aircraft and general aviation. In the United States, the FAA monitors airworthiness via certification programs, postproduction inspections, and publication of airworthiness directives. There is a complex body of regulations regarding civil aircraft certification. Internationally, ICAO performs a similar function in conjunction with various national and international organizations.

Civil Aviation Medicine

The purpose of civil aviation medicine is to provide aeromedical support to civil aviation, including those flying in airlines, air taxis, private and business aircraft, and utility operations (cropdusters, law enforcement, etc). Air traffic controllers also fall under the purview of aeromedical specialists. The scope of operations has been expanding rapidly during the past 20 years, starting with classic civilian aviation operations and now encompassing civilian spaceflight.

Medical Standards

In licensing pilots and crews to fly, licensing agencies (FAA, ICAO, European Civilian Aviation Conference [with its affiliated training organization, Joint Aviation Authorities Training Organization], military aeromedical bodies, etc) have developed standards for physical and mental health, usually on the basis of primary flying duty (pilot vs engineer) and level of responsibility (commercial passenger carrying jet vs private aircraft, fighter aircraft vs transport). Additionally, most agencies have implemented regular medical surveillance and examination schedules to periodically monitor aviator health.

Preexisting health conditions may disqualify candidates, and acquired conditions may disqualify previously trained flyers. Variation exists among agencies on considerations and conditions for waivers for these medical issues. In all cases, flying is considered a privilege instead of a right, and aeromedical examiners assume the responsibility of assuring not only pilot safety, but public safety in evaluating and providing this specialized, occupational health care. Most agencies require specific training and experience for physicians involved in assessing aviator health as part of the licensing and renewal processes. In the military context, these specialists are termed flight surgeons. The FAA designates aviation medical examiners only after they have had specific training and proven appropriate logistical capabilities.

Waivers and Special Issuances

Pilots who do not meet all of the medical requirements may still be able to fly, although technically "disqualified." The terms "waiver" and "special issuance" are used interchangeably here, although the former is usually a military term and the FAA uses the latter. Three primary options exist:

1) **Waiver or special issuance route (FAA)**: the pilot may apply for permission to resume flying after a medical condition has been addressed sufficiently to convince the FAA that the pilot no longer represents a potential hazard to him or herself or to the public. A pilot with coronary artery disease, for instance, may be allowed to return to flying after it is shown that his condition is treated (revascularization, medications) and stable and that all risk factors (eg, hypertension, hyperlipidemia, diabetes mellitus, etc) are mitigated and controlled with acceptable interventions. These waivers typically are time limited, and the pilot is expected to report changes in medical condition if they occur before his or her next flight physical examination. A **statement of demonstrated ability** is a special type of FAA waiver. It may be obtained for a fixed deficit not expected to change (eg, loss of full motility of the knee, color blindness, hearing loss). After application and demonstration of satisfactory performance to an FAA inspector, a statement of demonstrated ability may be granted.
2) **Exception route**: the FAA decides on a specific case, as opposed to a category or disease; the condition is no longer a safety hazard, even though it is usually disqualifying. Regular follow-up is expected. In the US military, a nonmedical commander has the authority to override medical recommendations, given operational needs.
3) **Judicial route**: the National Transportation Safety Board or the courts may overturn an FAA denial on the basis of appeal information supplied by the pilot (plaintiff).

In all cases, pilots are expected to self-regulate (Federal Aviation Regulation 61.53); that is, they are expected to know the medical regulations and not fly if they develop conditions that might adversely affect flying safety. On the military side, aviators are also expected to self-report. Underreporting of medical conditions or medications is not unusual.

Disqualifying Conditions

The sine qua non of disqualifying medical conditions is their ability to suddenly incapacitate, subtly degrade performance, or distract from flying or controlling duties. Any exception or waiver consideration must show that the pilot or crewmember will be personally safe when flying, not have an impact on the safety of others when flying, and that there will be no impact on ability to perform flying duties properly so that the purpose of the flight is not affected.

There are **15 specific conditions that disqualify aviators** under FAA rules. These are history or diagnosis of

1) diabetes mellitus requiring hypoglycemic medication; 2) angina pectoris; 3) coronary heart disease that has been treated or, if untreated, that has been symptomatic or clinically significant; 4) myocardial infarction; 5) cardiac valve replacement; 6) permanent cardiac pacemaker; 7) heart replacement; 8) psychosis; 9) bipolar disorder; 10) personality disorder that is severe enough to have repeatedly manifested itself by overt acts; 11) substance dependence; 12) substance abuse; 13) epilepsy; 14) disturbance of consciousness and without satisfactory explanation of cause; and 15) transient loss of control of nervous system function(s) without satisfactory explanation of cause.

Over time, as aeromedical experience and science have evolved, the tendency has been to become more liberal on allowing aviators to fly with various medical conditions based on the demonstrated safety record. Some conditions are more highly scrutinized in all aeromedical services due to their potential for sudden incapacitation, severity, or unpredictability. Conditions of particular concern include cardiac, neurologic, neoplastic, and psychiatric diseases. Conditions affecting the special senses, particularly vision, are of special significance due to potential for affecting aircraft control.

Periodic Medical Assessment

Any aviator's encounter with an aerospace medicine specialist must produce an opinion on the aviator's health status as it relates to flying safety, health of the airman, and mission completion. Even healthy aviators develop illnesses or incur injuries, as would be expected in any adult population.

Periodic flight physical examinations vary in scope, depending on whether flyers are civilian or military, their age, their job (pilot vs flight engineer), the aircraft flown (high-speed jet vs crop duster vs helicopter), their nationality (FAA rules differ somewhat from ICAO rules and other international rules), and preexisting medical conditions. The basics usually include a history and physical examination, eye examination, dental examination, specific laboratory tests, and hearing examination. Specialty consults and further testing may be needed, as waivers or existing medical conditions dictate. Eye examinations typically include visual acuity, accommodation, depth perception, visual fields, color and night vision, and glaucoma screening.

Medical Disability

Most aviators develop illnesses or suffer injuries requiring temporary or permanent disqualification or waivers at some point in their careers. Permanent disqualifications create significant monetary losses by way of training resources invested in pilots (military and civilian). This is addressed by very strict entry criteria, followed by some degree of relaxation of standards after training. Medical waiver systems vary between civilian and military systems and from country to country. Many medical issues in trained aviators can be effectively treated or waived for return to flying duties. In the military, no formal process of appeal exists, should the airman not agree with the aerospace medicine specialist.

Self-Imposed Stressors

Self-medication is known to be one of the more common stressors that flyers add to the existing stressors of flying. Adverse effects of common, over-the-counter medications can affect flight safety. Pilots and crew are expected to self-monitor and report medication use, but underreporting is common, especially when flyers consult health care providers untrained in aerospace medical problems.

In fatal general aviation accidents, 10% to 30% of pilots had alcohol in the bloodstream. Even small amounts (20-77 mg/dL) can cause impairment. Hangovers produce headaches, impaired mentation, and fatigue. The rule of thumb is "8 hours bottle to throttle."

Public Health Concerns

The World Health Organization is responsible for regulating and monitoring conditions at international airports. Per regulations, all international and especially sanitary airports must have a bacteriological laboratory (or rapid access to such a facility), availability of yellow fever vaccination, dedicated medical staff, a quarantine facility, a 400-m zone around the boarding area that is free of vectors such as *Aedes aegypti* (the vector mosquito that causes yellow fever and dengue), and must be without rodents. Aircraft disinsection is performed by individual countries and agencies per World Health Organization international health regulations for passenger and cargo compartments.

- The goal of the International Civil Aviation Organization (ICAO) is to promote the safe, orderly, and efficient growth of international civil aviation. Safety is improved through standardization of operational practices. The World Health Organization is responsible for regulating and monitoring conditions at international airports.
- In the United States, the Office of Aerospace Medicine oversees physical fitness of airmen and other persons associated with safety in flight and medical certification. Pilots, first officers, flight engineers, and air traffic controllers require Federal Aviation Administration (FAA) certification to fly or work

legally. Flight attendants do not require FAA certification but undergo examinations on a schedule determined by individual airlines.

- FAA requires design, performance, and operational safety information from the manufacturers to certify aircraft for use. Internationally, ICAO performs a similar function in conjunction with various national and international organizations.
- Standards for physical and mental health usually are determined on the basis of primary flying duty and level of responsibility. Preexisting health conditions may disqualify candidates, and acquired conditions may disqualify previously trained flyers. Pilots who do not meet all of the medical requirements may still be able to fly, although technically "disqualified," if they receive a waiver or special issuance.
- The sine qua non of disqualifying medical conditions is their ability to suddenly incapacitate, subtly degrade performance, or distract from flying or controlling duties. Fifteen specific conditions disqualify aviators under FAA rules.
- Self-medication is one of the more common stressors that flyers add to the existing stressors of flying. Adverse effects of common, over-the-counter medications can affect flight safety.

Aircraft Accident Investigation

The primary purpose of aircraft mishap investigations is to prevent future accidents, injuries, and fatalities. For US civilian accidents, the responsible, independent, investigating agency is the National Transportation Safety Board, which defines aircraft accidents as ". . .an occurrence associated with the operation of an aircraft which takes place between the time any person boards the aircraft with the intention of flight and all such persons have disembarked, and in which any person suffers death or serious injury, or in which the aircraft receives substantial damage." Accident studies have shown a steady decline for years, and commercial flight is the safest form of transportation, behind scheduled buses. General aviation is least safe, and the accident rates are much higher than commercial aviation operations.

Accident Investigations

The National Transportation Safety Board, the ICAO, and other accident-investigating groups (eg, military) have multidisciplinary teams, including physicians, following standardized investigation guidelines. Aircraft accident investigations have 5 phases:

1) **Preliminary evaluation**: planning, preparation, resource use, and jurisdictional decisions are made here.

2) **Data collection**: critical and often time sensitive; includes eyewitness accounts, collection of preexisting records (eg, medical, maintenance), on-scene data collection, retrieval of voice and data recorders, autopsies and medical examinations.
3) **Data analysis**: may include aircraft reconstruction, computer simulations.
4) **Conclusion**: causal and contributory factors are detailed for the sequence of events.
5) **Recommendations**: to prevent future accidents.

There are 5 objectives in the medical investigation of aircraft accidents:

1) **Identification**: necessary for the notification of next of kin and establishment of a legal certificate of death.
2) **Reconstruction of crash circumstances**: careful data collection and analysis help reconstruct events leading to preventive measures and legal and political responses.
3) **Determination of medical issues that are causal or contributory to the event**: preexisting disease may help explain some of or all of the crash events.

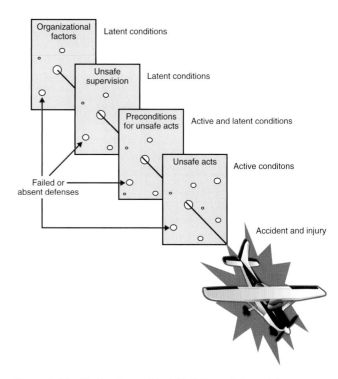

Figure 3 The "Swiss Cheese Model" of Error. (Adapted from Shappell SA, Wiegmann DA. The Human Factors Analysis and Classification System—HFACS. Washington [DC]: U.S. Department of Transportation. Federal Aviation Administration. 2000.)

4) **Analysis of structure and design in relation to injury and death**: assists planners and operators to prevent repeat incidents.

5) **Collection and preparation of data**: agencies compile statistics and train aircrew, accident investigators, and aviation medicine specialists.

Role of the Physician

The primary role of the physician in accident investigations is to prevent future accidents. Secondary or supporting roles of the flight surgeon and investigating physician include determining cause of injury and death, whether life support equipment functioned, and presence of physiologic or human factors. They also provide medical support to the team.

Systems Approach to Accident Investigations

Human factors combine the science and art of interfacing people and machines. There are human factor considerations in all phases of manned flight, from crew selection to flight. Human factors were causal in 40% to 60% of aircraft accidents. The Human Factors Analysis and Classification System (HFACS) uses a systematic approach to classify accidents (Figure 3). Based on Reason's taxonomy and expanded by Shappell and Wiegmann for use in investigations, HFACS constructs aid investigators in identifying potential preventive measures and provide industry and government with structured recommendations for improvement (Figure 4).

The HFACS construct uses 5 guiding principles:

1) Aviation is similar in nature to other complex productive systems.
2) Human errors are inevitable within such a system.
3) Blaming error on pilots is like blaming mechanical failure on the aircraft.
4) An accident, no matter how minor, is a failure of the system.
5) Accident investigation and error prevention go hand-in-hand.

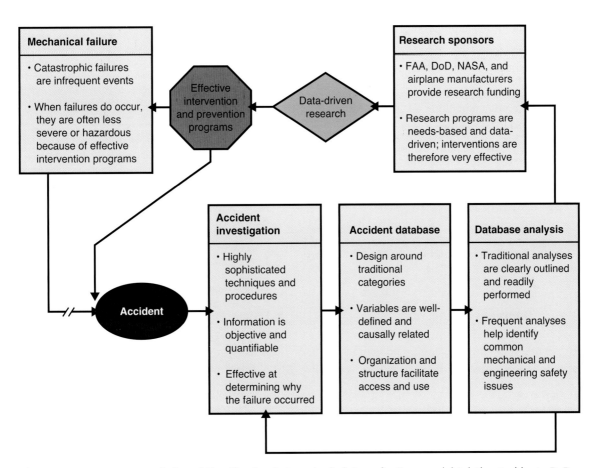

Figure 4 Human Factors Analysis and Classification System: Analysis Loop for Commercial Aviation Accidents. DoD denotes Department of Defense; FAA, Federal Aviation Administration; NASA, National Aeronautics Space Administration.

- The primary purpose of aircraft mishap investigations is to prevent future accidents, injuries, and fatalities. Accidents are investigated with multidisciplinary teams, including physicians, following standardized investigation guidelines.
- The National Transportation Safety Board conducts accident investigations of aircraft and other modes of transport in the United States.
- The flight surgeon and investigating physician determine cause of injury and death, whether life support equipment functioned, and presence of physiologic or human factors. They also provide medical support to the team.
- Human factors are causal in 40% to 60% of aircraft accidents. The Reason taxonomy of human error is often used as a foundation for the investigation.

SUGGESTED READING

Aerospace Medical Association Medical Guidelines Task Force. Medical guidelines for airline travel, 2nd ed. Aviat Space Environ Med. 2003 May;74(5 Suppl):A1-19.

Barratt MR, Pool SL. Principles of clinical medicine for space flight. New York: Springer. c2008.

Clement G. Fundamentals of space medicine. Space Technology Library. El Segundo (CA):Springer, Microcosm Press; c2005.

Davis JR, Johnson R, Stepanek J, Fogarty JA. Fundamentals of aerospace medicine. 4th ed. Philadelphia (PA): Wolters Kluwer Health/Lippincott Williams & Wilkins. c2008.

Previc FH, Ercoline WR. Spatial disorientation in aviation. Reston (VA): American Institute of Aeronautics and Astronautics, Inc. c2004.

Rainford DJ, Gradwell DP. Ernsting's aviation medicine. 4th ed. London: Hodder Arnold. c2006.

Rayman RB. Clinical aviation medicine. 4th ed. New York (NY): Professional Publishing Group. c2006.

Rayman RB, Zanick D, Korsgard T. Resources for inflight medical care. Aviat Space Environ Med. 2004 Mar;75(3): 278-80.

Shappell SA, Wiegmann DA. The Human Factors Analysis and Classification System—HFACS. Washington (DC): U.S. Department of Transportation. Federal Aviation Administration. 2000.

Questions and Answers

Questions

1. Which of the following is the only effective source of orientation information for a pilot?
   a. Semicircular canals
   b. Otolith organs
   c. Proprioceptors
   d. Vision
   e. Hearing

2. Commercial passenger airline aircraft cabins are normally pressurized to what maximum altitude in cruise flight?
   a. Mean sea level (MSL)
   b. 5,000 ft (1,500 m) above MSL
   c. 8,000 ft (2,400 m) above MSL
   d. 12,000 ft (3,700 m) above MSL
   e. 13,000 ft (4,000 m) above MSL

3. Human factors in aircraft accidents include such areas as physical disability, errors of judgment, crew coordination, and man-machine interface. Although sources and statistics vary, human factor elements appear to be responsible for what percentage of aircraft accidents?
   a. 0% to 20%
   b. 21% to 40%
   c. 41% to 60%
   d. 61% to 80%
   e. 81% to 90%

4. What specific organization or group is held responsible by federal law for determining the cause of all US civil aircraft accidents?
   a. The Department of Transportation
   b. The Aircraft Accident Investigation Branch of the Federal Aviation Administration
   c. National Transportation Safety Board
   d. The Department of Transportation–Federal Aviation Administration Conjoint Task Force on Aviation Accident Investigation
   e. The Safety Task Force for the US Department of Agriculture

5. Space motion sickness is a condition that affects what percentage of astronauts that travel into low-Earth orbit?
   a. 30%
   b. 50%
   c. 60%
   d. 70%
   e. 95%

6. Hypoxia can cause significant hyperventilation; subsequent hypocapnia will result in which of the following?
   a. Improved tissue oxygen delivery and cerebral vasoconstriction
   b. No effect on tissue oxygen delivery and cerebral vasodilatation
   c. Decrease in tissue oxygenation and cerebral vasoconstriction
   d. Decrease in tissue oxygenation and cerebral vasodilatation
   e. Improved tissue oxygen delivery and cerebral vasodilatation

7. The most serious threat to health on long-duration, exploration-class spaceflight missions is which of the following?
   a. Cardiovascular deconditioning
   b. Bone loss
   c. Radiation exposure
   d. Space motion sickness and neurovestibular problems
   e. Inability to absorb vital nutrients via the gastrointestinal tract due to microgravity-related change

8. An aviator is going to be exposed to an altitude of 42,000 ft (12,800 m). As the flight surgeon, which appropriate oxygen system should you recommend?
   a. High-flow oxygen at 50% fraction of inspired oxygen by rebreather mask
   b. Full-pressure suit
   c. 100% oxygen without positive-pressure breathing
   d. 100% oxygen with positive-pressure breathing
   e. 50% oxygen with positive-pressure breathing

9. Key tenets that encompass treatment of serious decompression sickness (severe and progressive neurologic signs) include which of the following?
   a. Immediate, high-dose, corticosteroid therapy, administered intravenously
   b. Hyperbaric oxygen therapy
   c. Calcium channel blockade
   d. High-flow, 100% oxygen therapy at sea-level pressure
   e. Intravenous perfluorocarbon emulsions combined with high-flow oxygen by closed face mask

10. Which of the following is an absolute contraindication to flight as a passenger?
    a. Upper respiratory infection
    b. Glaucoma
    c. Presence of an untreated pneumothorax
    d. Presence of a colostomy
    e. Uncomplicated pregnancy in the beginning of the second trimester

Answers

1. Answer d.

Vision is the primary source of information for the pilot because it not only relays the most reliable spatial information but also can be used to scan flight instruments that will provide accurate orienting information. Vestibular and kinesthetic signals, often provide inaccurate information in flight environments. Human hearing, while important for communication, does not allow for meaningful support in spatial orientation in the flight environment.

2. Answer c.

The stated maximum altitude for commercial airliners carrying passengers is 8,000 ft (2,400 m) above MSL (Federal Aviation Administration and International Civil Aviation Organization). Variations may occur based on aircraft systems and operational requirements.

3. Answer c.

Statistics do vary, but about 40% to 60% of aircraft accidents are due to human factors. Dhenin reports that in one study, 62 of 124 accidents (50%) were due to crew-human failures, and in another study, 42% were due to "pilot error." Rayman reports 55% of US Air Force accidents are due to personnel error.

4. Answer c.

The National Transportation Safety Board is a designated, independent US government organization dedicated to the investigation of accidents.

5. Answer d.

Space motion sickness affects 70% of astronauts. Most symptoms subside within 72 hours.

6. Answer d.

Hypocapnia causes significant cerebral vasoconstriction; by shifting of the oxygen-hemoglobin dissociation curve to the left, a decrease in tissue oxygenation results.

7. Answer c.

The most serious threat for long-duration space missions is the threat of radiation exposure, which can be markedly accentuated with solar flare activity. Shielding of the crew from radiation is one of the life-support functions that needs to be accomplished by the space vehicle.

8. Answer d.

At 39,000 ft (12,000 m), the mere breathing of 100% oxygen will not suffice to maintain adequate oxygenation, addition of positive-pressure breathing will be necessary.

9. Answer b.

Severe decompression illness should be promptly treated with hyperbaric oxygen. An environment of higher pressure and oxygen content allows for inert gas washout via the oxygen gradient and compression of any clinically significant vascular or extravascular bubble burden. Use of perfluorocarbon emulsions is not current clinical practice, although research into use of these oxygen-transport systems is ongoing.

10. Answer c.

There are few absolute contraindications to aeromedical transport of the ill or injured patient. Untreated pneumothorax, because of the potential gas expansion problems with flight to higher altitudes (Law of Boyle-Mariotte), can be deadly. The difficulty of monitoring breath sounds and impending respiratory compromise in a flight environment make this diagnosis a nearly 100% contraindication to flight. Pregnant women without pregnancy-related complications can travel by air without difficulty until the 36th week of gestation.

16

PUBLIC HEALTH PRACTICE, LEADERSHIP, AND HEALTH CARE LAW

Robin G. Molella, MD, MPH

One of the earliest definitions of public health as a discipline comes from the American public health leader, Charles-Edward A. Winslow. He defined public health as

> the science and art of preventing disease, prolonging life, and promoting physical health and efficiency through organized community efforts for the sanitation of the environment, the control of community infections, the education of the individual in principles of personal hygiene, the organization of medical and nursing service for the early diagnosis and preventive treatment of disease, and the development of the social machinery which will ensure every individual in the community a standard of living adequate for the maintenance of health.

This definition is still widely used today. A more concise definition of discipline has been coined by the Association of Schools of Public Health: "the strategic, organized, and interdisciplinary application of knowledge, skills, and competencies necessary to perform essential public health services and other activities to improve the population's health."

Regardless of the specific definition used, it is important to recognize that public health is focused on **health at the population level**. This does not mean that individuals are ignored; rather, the goal of improving the health of an entire population is bigger than focusing on an individual.

This broad focus allows public health officials to use strategies and tools that differ from those used by health care providers, who focus on individual patients. Even strategies that have only a small effect on an individual's health can have large effects when applied to a population.

Public Health as a Government Service

The core functions of public health were first outlined in the Institute of Medicine report, *The Future of Public Health*, and marked a significant change in the emphasis in public health. In this report, the focus on the direct provision of services was decreased and more efforts were directed toward establishing the processes, partnerships and practices necessary for maintaining public health. The core functions of assessment, policy development, and assurance encompass a number of essential public health activities, as detailed in Figure 1. These activities form the basis for standards of public health practice. System management, epidemiology, and biostatistics are central to most activities.

Although medicine and public health share many common goals, including preventing disease, prolonging life, and promoting physical health, public health is a government service. Like other public services (eg, law enforcement, fire protection, garbage collection), public health is not a service that individuals can provide for themselves; public health depends on community efforts

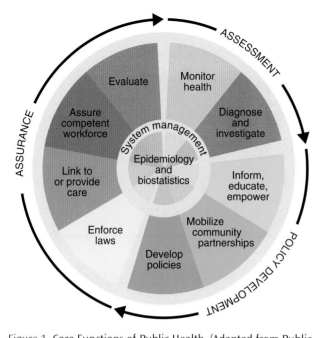

Figure 1 Core Functions of Public Health. (Adapted from Public health in America [Internet]. [cited 7 Oct 2009]. Available from http://www.health.gov/phfunctions/public.htm.)

and requires development of community resources. However, as a government service, public health programs and policies necessarily are subject to the political constraints of the day. Public health professionals answer to political leadership, and when that leadership changes, so do the priorities. These changes can affect funding levels and the capacity of public health activity.

- Public health focuses on the population level and uses strategies and tools that differ from those used to treat individuals.
- The core functions of public health are assessment, policy development, and assurance.
- Public health depends on community efforts and community resources. However, public health priorities may shift with changes in political leadership.

Determinants of Health and Health Disparities

The most widely accepted definition of health in the public health field is found in the preamble of the constitution of the World Health Organization: "Health is a state of complete physical, mental and social well-being and not merely the absence of disease or infirmity." This broad definition encompasses the objectives of public health programs. Its breadth acknowledges that the determinants of health are more than exposure to contagion or access to modern medicine; included are access to education, safe working environments, and safe and reliable sources of nutrition. Thus, a web of services and social constructs protect the health of communities (Figure 2).

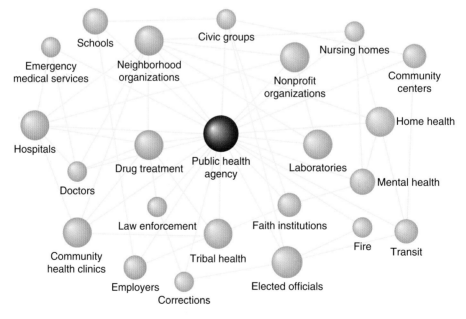

Figure 2 Web of Services and Social Constructs That Protect Public Health. (Adapted from Camden County Health and Human Services [Intranet]. Camden County Mobilizing for Action Through Planning and Partnership Coalition [MAPP] assessments and community health improvement plan. Camden [NJ]: Camden County Board of Freeholders; c2001. [cited 2009 Oct 21]. Available from http://www.camdencounty.com/health/healthserv/mapp.html. Used with permission.)

Population models of health determinants potentially can identify opportunities for intervention; they are used by public health officials when estimating the impact of a potential policy or program intervention on the overall health of a community (Figure 3). Although most experts agree about the determinants of health in principle, models of these determinants vary in numerous ways. For example, they may differ in how they define health, how they categorize factors affecting population health, and how they assume causal relationships between the factors affecting health.

Social determinants of health can create health disparities by contributing to or detracting from the health of individuals and communities. These factors include socioeconomic status, transportation, housing, access to services, discrimination by social grouping (eg, race, sex, or class), and social or environmental stressors. As an example, consider life expectancy in the United States (Figure 4). Although the data here are stratified by race and sex, other factors such as income, geographic location, and sexual orientation also can affect life expectancy. The social determinants of health have long been recognized by public health practitioners, who observed that improvements in living conditions and reductions of poverty could improve health status. However, these considerations were overshadowed during the 20th century by biomedical and behavioral approaches.

In 2000, for the first time in the history of the "Healthy People" initiative, the US government acknowledged the imperative of addressing health disparities. This approach recognized that most disparities were not caused by immutable factors such as genetics but were due to factors that could be changed to achieve health equity. Measuring and addressing health disparities became a national priority; this was a dramatic step in the direction of eliminating those disparities. The current understanding of health disparities acknowledges that without changes in social conditions, true health equity cannot be achieved.

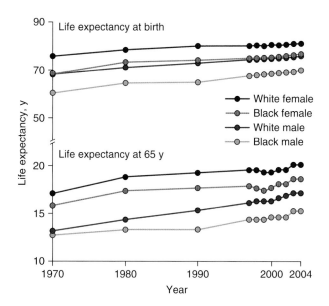

Figure 4 Life Expectancy at Birth and at 65 Years of Age, United States, 1970-2004. Data are stratified by race and sex. Life expectancies before 1997 are from decennial life tables that were based on census data and deaths for a 3-year period around the census year. Therefore, the middle year in each 3-year period is plotted in this figure. Beginning in 1997, the annual life tables are complete life tables based on a methodology similar to that used for decennial life tables. (Available from National Center for Health Statistics. Health, United States, 2007: with chartbook on trends in the health of Americans. Hyattsville [MD]: US Government Printing Office.)

- Determinants of health include access to education, safe working environments, and safe and reliable sources of nutrition.
- Social determinants of health can create health disparities by contributing to or detracting from the health of individuals and communities.
- The current understanding of health disparities acknowledges that without changes in social conditions, true health equity cannot be achieved.

Community Factors and Public Health

Community Assessment

Community assessment is a formal process of evaluating strengths and weaknesses in a community for the purpose of identifying opportunities to improve public health. When the assessment is done well, the information gathered can be used to accomplish the goals of community empowerment. This process may be initiated by public health officials or by other interested stakeholders. Identifying and engaging the major stakeholders during assessment is critical. In addition, community engagement creates a sense of

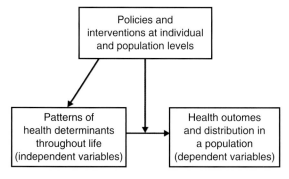

Figure 3 Impact of Policies on Public Health. (Adapted from Kindig D, Stoddart G. What is population health? Am J Public Health. 2003 Mar;93(3):380-3. Used with permission.)

ownership of the assessment results and provides the opportunity to address stakeholder interests.

A community-wide strategic planning process for health improvement, named Mobilizing for Action through Planning and Partnerships, was released in 2001 by the National Association of County and City Health Officials and by the Centers for Disease Control and Prevention (CDC). It is intended to guide system partners and community members through a process that includes assessment of 4 community factors (Figure 5). These factors are 1) community perceptions of strengths, assets, and needs; 2) forces of change in the community, eg, changes in legislation, funding shifts, or recent natural disasters; 3) community health status through the collection and analysis of health data; and 4) the performance and capabilities of the local public health system. The tool used for these assessments is from the National Public Health Performance Standards Program (NPHPSP).

In 1977, by the authority of the Stafford Amendment to the Health Services Extension Act (PL 95-83, Sec 341), the Department of Health, Education, and Welfare was instructed to develop model standards for preventive health services. Developing the standards of public health practice led to the creation of the NPHPSP. This collaborative effort to enhance the country's public health systems includes 7 national partners—among them are the American Public Health Association, the Association of State and Territorial Health Officials, and the CDC. The model standards are designed around the 10 essential public health services (Box 1) and focus on the overall public health system. They have been devised to improve the quality and accountability of public health practice. The NPHPSP model standards for developing policies and plans that support individual and statewide health efforts are depicted in Box 2.

Community Empowerment

Communities are a sociological construct consisting of interactions between individuals and of consequences that are based on violations of shared expectations, values, and beliefs. An important tool in public health is empowerment, the process of raising the critical consciousness of individuals or groups to make choices. Furthermore, it raises the capacity of these individuals or groups to transform choices into desired actions and outcomes. Central to this process are actions that build individual and collective assets and actions that improve the efficiency and fairness of the organizations and institutions that govern asset use. Community empowerment is about increasing the wealth, capacity, and resilience of the population as a whole. Although individuals may gain from this intervention, they are not intended as the primary beneficiary.

At its heart, empowerment aims to create sustainable change within the community. This is a much bigger and more difficult task than providing charitable sustenance. For example, aid in terms of food, medicine, and other supplies is a short-term emergency response. In contrast, empowerment aims for self-sufficiency, self-reliance, and sustainable increases in community resources through vocational training, health education, policy changes, and

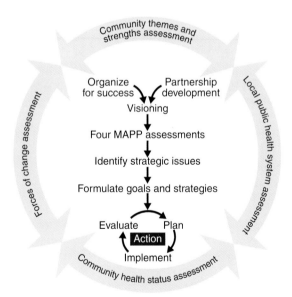

Figure 5   National Public Health Performance Standards Program Assessment Tool. MAPP denotes Mobilizing for Action through Planning and Partnerships. (Adapted from National Association of County & City Health Officials [Internet]. Mobilizing for action through planning and partnerships: a community approach to health improvement. Washington [DC]: NACCHO. [cited 7 Oct 2009]. Available from http://www.naccho. org/topics/infrastructure/mapp/upload/MAPPfactsheet-systempartners.pdf.)

Box 1 Essential Public Health Services

1. Monitor health status

2. Diagnose and investigate health problems

3. Inform, educate, and empower people

4. Mobilize communities to address health problems

5. Develop policies and plans

6. Enforce laws and regulations

7. Link people to needed health services

8. Assure a competent public health and personal care workforce

9. Evaluate health services

10. Conduct research for new innovations

Adapted from Centers for Disease Control and Prevention [Internet]. 10 Essential public health services. Atlanta (GA): CDC. [cited 2009 Oct 20]. Available from http://www.cdc.gov/od/ocphp/nphpsp/EssentialPHServices.htm.

Box 2 State Public Health System Model Standards for Developing Policies and Plans That Support Individual and Statewide Health Efforts

Planning and Implementation

The SPHS conducts comprehensive and strategic health improvement planning and policy development that integrates health status information, public input and communication, analysis of policy options, and recommendations for action based on the best evidence. Planning and policy development are conducted for public health programs, for organizations, and for the public health system, each with the purpose of improving public health performance and effectiveness.

To accomplish this, the SPHS:

- Develops statewide health improvement processes that include convening partners, facilitating collaborations, and gaining statewide participation in planning and implementation of needed improvements in the public health system.

- Produces a state health improvement plan(s) that outlines strategic directions for statewide improvements in health promotion, disease prevention, and response to emerging public health problems.

- Establishes and maintains public health emergency response capacity, plans, and protocols for all hazards, addressing 24/7 readiness, multi-agency coordination, emergency operations, and the special needs of vulnerable populations in an emergency.

- Engages in health policy development activities and takes necessary actions (including communication with advocacy groups and advocating to policy makers) to raise awareness of policies that affect the public's health.

State-Local Relationships

The SPHS works with local public health systems to provide assistance, capacity building, and resources for their efforts to develop local policies and plans that support individual and statewide health efforts.

To accomplish this, the SPHS:

- Provides technical assistance and training to local public health systems developing community health improvement plans.

- Supports development of community health improvement plans and provides assistance in adapting and integrating statewide improvement strategies to the local level.

- Provides assistance to local public health systems in the development of local all-hazard preparedness plans.

- Provides technical assistance and support for conducting local health policy development.

Performance Management and Quality Improvement

The SPHS reviews the effectiveness of its performance in policy and planning. SPHS members actively use the information from these reviews to continuously improve the quality of policy and planning activities in supporting individual and statewide health efforts.

To accomplish this, the SPHS:

- Regularly monitors the state's progress toward accomplishing its health improvement objectives.

- Reviews new and existing policies to determine their public health impact.

- Conducts exercises and drills to test preparedness response capacity outlined in the state's all-hazard preparedness plan.

- Manages the overall performance of its policy and planning activities for the purpose of quality improvement.

Public Health Capacity and Resources

The SPHS effectively invests in and uses its human, information, organizational, and financial resources to assure that its health planning and policy practices meet the needs of the state's population.

To accomplish this, the SPHS:

- Commits adequate financial resources to develop and implement health policies and plans.

- Aligns organizational relationships to focus statewide assets on health planning and policy development.

- Uses the skills of the SPHS workforce in long-range, operational, and strategic planning techniques.

- Uses the skills of the SPHS workforce in health policy development, including skills in policy analysis and in obtaining public participation in the policy-making process.

Abbreviation: SPHS, state public health system.
Adapted from National Public Health Performance Standards Program [Internet]. State public health system performance assessment: version 2.0. Model standards. US Department of Health and Human Services/Centers for Disease Control and Prevention. [cited 7 Oct 2009]. Available from http://www.cdc.gov/od/ocphp/nphpsp/documents/FINAL%20State%20MS.pdf.

other actions. The 7 key factors known to contribute to community empowerment are shown in the Table.

- Community assessment is a formal process of identifying opportunities to improve public health.
- "Mobilizing for Action through Planning and Partnerships" is a community-wide strategic planning process that guides system partners and community members through a community health improvement process.
- Model standards of public health practice have been developed by the US government in collaboration with other national health organizations. The overall goal is to improve the quality and accountability of public health practices.
- Community empowerment aims to create sustainable change (eg, self-sufficiency, self-reliance, and increased community resources) through vocational training, health education, policy changes, and other actions.

Public Health Law

Federal, State, and Local Responsibilities

Laws are a system of conduct that rely on the power of a government that establishes them and has the capability of enforcing them. Inherent in this system is the understanding that individuals transfer certain rights to the government for the purpose of maintaining order. Individuals willingly give up some of their rights because they gain more by having a government than they lose by surrendering their rights.

In the United States, individuals are governed and laws are established by 2 levels of government (federal and state). The powers of the federal government and those of the states are outlined in constitutions, which describe the general functions of government and allocate power to the different government branches. The US Constitution gives Congress the right to collect taxes to provide for the general welfare of the United States; this right is commonly known as the **welfare clause**. In combination with the right to regulate interstate and foreign commerce, the welfare clause provides the legal basis for establishing public health agencies (eg, the CDC, the Public Health Service) and for regulating and licensing biologically active products (eg, drugs, medical devices). When the US Congress or a state legislature enacts a law that creates an agency with ongoing responsibilities for regulatory oversight, these agencies have the full force of law if they act in accordance with a valid statute and if the agency's policies and rules were enacted directly by a legislative body. Administrative rules and regulations are issued at all levels of government (federal, state, and local). These regulations from agencies such as the Department of Health and Human Services, health care financing organizations, and state boards of health are myriad, complex, and likely to increase.

The US Constitution restricts the powers of the states in areas of national importance (eg, immigration, national taxation, interstate commerce, and maintaining an army). Notably, the tenth amendment to the US Constitution grants states extensive powers by specifically reserving all powers not expressly granted to the federal government and not expressly prohibited by the Constitution to the states. Much of what is litigated at the level of the US Supreme Court concerns conflict between state and individual rights

Table Factors That Contribute to Community Empowerment

Methods[a]	Primary Aim	Activities
Empowerment training and leadership development	Educate individuals about rights and opportunities; develop leadership	Training, conference, symposia
Media use by advocates to gain support	Influence public policy	Media events
Public education	Promote public and leader awareness	Speakers bureau, newsletters, community advisory board
Organizing partnerships	Enhance negotiating power, self reliance, resources, and facilities	Labor unions, associations, cooperatives, coalitions, mothers' clubs
Work or job training	Promote economic self-reliance and employable skills	Vocational training, income-generating projects; microenterprise
Enabling service and assistance	Provide relief and critical services	Medical, legal, or financial assistance; counseling and support groups; community outreach
Rights protection and social action or reform	Protect from abuse, promote rights to reform laws, policies, and programs	Lobbying; strikes, marches, and picketing; delegation to see government officials

[a] The acronym for these methods is EMPOWER.
Adapted from Kar SB, Pascual CA, Chickering KL. Empowerment of women for health promotion: a meta-analysis. Soc Sci Med. 1999 Dec;49(11):1431-60. Erratum in: Soc Sci Med 2000 Jun;50(11):1701. Used with permission.

or between state and federal law. The power and responsibility to protect the health of the citizens generally are state matters. State powers are limited by safeguards for due process, as described in the US Constitution. States may delegate power to counties or to local agencies.

The rights of sovereign governments to regulate private interests for public good are termed police powers. In this regard, public health powers may be classified into 2 broad categories: 1) regulation of persons to prevent transmission of communicable disease and 2) regulation of professions and businesses. The ability of a superior government to block more stringent regulation by a lower level of government in a particular area is termed preemption. Preemption is an important aspect of balancing federal and state authority, and it is a means of maintaining some legal uniformity across states. Preemption also prevents local authorities from enacting more stringent regulations than the state. The strategy of inserting preemption clauses into state legislation is a way for special-interest groups to combat stringent local regulation. Such preemption practices often reduce public protection. Preemption prevents local governments from meeting the needs of the community and decreases debate at the local level, which usually is a key factor in increasing awareness of a public health threat.

Coercive Measures

Coercive measures of disease control are the most extreme measures in public health practice. The courts have upheld the right of public health agencies to exert these powers, but they repeatedly hold that such powers are not without limitation and that due process must be provided. Often, public health officials must meet the standard of providing proof of an actual danger to the community before coercive measures are allowed.

Quarantine and isolation orders may be given when necessary to protect the public health, but affected individuals are protected by due process. These safeguards include the right to a hearing, the right to counsel, and the right to an appeal. Specific statutes allow incarceration of individuals who refuse treatment for a disease or are not compliant with treatment when such behaviors pose a serious public health threat (eg, tuberculosis). Another coercive measure is forced treatment (eg, mandatory, directly observed therapy).

Mandatory vaccination has been upheld constitutionally by the Supreme Court since the 1905 case of *Jacobson v Massachusetts*. That case held that states could have compulsory vaccination laws but could not enact them in an arbitrary or unreasonable manner. Many state laws permit exemptions for religious reasons, and some states also allow a conscientious objection exemption.

Because of the nature of the US legal system, many of the current compulsory public health measures may be outdated or of limited value because they were enacted in the context of specific threats. Consequently, they may not be as meaningful in the present environment of threats from bioterrorism, natural disasters, and pandemic illness. Recognizing the need to clarify and revise state statutes pertaining to serious public health emergencies, the Center for Law and the Public's Health was established by the CDC, Georgetown University, and Johns Hopkins University to draft model legislation. This draft legislation, the Model State Emergency Health Powers Act, provides states with strong powers to act in the event of a serious public health threat. Many states and other jurisdictions have passed bills or resolutions that include provisions from or similar to those in the Act.

Public Health Licensure

The power to regulate businesses and professions ensures that these individuals and entities act in reasonably safe ways. Licensure, established by the legislature, authorizes an agency such as a board of health, board of regents, or a special professional or occupational board to create rules relating to the activities of the professional or entity. Public health licensure is used to regulate 3 general areas: 1) professionals in public health or health care; 2) health care institutions; and 3) businesses that affect public health (eg, milk or food production, waste management, water treatment). One extension of the power of licensure is the ability to mandate medical examinations such as routine examinations for commercial drivers and airline pilots, for immigrants, before marriage, or for health care employees in some states. At the federal level, the legal authority usually is derived from the interstate commerce clause.

Licensure has 2 major drawbacks: it can be used to restrict entry into a profession, and it provides licensees with a monopoly on services. However, once granted, a license cannot be revoked without due process.

Regulation of Property, Searches, and Inspections

Public health has the power to regulate the use of private property in a number of ways. One such power is the right to manage and abate public nuisances, defined as a condition that prevents the public from safely performing normal activities of daily living. Such nuisances include toxic chemicals in a homegrown methamphetamine laboratory or conditions that bring rodents or insects or create foul stenches. Abatement involves invasion of private property, but without clear justification, it may be considered seizure of private property without due process, a violation of the fourth amendment of the US Constitution. Many of these actions are carried out with guidance from local statutes.

Searches and inspections are the final tool used to regulate professions and businesses. Legally, these inspections are considered a type of search; as such, they must be conducted with constitutional safeguards. Thus, when an inspection is not permitted voluntarily, a warrant must be obtained. An exception to the warrant requirement is for businesses that are so commonly regulated that no expectation of privacy exists. For example, restaurants undergo regular food safety inspections and fire inspections without requirement of a warrant.

Data Collection, Data Access, and Research

One of the most well-known public health powers is that of data collection (see Chapter 3). Public health surveillance systems are established through state powers. Community surveillance and the subsequent investigation of disease outbreaks are essential components of the public health mission. Central to this practice are the collection of vital statistics (including birth and death rates), causes of death and injury, and rates of reportable infectious diseases. For many years, such surveillance systems were invisible to the general public, but with the globalization of the food supply, the ease and rapidity of travel, and the threat of bioterrorism, the general public has become more aware of these systems in the control of infectious and noninfectious illness.

Data gathered by these surveillance systems generally are available to the public. The federal **Freedom of Information Act** requires all documents in the hands of federal employees, on federal premises, or within the control of federal employees to be made available to the public unless they are specifically exempted. Nondisclosable reports include personnel and medical records, trade secret and commercial or financial information, and interagency and intra-agency communications. Information can be exempt from disclosure by statute, which allows federal agencies to protect confidentiality during the conduct of a federally authorized investigation. State and federal privacy laws also help determine what information will be stored and released. These provide protection for name-identified records that contain medical or other confidential information, but additional protections allow name-identified individuals to access that information. These protections are delineated in the federal Privacy Act (5 USC Sec 552a).

Many essential public health functions cannot be carried out in a timely fashion if relevant research efforts are held to the same standard as traditional biomedical research. Conduct of biomedical research is governed by strict rules, and research projects typically require approval by institutional review boards and must adhere to other practices such as informed consent. It is generally accepted that if disease surveillance data are collected by a public health agency with the intent of providing care to the community, rather than advancing scientific knowledge in general, then the authority for participant protection derives from public health codes, not from research regulations. Statutes determine which information must be reported and recorded, and penalties may be assessed for failing to comply with statutes. Similarly, the ability to conduct investigations and take actions for disease control is based on statutes created under the power of a state health authority. These allow epidemiologic activities such as contact tracing and outbreak investigation. Cooperation with investigations can be compelled with due process.

- In the United States, the welfare clause provides the legal basis for Congress to establish federal public health agencies. However, the power and responsibility to protect the health of the citizens generally are state matters.
- Coercive measures of disease control (eg, quarantine, incarceration, forced treatment) can be used by public health agencies if they provide proof of danger to the community without such measures. Compulsory vaccination programs are supported constitutionally, but many states allow exemptions.
- Licensure authorizes an agency to create rules that regulate the activities of the professional or entity. Through this power, medical examinations can be mandated.
- Public health agencies have the power to manage and abate public nuisances and to search and inspect businesses. Usually, a warrant must be obtained when an inspection is not permitted voluntarily.
- Disease surveillance data, collected by a public health agency for the purpose of providing care to the community, does not require institutional review board approval or informed participant consent.
- The Freedom of Information Act requires virtually all federal documents to be made available to the public unless they are specifically exempted.

Public Health Ethics

The ethical principles underlying public health and medicine have common roots. The earliest ethical principles are that of **nonmaleficence** (do no harm) and **beneficence** (help the patient); these date back to Hippocrates and focus primarily on the relationship between an individual provider and a patient. These principles have been extended to public health research and practice and now also include the principle of **autonomy** (the patient's right to make informed health decisions and be a partner in the decision-making process), which became a common bioethical expectation in the 1960s.

Most physicians can disregard population health needs and focus entirely on what is best for their patients. However, because public health organizations are charged with maintaining and improving the health of populations, they cannot avoid these ethical dilemmas. Public health officials must consider the ethics of serving the needs of the population over the needs of the individual, allocating limited resources, and answering questions of equity. For example, consider the preparations for epidemic influenza. When a vaccine is first available, it will be in limited quantity. How should immunizations be prioritized? Should health care workers, firefighters, and police personnel be immunized so that the safety of the community and the needs of individuals are protected? Or should those with greatest risk of death be immunized first? For most ethical challenges, no single answer is absolutely correct; simply, the best answer is selected on the basis of shared values and the facts as they are known at the time.

Two concepts that must be reviewed in a discussion of ethics are nihilism and relativism. In **nihilism**, morality is considered an illusion; stated differently, morality reflects the self-interests of those in power (termed conventional morality). The nihilist chooses not to engage in discussions of morality because of the influence that those in power have on the mores of the day, yet conventional morality can only be modified or checked by others who rigorously compare it with higher ideals and basic principles. In **relativism**, morality is based on culture; no single path is always right, and the path chosen is consistent with the prevailing culture. On the surface, relative morality seems superior to absolute morality because it explains differences in the morality of diverse cultures. However, it also can lead to acceptance of acts, beliefs, and behaviors that generally are considered unethical. For example, Nazis believed they were morally superior and used this belief to justify genocide. If one accepts that a belief in a moral position makes that position morally correct, then no behavior, practice, or policy can ever be condemned as immoral.

Legal Aspects

Public health ethicists use factual information and widely accepted ethical principles to inform policy making and programmatic intervention such that the health of the population is improved. Importantly, health laws both inform our ethical decision making and are informed by it. For example, ethical regulations on research can be codified into law; thus, the society's consensus about a moral issue determines the limits of permissible research.

One of the most common challenges of public health interventions is controversy over interfering with individual freedoms to improve the common good. However, some limits on individual rights are expected and necessary to preserve safety (eg, driving conventions such as speed limits). A strategy to protect fetuses from neural tube defects balanced personal rights (the right to consume nonfortified foods) against the need to protect the population (neural tube defects can be devastating for the individual and costly and problematic for society) and resulted in a new statute that required fortification of cereal products with folic acid. Other conflicts in public health between individual and community rights include recent legislation about clean air and protection from the harmful effects of secondhand smoke.

Epidemiology and Other Research

Although much of public health research is fundamentally observational and unlikely to cause harm, ethical dilemmas still are faced in a number of areas during the course of public health functions. Medical ethics in research underwent great scrutiny at the end of World War II as the abuses of concentration camp prisoners by Dr Josef Mengele came to light. But ethical abuses historically are not limited to Nazi war criminals.

In 1972, information emerged about a long-term syphilis research program that was being conducted by the US Public Health Service. This study began in 1932 and enrolled 400 black men from the Tuskegee area in Macon County, Alabama, a county in which 40% of the population were infected with the disease. The intent of the study was to observe the natural course of syphilis without treatment. At the inception of the study, some evidence suggested that the available therapy was worse than the disease itself, but by the 1940s, penicillin had become the first-line treatment for syphilis. However, none of the men were offered treatment until 1972. Furthermore, investigators did not explain the objective of the study to participants, nor were participants given the opportunity to provide informed consent. Although informed consent is now held as a paramount ethical principle, it was not always considered essential in the era of paternalistic health care.

The outcry in the aftermath of the Tuskegee study led directly to the establishment of rules of conduct for human experimentation. Today, every subject must be informed of the intent of the research, the risks of participation, and the benefits of participation (if any). Research subjects must consent to participate without any coercion. Additionally, research protocols must be reviewed by an institutional review board, which will confirm that the study plans are ethical. The board must include community members and scientists. Mechanisms must be in place to review intermediate outcomes so that a study may be stopped if participation appears to cause significant harm. All institutions that receive federal funds must follow these rules. (Further details of conducting studies are described in Chapter 3).

Religious and Secular Ethics Frameworks

The major world religions all include ethical tenets as part of their teachings, and many individuals receive moral education through their religious studies. Thus, many individuals connect moral decision making with religion. However, a secular ethical framework is possible, and religion is not a prerequisite for ethical decision making.

Managing Limited Resources

One of the most daunting challenges of public health is the distribution of limited resources. Within the US health care system, these distribution questions often are avoided by using the ability to pay as a means of rationing access to services. Allocation questions in public health likely will continue, and as these may require redistribution of wealth or allocation decisions based on criteria other than wealth, these choices are expected to be controversial.

Expert Consensus

Sometimes, the necessary facts are uncertain, unclear, or unreliable. Epidemiologic studies do not prove causal relationships, and studies to clarify factual data may not be possible because of financial, ethical, or time constraints. When the facts are uncertain but a consensus of experts exists, public health activities may proceed, although perhaps not with full force. For example, with data on secondhand smoke leading to a clear expert consensus, public health organizations have recommended restriction of smoking in public places. In another example, an approved vaccine with proven protective activity may, in a cost-benefit analysis, show uncertain benefits if provided through a community-wide vaccination program. Although evidence of a clear economic benefit is lacking, the consequence of the disease might be serious enough that a public health organization would encourage vaccination but not require it for school entrance.

- The ethical principles of nonmaleficence and beneficence are the same for public health and medicine. Ethics in public health also consider the needs of the population and how that may interfere with individual freedoms.
- Ethical regulations on research can be codified into law, thereby allowing society's consensus about a moral issue to determine the limits of permissible research.
- Although many connect moral decision making with religion, a secular ethical framework is possible and religion is not a prerequisite for ethical decision making.
- The distribution of limited public health resources raises questions about rationing access to services. Appropriate allocation may require redistribution of wealth or other controversial choices.
- When studies are limited by financial, ethical, or time constraints, public health activities may proceed by using a consensus of expert opinions as its foundation.

Leadership and Management

Effectiveness in public health requires good leadership and management. It is useful to consider leadership and management as 2 different but related skill sets, and although some debate exists about which is more important to an organization, truly both are essential and in fact are complementary. Managers focus on accomplishing specific tasks, problem solving, allocation of resources (eg, money, time, materials, and equipment), and record keeping. Supervisory management roles require an ability to establish expectations, give feedback, and manage poor performance. In contrast, what skills should an effective leader have? Leaders influence people; thus, leadership skills must be based on vision, inspiration, and persuasion. An effective leader is typically well-versed in managing power and influencing individuals through inspiration, coaching, counseling, delegating, mentoring, and goal setting. Leaders carry out their roles in a wide range of styles: autocratic, democratic, participatory, and laissez-faire (ie, hands off), to name just a few. Often, leadership style depends on the situation, including the life cycle of the organization.

Many of the skills needed for group leadership are part of the day-to-day practice of public health, including group facilitation and decision making, meeting management and facilitation, group dynamics, and systems thinking. Some of the key skills needed for successful public health leadership include working with groups, effective communication, financial management, and decision analysis.

Working With Groups

To gather the broadest support from stakeholders, public health officials need to work with groups. Perhaps one of the most well-known group-process techniques is **brainstorming**. In this method, used to generate a large number of ideas in a short time, individuals are asked to offer suggestions for solving the question at hand. **The nominal group technique**, developed by Delbecq and Van de Ven, asks individuals to work in groups of less than 10. They brainstorm individually and write down solutions to the problem. Suggestions are shared among members, with each participant offering one suggestion at a time. No criticism is allowed in this process, although questions and clarifications are encouraged. The individuals then rate and vote on the ideas, votes are tabulated, the subgroups report to the whole group, and further ratings and decisions on the top choices can be made.

Another group technique that is useful for managers and leaders is the **Delphi method**, used when attempting to obtain a consensus from a panel of independent experts. In this systematic, interactive forecasting method, carefully selected experts answer questionnaires in 2 or more rounds. After each round, a facilitator provides an anonymous summary of the experts' forecasts from the previous round and the reasons provided for their judgments. Participants are encouraged to revise earlier answers after reviewing the replies of other group members. During this process, the range of the answers should decrease, and the group should converge toward the best (or "correct") answer. Finally, the process is halted after reaching a predefined stopping criterion (eg, number of rounds, achievement of consensus, stability of results), and the mean or median scores of the final rounds are used to determine the results.

- Strong leadership and management skills are necessary for day-to-day practice of public health. Often, leadership style depends on the situation, including the life cycle of the organization.
- To gather the broadest support from stakeholders, public health officials often need to work with groups to solve problems and develop a consensus of expert opinions.

Effective Communication

A key skill in public health is effective communication. For public health officials to advance an agenda that improves health in a population or community, they must be able to describe why that agenda is appropriate and valuable. They must be able to handle controversies that arise as the agenda is advanced, and they must know when to retreat if an agenda is so controversial that it endangers other programs. An example of such a communication challenge occurred in Minnesota when a statewide vaccination registry was being considered. The proposed registry would have notified parents and providers when immunizations were needed. State legislation was required to establish the registry, but when the proposal was brought forward, questions were raised about informed consent and privacy. The magnitude of concern was so great that the practices of existing registries also were questioned. Ultimately, rather than risk affecting the existing programs, the proposed legislation was withdrawn from consideration. Currently, Minnesota has only local immunization registries that are developing ways to work together.

Public health officials interested in a particular agenda will often look for opportunities to systematically present their case over time. Termed **agenda building**, this strategy is used to increase awareness of an important public health issue. Sometimes, greater attention is achieved with the help of a celebrity spokesperson or if the agenda is presented in conjunction with a notable, relevant event. For example, if the agenda concerns new food safety legislation, the media may be uninterested until an outbreak of foodborne illness occurs. When the spotlight is on, politicians may feel more pressure to act.

Agenda building is separate from a related media activity, agenda setting. In **agenda setting**, the media often creates ideas and expectations through their reporting, and the 24-hour news cycle magnifies this effect. For example, studies have shown that the extent to which the media

covers certain events greatly influences the public perception of the severity of a given problem, although the actual severity often is unrelated to the perceived severity. It helps to recognize that mainstream media outlets are for-profit ventures with incomes that are based on circulation and viewership. Thus, the media benefits from a reporting format that describes extreme positions, not centrist views. Simply stated, controversy sells—but this is in direct conflict with the public health mission of collaborating and creating consensus.

Nevertheless, public health efforts depend on the media to inform and educate the public and policy makers. One specific form of public health communication is risk communication (see Chapter 13). **Risk communication** is intended to inform and has the goal of affecting behavior. Simple risk communication messages include the importance of physical activity and sensible eating habits for good health or hand washing as a disease-prevention strategy. Other risk-communication strategies are used to communicate imminent threats to safety. In all instances, messages need to be carefully crafted, with clear action steps that remedy the risk. For imminent-threat communications, public health officials must honestly describe what is and is not known.

Maintaining public trust is essential. The media may attempt to get the most dramatic sound bite or quote and will often try to lead an interviewee to speculate or make a comment that, when quoted out of context, is misleading or even inflammatory. Early communication can effectively quell panic. Effective public health officials use communication and the media with skill to assure that the public remains informed and engaged in the public health agenda.

- Agenda building is the systematic presentation of an important public health issue over time to increase awareness.
- Agenda setting is the creation of ideas and expectations through media reporting.
- Risk communication is intended to inform and has the goal of affecting behavior. These can be disease-prevention messages or warnings pertaining to imminent threats.

Financial Management and Decision Analysis

Financial stewardship is an essential part of public health leadership. The more financially savvy a public health professional, the better that person can guide policy making and programming to apply available funds where they may do the most good.

Public health is funded at the federal level by tax dollars. However, because the federal government is not constitutionally charged with public health oversight, it uses funding to influence public health policy. It can either withhold funding (eg, the 1984 National Minimum Drinking

Age Act prohibited alcohol sales or possession to persons younger than 21 years as a condition of receiving state highway funds) or offer grants and other funds to those who provide local services or programming (eg, the Women, Infants, and Children program is federally funded but locally administered).

State budgets for public health also are funded largely from tax dollars, although state departments of health frequently receive federal funds to support programs. Some federal funds allocated to states are intended to be passed through or awarded to local agencies. In addition, states may collect fees for licenses and other services that are performed by an agency and its subsidiaries. At the local public health agency level, budgets are extraordinarily complex in terms of revenue sources and expenses. Local tax dollars usually provide only part of the revenue needed to operate. Fees and contracts cover a very small portion of services. The remaining operating budget comes from grants and pass-through funding (ie, federal funds that are administered locally).

Because public health leaders must be good stewards of limited resources, it is essential that they understand basic economic concepts to evaluate programs and policies. A leader must be able to interpret data and determine which programs and policies should be funded. For example, if 2 programs are known to have the same outcomes or benefits, a simple cost analysis, termed a **cost-minimization** study, could be performed. This is analogous to "comparison shopping." However, implicit in such a study is the assumption that the 2 products or outcomes are exactly the same, and this is rarely the case.

If similar outcomes are being compared (eg, years of life gained or cases correctly identified), a **cost-effectiveness** analysis can be performed. In cost-effectiveness analysis, costs are calculated in dollars and outcomes are calculated in the most natural and meaningful units. Cost-effectiveness studies excel at identifying the best option for achieving a specific goal. For example, 2 strategies have the goal of decreasing teen pregnancy rates—strategy A provides free condoms in high schools and strategy B provides abstinence education. Which strategy decreases teen pregnancy in the most cost-effective manner? The direct, indirect, and intangible costs must be calculated and the outcomes measured. The cost per pregnancy prevented could then be determined.

Consider that costs and benefits are always relative to the perspective. Premature death is not a cost to a health insurer, which now has one fewer individual requesting benefits, but it is a cost to society. Thus, a comprehensive, societal perspective is critical in an economic analysis because the value of an outcome (eg, lives lost and saved) is appraised more completely. Another common perspective is that of the insurer, which bears the brunt of direct costs. As long as the perspective is clearly stated, the analysis is valid, although not perhaps as relevant to the public health questions being raised.

Often, public health agencies have to choose between 2 unrelated options (eg, childhood vaccinations vs a program to improve air quality); in such circumstances, it can be difficult to make a choice. If a value can be placed on the quality of years of life saved or improved, programs that do not have a common natural unit of outcome can be compared with a **cost-utility analysis**. This analysis is broader than a cost-effectiveness analysis. Cost-utility analysis may evaluate outcomes in terms of costs per quality-adjusted life year. It should be performed when quality of life is one of the most important outcomes, when reductions in morbidity and mortality are being examined, or when programs have numerous, differing outcomes and a common unit of comparison is needed. This strategy is not useful if the process of determining outcomes for comparison is itself not cost effective.

Cost-benefit analysis uses currency values to measure costs and benefits. That is, a natural outcome such as deaths prevented or blood pressure lowered by 1 mm Hg must be assigned a monetary value. Although cost-benefit analysis theoretically is the broadest analytic tool, assigning monetary values to outcomes makes the analysis very difficult to conduct. For example, consider a strategy that reduces morbidity and allows individuals to work longer than they might without treatment. How much are those preserved work years valued? Does it matter in the analysis if these workers receive high or low pay? What is the dollar value of self-esteem gained by earning a living instead of relying on charity? Obviously, many benefits are not easily assigned a monetary value; thus, economists tend to prefer cost-utility analysis over cost-benefit analysis.

Markov models can be used to examine related, random events over time and model the costs and outcomes in the future. This type of analysis has value in public health because interventions are implemented over time, and although events affecting outcomes may happen randomly, they are often related to what has happened before. To create a Markov model, a limited set of possible outcomes is defined. Each member of the hypothetical cohort can be in only one state at a time. Probabilities are assigned to reflect the likelihood of changing from one state to another. The costs or benefits of each transition have also been defined. The model, once built, is then cycled for either a predetermined number of cycles (eg, 10 cycles representing 10 years) or until all members of a cohort have reached an end point. At the end of the process, the different transition costs and benefits are added for each end point and then can be compared.

Consider the example of colon cancer screening. One hundred hypothetical, generally healthy individuals undergo colonoscopy and are cycled through a model in which some have polyps, some have cancer, some have complications from the test, and the test itself can produce false-negative and false-positive results. A second model, built for a second hypothetical cohort, examines occult

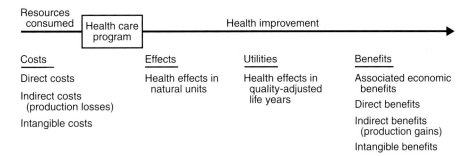

Figure 6 Methods for Economic Evaluation of Health Care Programs. (Adapted from Drummond MF, Stoddart GL, Torrance GW. Methods for the economic evaluation of health care programmes. Oxford: Oxford Medical Publishers; 1987. Used with permission.)

blood testing. When both models are cycled the same number of times, the costs of the different screening methods can be compared. Figure 6 summarizes various costs and outcomes used in economic evaluation of health care programs.

Decision analysis is a formal method of approaching the decision making process. Graphic representations of decision analysis problems commonly include influence diagrams and decision trees. Both tools represent available alternatives and the uncertainty of the various outcomes of each possibility. Uncertainties are represented by probabilities and by probability functions (mathematical representations of the interactions between uncertainties). Risk aversion is also represented by a mathematical value, termed the utility factor, and for each node on the decision tree, outcomes can be calculated and compared. Whether such structured decision making processes truly result in better, more reliable decisions is still a subject of controversy.

- Various types of cost analyses can be performed to determine where best to apply available public health funds. Because costs and benefits are always relative, the perspective of the analysis must be detailed to provide context when interpreting results.
- A cost-minimization study assumes that the 2 outcomes being compared are exactly the same. A cost-effectiveness analysis is performed when the 2 outcomes are similar. A cost-utility analysis is used when comparing programs that do not have a common natural unit of outcome. A cost-benefit analysis assigns currency values to outcomes.
- Markov models can be used in public health to analyze interventions implemented over time and related, random events that may affect outcome.
- Decision analysis uses graphic representations such as influence diagrams and decision trees to show available alternatives and the uncertainty of the various outcomes.

SUGGESTED READING

Bayer R, Gostin LO, Jennings B. Public health ethics: theory, policy, and practice. New York: Oxford University Press; c2007.

Delbecq AL, Van de Ven AH. A group process model for problem identification and program planning. J Appl Behav Sci. 1971;7(4):466-91.

Delbecq AL, Van de Ven AH, Gustafson DH. Group techniques for program planners: a guide to nominal group and Delphi processes. Glenview (IL): Scott, Foresman; c1975.

Detels R, McEwen J, Beaglehole R, Tanaka H. Oxford textbook of public health. 4th ed. Oxford: Oxford University Press; c2002.

Drummond MF, Stoddart GL, Torrance GW. Methods for the economic evaluation of health care programmes. Oxford: Oxford University Press; c1987.

Friedman DJ, Starfield B. Models of population health: their value for US public health practice, policy, and research. Am J Public Health. 2003 Mar;93(3):366-9.

Goodman RA, Hoffman RE, Lopez W, Matthews GW, Rothstein MA, Foster KL. Law in public health practice. Oxford: Oxford University Press; c2007.

Kar SB, Pascual CA, Chickering KL. Empowerment of women for health promotion: a meta-analysis. Soc Sci Med. 1999 Dec;49(11):1431-60. Erratum in: Soc Sci Med 2000 Jun;50(11):1701.

Metzler M. Social determinants of health: what, how, why, and now. Prev Chronic Dis. 2007 Oct;4(4):A85. Epub 2007 Sep 15.

Novick LF, Morrow CB, Mays GP. Public health administration: principles for population-based management. 2nd ed. Sudbury (MA): Jones and Bartlett; c2008.

Rowitz L. Public health leadership: putting principles into practice. 2nd ed. Sudbury (MA): Jones and Bartlett Publishers; c2009.

Schneider MJ. Introduction to public health. Sudbury (MA): Jones and Bartlett; c2006.

US Department of Health and Human Services. Healthy people 2010: understanding and improving health. 2nd ed. Washington (DC): US Government Printing Office. November 2000.

Wallerstein N, Bernstein E. Empowerment education: Freire's ideas adapted to health education. Health Educ Q. 1988 Winter;15(4):379-94.

Questions and Answers

Questions

1. Which economic evaluation method should be used when assessing intermediate outcomes such as the degree to which blood pressure is lowered or the number of pounds lost?
   a. Cost-benefit analysis
   b. Cost-effectiveness analysis
   c. Cost-minimization analysis
   d. Cost-utility analysis
   e. Markov model

2. All of the following are considered social determinants of health *except*:
   a. Race
   b. Socioeconomic status
   c. Genetics
   d. Sex
   e. Community resources

3. Of the choices listed below, which method is the best for establishing expert consensus?
   a. Nominal group technique
   b. Brainstorming
   c. The Delphi method
   d. Risk communication
   e. Decision analysis

4. Which of the following is *not* one of the essential public health services?
   a. Mobilize community partnerships
   b. Assess the health of communities
   c. Form public policies
   d. Assure that populations have access to appropriate and cost-effective care and services
   e. Run and manage a clinic for the underserved

5. The systematic approach of drawing public attention over time to an important community health issue is termed:
   a. Agenda setting
   b. Risk communication
   c. Agenda building
   d. Health education
   e. Establishing consensus

6. Which of the following is true about public health powers?
   a. Public health has the right to take whatever actions necessary to protect public health, as was decided in *Jacobson v Massachusetts*.
   b. Coercive measures in the name of public health are never justified. Alternate strategies for managing public health must be sought.
   c. States have broad powers for improving public health, but individual freedoms may not be limited without due process.
   d. Public health powers include the right to obtain personal medical information but only with informed consent.
   e. Public health officials must have a warrant to search private businesses.

7. Which ethical principle or view suggests that morality is an illusion created by those in power?
   a. Nonmaleficence
   b. Beneficence
   c. Autonomy
   d. Relativism
   e. Nihilism

Answers

1. Answer b.

Cost-effectiveness analysis is useful when the effects measured are simple and the same for both options being compared. It does not require economic valuation of the outcomes (as it would be in a cost-benefit analysis), nor does it require evaluation of utility or quality of life (as it would be in a cost-utility analysis). Such studies can give extremely useful information, but they are limited if the outcomes are complex. A Markov model is a mathematical approach to predicting what outcomes might occur, given a set of assumptions.

2. Answer c.

Genetic predisposition to illness is not a social determinant of health. Race, socioeconomic status, community resources, and sex are considered social determinants of health. Although race and sex are fixed by genetics, they are considered social determinants because health disparities can occur through discrimination by social grouping.

3. Answer c.

The Delphi method is a systematic method of asking individual experts to record their opinions and respond to the opinions of other experts. Theoretically, this systematic approach allows expert opinions to converge on the single best answer. The nominal group technique is a group approach to decision making that encourages all members to contribute ideas. Brainstorming is a simple method of gathering ideas from groups; however, some individuals may self-censor their ideas and limit the breadth and depth of options presented. Risk communication is a technique used to communicate to the public. Decision analysis is a formal and systematic approach to considering the various consequences of possible policies.

4. Answer e.

Although it is still common for public health agencies to provide direct health services, the direct provision of services is not an essential public health service.

5. Answer c.

Agenda building is a strategy used to increase awareness of an important public health issue. Education is certainly a part of agenda building, but agenda building specifically seeks to increase the sense of urgency about taking action and to increase consensus about the necessary actions.

6. Answer c.

States powers for public health are broad and are considered part of the police powers granted by government. However, even with emergency powers such as quarantine and mandatory treatment, the state is limited by constitutional protections and the requirement of due process. *Jacobson v Massachusetts* established that states could pass laws mandating vaccination; however, mandates cannot be decided arbitrarily, and due process must be provided. Some personal health information can be collected without informed consent (eg, collection of infectious disease data). Some businesses have been regulated so commonly and for so long that inspections can be performed without warrants.

7. Answer e.

Nihilism is an ethical view that suggests that there is no absolute morality, only the moral view in vogue by those in power. Nihilists often disengage from discussions of ethical challenges because of this view. Relativists believe that there are no absolute mores; rather, they believe morality is relative to culture. Public health shares all of the basic ethics principles with medicine. However, in addition to these basic principles, public health ethics address population health and consider questions about limited resources, redistribution of wealth and power, and conflicts between individual rights and what is best for the community.

17

HEALTH CARE MANAGEMENT AND FINANCING

William J. Litchy, MD; Mark A. Matthias, BA; Kurtis M. Hoppe, MD; and
Kyle J. Kircher, MD

Introduction

Health care financing and health care management in the
United States have been intricately intertwined in their
evolution and have been dependent on technology, on
public and private policy and funding, and the needs of
employers and employees. Virtually all major changes in
health care management in the United States have occurred
in the last century.

In 1918, the US Bureau of Labor Statistics reported that
the cost of hospital care accounted for only 7.6% of personal annual medical expenditures. In fact, a 1919 State of
Illinois report noted that the financial burden to the individual or the individual's family was not the cost of medical care. The true burden for individuals resulted from lost
work time and lost wages, estimated to be 4 times the cost
of medical care.

Little has changed over the decades; the cost of health
care today is still only one-third the estimated cost of absen-
teeism and presenteeism in the workplace. The difference
is that the individual's burden in many cases is now carried
by employers and by state and federal governments.

Movement toward other reimbursement mechanisms
for health care was advanced as medical technology
improved and health care costs increased. By 1920, many
European countries had some form of compulsory nation-
alized health care insurance. A proposal for similar coverage presented in the United States by the American
Association of Labor Legislation failed to be enacted, prin-
cipally because there was still a low demand for health

insurance by individuals, and providers opposed it because
of the belief that it would interfere with how health
care was delivered. By 1929, as a result of the continuing
increase in health care costs, Baylor College in Dallas,
Texas, offered the first health insurance policy to employees. The coverage was for hospital care only and covered
up to 21 days of care per year. The Blue Cross health plan
was started in 1932 in Sacramento, California, as the first
not-for-profit health plan in the United States. It too covered only hospital care, and as a result, much health care
was delivered in the hospital setting. It was not until 1939
that California Physician Services organized the first pre-
payment plan to cover physician services, Blue Shield.
Eventually, these 2 plans joined, forming Blue Cross Blue
Shield.

Between 1940 and 1960, the demand for health insurance increased. Commercial insurance companies, until
this time involved with property and life insurance, entered
the health care market and grew rapidly. There were several
reasons why this segment of health insurance grew quickly.
Unlike Blue Cross Blue Shield, the commercial companies
were for-profit entities and were able to select the people
they were willing to insure. This ability to select patients
allowed the commercial companies to avoid patients with
high-cost health care needs. In 1942, when it was difficult
to maintain a work force during wartime, the Stabilization
Act limited wage increases but permitted the adoption
of employer-based insurance plans. The Stabilization Act
was, in essence, a pay increase, providing a new benefit and
helping to attract and retain workers. Further government

tax regulations helped establish employee-based insurance. Employers did not have to pay taxes on employer-provided contributions to health insurance plans, and subsequently, tax breaks were introduced for other health insurance benefits. By 1958, as the result of both the demand by the work force and the government regulations, 75% of all persons in the United States had some form of health insurance coverage.

The 1960s brought the involvement of the federal government in health care. The signing of the Social Security Act of 1965 enacted Medicare (Title XVIII) and Medicaid (Title XIX), which today are under the auspices of the Centers for Medicare and Medicaid Services (CMS). Medicare is a federal health insurance plan for people age 65 years or older, as well as for certain people younger than 65 years who have disabilities, and for persons of all ages who have end-stage renal disease. Medicaid, administered by the states individually, is a program for people with low incomes or very costly medical bills.

Initially, enrollment in Medicare was 19 million persons; in 2008, it exceeded 42 million persons. Since the beginning of Medicare, there have been numerous additions to the CMS programs, including the Balanced Budget Act of 1997, which enacted new care and payment systems.

Since the 1970s, health care issues have revolved less around who pays for health care and more around how health care is managed and delivered. The Health Maintenance Act of 1973 enacted the laws for health maintenance organizations (HMOs), an attempt to control cost and improve quality of care. Networks of providers (preferred provider organizations [PPOs]) and sites of care (point of service [POS]) were introduced as another way to control cost and quality. In the decade of 2000, universal health care for everyone in the United States is once again being considered as the way to make low-cost, high-quality care available to all persons.

- The delivery of health care insurance has changed dramatically since the early 1900s, including employer-based plans and the introduction of Medicare and Medicaid in 1965.

Organizational Structures of Health Care Systems: Public Sector

World Health Organization

The World Health Organization (WHO), headquartered in Geneva, Switzerland, was officially empowered on April 7, 1948, a date commemorated each year as World Health Day. As the chief agency of the United Nations charged with **coordinating international health efforts**, WHO assists member countries in addressing the public health needs of their citizens. Besides its headquarters, the health organization maintains 6 regional offices—Brazzaville,

Congo; Cairo, Egypt; Copenhagen, Denmark; Manila, Philippines; New Delhi, India; and Washington, District of Columbia, United States—as well as 147 country offices. While WHO partners with countries to improve public health, its international status, neutrality, and nearly universal membership ensure more ready acceptance of its assistance and standards, especially during health crises caused or worsened by natural disasters, armed civil strife, or economic difficulties.

WHO's role in preventing the spread of infectious disease is well known. Through its Global Outbreak Alert and Response Network, the organization and its member partners monitor and prepare for epidemics, such as the severe acute respiratory syndrome (SARS). Yaws (caused by the spirochetal bacterium *Treponema pertenue*), onchocerciasis (river blindness), polio, and smallpox (the first and only infectious disease eradicated) have received sustained, multiyear, coordinated attention by WHO. Human immunodeficiency virus–AIDS, malaria, and tuberculosis are receiving similar intensive efforts aimed at disease treatment, control, and eventual suppression, if not eradication. However, acknowledging the role that health security has in maintaining civil societies that adequately serve the needs of their citizens, WHO developed **International Health Regulations** (IHR), which establish methods and procedures used by member countries to identify disease outbreaks, including the more established diseases, such as polio, and halt their spread. More recent IHR mandates require countries to improve their capacity for prevention and management of disease outbreaks.

Although WHO programs to control infectious diseases have received greater recognition, WHO also sets standards for disease classification, such as the **International Classification of Diseases** (ICD), used by clinicians, epidemiologists, and governments throughout the world. WHO publishes reports on international travel and health, as well as *World Health Report*, which since 1995 has provided global health assessments to aid in policy formulation and contribution decisions. Its 2008 *World Health Report*, "Primary Health Care: Now More Than Ever," details the failings of today's health systems to deliver expected health benefits and outcomes. Through its Essential Medicines and Pharmaceutical Policies Department, WHO develops programs and policies to assist member countries in ensuring access and delivery of safe and effective medications, sets standards for pharmaceutical quality and dosage through The International Pharmacopoeia, and, in the WHO Model Lists of Essential Medicines, recommends medicines that at a minimum are essential for basic health care system functioning or are for priority diseases.

Department of Health and Human Services

In the United States, health care is organized into public and private sectors. In the public sector, funding for health care is overwhelmingly appropriated by the federal government and is directly funded locally through state, county, or municipal agencies or awarded to the private sector in the form of grants.

As the primary federal department charged with the protection of health, the US Department of Health and Human Services (DHHS) oversees numerous agencies (Box). After restructuring in the late 1990s, the Social Security Administration (SSA) became an independent agency, no longer part of DHHS. The Office of Public Health and Science (OPHS) was formed and includes the Office of the Surgeon General.

Although each agency may regard certain aspects of health issues as its main purview, the mission, administration, and funding of these agencies may overlap, especially as the US population ages. In 2003, the newly established Department of Homeland Security subsumed several emergency preparedness and response activities, though the Office of Public Health Emergency Preparedness and Response remained at DHHS and coordinates the public health response to bioterrorism, as well as other emergencies managed by other federal agencies.

Centers for Medicare and Medicaid Services

The CMS administers the 2 largest health care programs in the United States, Medicare and Medicaid. It also administers the State Children's Health Insurance Program (SCHIP). The Medicare program, a federally administered program, provides insurance for hospital and physician care and oversees outpatient prescription drug coverage in partnership with private insurers. Medicaid is a state-administered program partially reimbursed by the federal government.

Box Agencies Overseen by the US Department of Health and Human Services

Administration for Children and Families (ACF)

Administration on Aging (AoA)

Agency for Healthcare Research and Quality (AHRQ)

Agency for Toxic Substances and Disease Registry (ATSDR)

Centers for Disease Control and Prevention (CDC)

Centers for Medicare and Medicaid Services (CMS)

Food and Drug Administration (FDA)

Health Resources and Services Administration (HRSA)

Indian Health Services (IHS)

National Institutes of Health (NIH)

Substance Abuse and Mental Health Services Administration (SAMHSA)

Centers for Disease Control and Prevention

The Centers for Disease Control and Prevention (CDC) is the **main federal agency for promoting public health activities in the United States**. It is organized into coordinating centers for environmental health and injury prevention, health information services, health promotion, infectious diseases, global health, and terrorism preparedness and emergency response. Workplace health and safety research and prevention are coordinated through the National Institute for Occupational Safety and Health (NIOSH), a part of the CDC. Although it is headquartered in Atlanta, Georgia, the CDC operates offices in more than 50 countries around the world to fulfill its broad mission.

Food and Drug Administration

The Food and Drug Administration (FDA) is charged with ensuring the safety of the human and animal drugs, biologics, foodstuffs, cosmetics, and devices used for medical purposes in the United States. However, meat and poultry products are regulated by the US Department of Agriculture.

FDA also oversees products that produce radiation, which include cell phones and household microwave ovens, as well as diagnostic and therapeutic radiologic equipment. In addition, the FDA inspects manufacturing facilities and guarantees the safety of vaccines and the integrity of the nation's blood supply.

The Role of the States

State administration of public health programs varies considerably across the country in both organization and structure, as well as the extent of official participation and oversight in public health initiatives and regulations. For example, some state health departments administer Medicaid, mental health programs, and health professional licensure, but most state health departments do not. Most states have not assigned the implementation of federal environmental protection statutes to state health departments. The preeminence of environmental protection over environmental health activities has been reflected in budgetary considerations favoring the former over the latter.

Local public health departments are organized most frequently at the county level rather than at other local governmental entity levels (eg, municipalities) and are typically governed by local health boards. Responsibilities differ from state to state, although most state health departments administer many preventive services in local communities. Many local public health departments also directly provide health care services through local hospitals, mental health clinics, and long-term care facilities. However, an increasing number of departments contract for services or, instead of running certain local entities, contribute financially to them. Funding is mainly local, with state funding, pass-through federal monies, or direct federal funding supplying most of the rest of needed operational dollars.

- The World Health Organization (WHO), the chief United Nations agency charged with coordinating international health efforts, assists member countries in addressing the public health needs of their citizens.
- The Department of Health and Human Services (DHHS) is the primary federal department charged with health protection and oversees numerous agencies, including the Food and Drug Administration (FDA) and the Centers for Disease Control and Prevention (CDC), the main federal agency for promoting public health activities.
- State roles in the administration of public health programs vary considerably across the United States, and public health departments differ from state to state in their organization, structure, and responsibilities.

Organizational Structures of Health Care Systems: Private Sector

Many different organizational structures have been developed to deliver health care in the United States. During the 1990s, the growth of managed care spurred the widespread use of a number of these models to curb rising health care costs. These health care models are confusing because various acronyms are used. However, on a simplistic level, this maze of jargon can be sorted out by simply remembering that it all comes down to 3 parties where health care delivery is concerned: the patients, the providers, and the payers (Table 1). From the standpoint of providers, it is helpful to remember that the model can be as simple as 1 physician or independent practitioner providing care to 1 patient in an office setting. However, in the reality of today's health care world, few medical care providers choose to go into individual practice; most join organizational structures of various sizes. With these larger organizations also come various practice and payment arrangements.

Health Maintenance Organizations

Much has been written about this organizational structure. The term "HMO" is often mistakenly considered to be a synonym for managed care because the growth of HMOs occurred during the time of growth in all managed-care entities. But, in truth, the idea of HMOs, or prepaid medical care, is not new. It goes back more than 100 years when the mining, lumber, and railroad industries developed the idea of prepaying for the health care of their workers. The history of the growth and development of HMOs over the past century is well documented in *Managed Care Primer*, which notes that perhaps the greatest growth of HMOs was stimulated by congressional approval of the Health Maintenance Act of 1973. This legislation required that employers contribute toward the HMO premium an amount equal to that contributed toward indemnity plan premiums for employees. The basic concept behind HMOs is that health care be prepaid and include a specified set of services.

The limitations found in HMO coverage can be highly frustrating to physicians who expect insurance to cover all costs. But in reality, these very coverage limitations allow an HMO to offer services at a reasonable rate without having to rely on large deductibles or other types of co-pays that

Table 1 Different Organizational Structures for Health Care Delivery and the Relationship With People, Payments, and Services Delivered

Relationship	Organizational Structure			
	HMO	IPA	PPO	POS
Payer	HMO	Managed care organization, employer or insurer	Managed care organization; employer, insurer, government	HMO or PPO
Provider	HMO-contracted providers	Large pool of participating providers	Providers in or out of network	Providers in or out of network
Patient payment	None or small	Small co-pay	None, or co-pay when provider outside the network	None, or large co-pay when provider outside the network
Services	Limited to the HMO network	Limited to the network of participating providers	Not restricted as long as patient is willing to pay co-pay	Limited to a defined provider network or outside the network

Abbreviations: HMO, health maintenance organization; IPA, independent practice association; POS, point of service; PPO, preferred provider organization.

pass along costs to members. HMOs have various approaches to control costs, including the management of use, cases, and network.

Preferred Provider Organizations

A PPO is a managed care organization of medical doctors, hospitals, and other health care providers who have contracted with an insurer to provide health care at reduced rates to the insurer's members. The idea behind the PPO is that providers **offer health care services to group members at a substantial discount** from their usual rates. This provision benefits the insurer, who receives reduced rates when its insured members use the services of the preferred provider. The providers also benefit as they see an increase in the use of services because almost all of the insured members use only the providers who participate in the preferred organization. Even the insured member should benefit because lower costs to the insurer should result in lower rates of increase in the premium.

PPOs earn money by charging an **access fee** to the insurance company for the use of their network. They negotiate with providers to set fee schedules and handle administrative issues between insurers and providers. PPOs can also contract with one another to strengthen their position in certain geographic areas without needing to form new relationships directly with providers.

Independent Practice Association

An independent practice association (IPA) is made up of **independent physicians who are typically in solo or small practice settings**. The IPA then contracts to provide services to managed care organizations, employers, or insurers on a negotiated capitated rate or negotiated fee for service (FFS). The typical IPA encompasses all specialties, but an IPA can be solely for primary care or for a single subspecialty.

IPAs are usually formed as a limited liability company, S corporation, C corporation, or other stock entity. They assemble physicians in self-directed groups within a geographic region to create and implement novel health care solutions, to form collaborative efforts among physicians to implement these programs, and to exert political influence upward within the medical community to effect positive change.

Point-of-Service Plans

POS plans are a hybrid option similar in many respects to both PPOs and HMO plans. Through an operational method like that of the HMO structures, POS plan participants must **designate a network-based physician as their primary health care provider**. However, POS members are free to go outside their designated provider networks to

seek health care services within a structure similar to the PPO. Unfortunately, patients who choose to venture outside their networks have to pay an increasing portion of the costs. Because POS plans **allow members to choose how and where to receive benefits** and what their out-of-pocket expenses will be, the plans have become a popular health care coverage option. Even so, POS plan insurance differs from the alternatives, and prospective consumers must appreciate the nuances of this choice.

Participants must select their primary care physician when they first enroll in a POS plan. When members receive covered services from the primary care physician they originally selected or through referrals from that primary care physician, they receive in-plan benefits. However, when members choose to receive those same services from a provider other than the original primary care physician or without a referral from that primary care physician, they receive out-of-plan benefits and may end up paying far more in out-of-pocket expenses. It is an important distinction for POS plans that participants are not strictly limited to the health care services provided within the network. POS plan members also have the option of visiting specialists, as well as physicians from outside their primary care provider's network of doctors and medical physicians, albeit at increased cost.

- The basic concept behind health maintenance organizations (HMOs) is that care is prepaid and includes a specified set of services, and these organizations control costs through various approaches, including the management of use, cases, and network.
- The idea behind the preferred provider organization (PPO) is that providers offer health care services to group members at a substantial discount from their usual rates.
- An independent practice association (IPA) consists of independent physicians, typically in solo or small practice settings, with whom the association contracts to provide services to managed care organizations, employers, or insurers on a negotiated capitated rate or negotiated fee for service (FFS).
- Point of service (POS) plans are a hybrid option similar in many respects to PPOs and HMOs and in which participants must designate a network-based physician as their primary health care provider and yet may go outside their designated provider network to seek health care services.

Finance and Delivery of Health Care: Public Sector

In the United States, the financing and delivery of an individual's health care may involve both public and private sectors, with numerous different levels of governmental oversight and participation.

Medicare

Medicare—enacted as Title XVIII of the Social Security Act, begun in 1965, and administered by the CMS—serves more than 40 million persons today. Although this federal health insurance program was initially intended for all persons aged 65 years or older, it was expanded in 1975 to include persons permanently disabled who are younger than 65. Medicare consists of 4 parts:

1) **Part A (hospital insurance)** covers health and hospice care in a hospital, skilled nursing facility, or the patient's home. It is primarily funded by employers and employees as a dedicated tax on earnings. Except for patients who are disabled with amyotrophic lateral sclerosis, all other patients who have a disability and are younger than 65 years receive Part A 24 months after Social Security payments begin. This part of Medicare accounts for most of the spending in the program.

2) **Part B (medical insurance)** covers physician services, as well as outpatient care and some preventive services. Unlike Part A, Part B is voluntary and requires a monthly premium that is in turn income adjusted. However, like Part A, it contains cost-sharing elements, including a deductible and co-insurance. This part of Medicare is funded by general revenues in addition to beneficiary premiums.

3) **Part C (Medicare Advantage)** refers to private health plans approved by Medicare. Managed care plans (eg, HMO, PPO) or private FFS plans provide services similar to those of Part A, Part B, and, often, Part D but may also cover services not covered by traditional Medicare, such as vision, hearing, and dental care. However, each plan may enact different levels of cost-sharing and may restrict beneficiaries to networks of contracted providers.

4) **Part D (prescription drugs)** covers outpatient prescription medications. The program is delivered through contracted private plans. Each plan may differ in the drugs covered and the costs. Monthly beneficiary premiums, general revenues, and payments by states fund the plans, and deductibles, co-payments, and co-insurance apply. Part D has a coverage gap at which all costs are paid out of pocket until the total expenditure of the beneficiary qualifies him or her for catastrophic coverage.

Medicaid

Medicaid, enacted as Title XIX of the Social Security Act, was likewise initiated in 1965 but is administered jointly by federal and state governments. It is the largest long-term–care program in the United States.

Although participation is voluntary, all states currently take part in Medicaid and are required to adhere to federal standards regarding reimbursement, eligibility, administration, and services. Thereafter, states have considerable flexibility in program administration and care delivery. Funding for the program is a partnership in which the federal government reimburses a share of the care delivery and administration costs through a formula that varies from state to state.

Generally covered are populations regarded as "mandatory categorically needy": children from low-income families, pregnant or postpartum women, aged persons, blind persons, disabled persons, low-income families with children who qualify for federal assistance, and low-income Medicare beneficiaries. However, optional categories, such as medically needy or special groups, may be covered depending on the state; many individuals in these groups have too many financial resources to qualify as mandatory categorically needy. In addition, some individuals may qualify under certain waiver programs.

Title V of the Social Security Act, originally enacted in 1935, was intended to pay for women's and children's health care. Today, although administered by the Health Resource and Services Administration, Title V grants require close coordination with Medicaid for coverage of the special physical, emotional, and developmental needs of low-income children through the Early and Periodic Screening, Diagnosis, and Treatment (EPSDT) program. Prenatal care is also provided through Title V partnerships with state maternal and child health programs.

Title X of the Public Service Act, administered by OPHS, is the only federal grant program dedicated solely to providing comprehensive family planning and access to contraceptive services. Related preventive health services are also provided through supported clinics, including human immunodeficiency virus counseling, testing, and referral. The law states that programs that use abortion as birth control are ineligible for grants.

Department of Agriculture

The Food and Nutrition Service of the US Department of Agriculture administers the **Special Supplemental Nutrition Program for Women, Infants, and Children** (WIC), a grant program to states. Eligible individuals include pregnant or postpartum women, infants, and children up to age 5 years who meet income and nutritional risk requirements. In addition to nutritious foods, the program also provides nutrition education, referrals for additional health and social services, and infant formula.

Department of Veterans Affairs

The US Department of Veterans Affairs administers health care benefits and care to eligible veterans at 155 medical centers, as well as more than 1,400 other sites of care, including outpatient clinics, nursing homes, and home health programs. The Veterans Affairs medical system provides backup for the US Department of Defense during wartime and for federal support organizations during disasters. Its programs for drug and alcohol addiction and posttraumatic stress disorder are well known. Less heralded, however, are its programs to assist homeless veterans, including transitional housing.

Military Health Service

The Military Health Service, administered by the Department of Defense, provides comprehensive medical care during military operations, natural disasters, and humanitarian crises worldwide. Through its **TRICARE** program—the triple-option benefit plan for military families—health care is delivered to active-duty service members, National Guard and Reserve members, their families, and retirees.

Indian Health Service

The Indian Health Service, an agency under the auspices of DHHS, is the federal health program for **American Indians and Alaska Native people**. The federal system includes 31 hospitals and 52 health centers, and its public health priorities include disease prevention, health promotion, and adverse health factor elimination.

- Medicare is a federal health insurance program of 4 parts, initially intended for all persons age 65 years or older but expanded to include persons permanently disabled who are younger than 65, that today provides service to 40 million persons.
- Medicaid, the largest long-term–care program in the United States, is a voluntary program with both federal and state funding, with all states currently taking part

and thus required to adhere to federal standards regarding reimbursement, eligibility, administration, and services.

- Department of Agriculture administers the Special Supplemental Nutrition Program for Women, Infants, and Children (WIC), a grant program to states for qualifying adults and children in need.
- Department of Veterans Affairs offers a medical system providing backup for the Department of Defense during wartime and for federal support organizations during disasters. It has well-known programs for drug and alcohol addiction and posttraumatic stress disorder.
- Military Health Service provides comprehensive medical care during military operations, natural disasters, and humanitarian crises worldwide and runs TRICARE, which provides health care for service members, their families, and retirees.
- The Indian Health Service is the federal health program for American Indians and Alaska Native peoples and includes 31 hospitals and 52 health centers.

Finance and Delivery of Health Care: Private Sector

Although many people in the United States receive health care through public funding mechanisms, the private sector has a major role in funding health care for the nonelderly population. But despite public and private health care funding, nearly 45 million people in the United States are uninsured (Figure 1), and even more are underinsured.

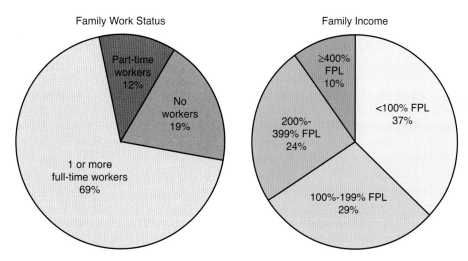

Figure 1 Characteristics of the 45 Million Nonelderly Uninsured Persons in the United States, 2007. FPL indicates the federal poverty level. (Adapted from Kaiser Commission on Medicaid and the Uninsured [Internet]. Washington [DC]: Kaiser Family Foundation. The uninsured and the difference health insurance makes. 2008 Sep. [Cited: 2009 Oct 5]. Available from http://www.kff.org/uninsured/upload/1420-10.pdf. Used with permission.)

The financial burden of uninsured persons is shared by all; both the public and private sectors absorb the cost of care when it is needed for this segment of the population.

Employer-Based Health Insurance

Employer-sponsored health insurance is the cornerstone of the health care system in the United States. Through this system, more than 60% of persons who are younger than 65 years have health care coverage. Employer-based health insurance means that the **employer pays for all or a portion** of health care coverage for the employee and the employee's dependents.

Employers may provide this insurance by either paying monthly premiums and avoiding risk or, as in many large companies, by being self-insured and taking the risk themselves. Between Medicare and Medicaid in the public sector and employee-based health insurance in the private sector, more than 75% of all people in the United States have insurance.

The emergence of employee-sponsored health insurance resulted from several events. First, President Franklin D. Roosevelt decided not to pursue universal health care coverage in the 1930s—coverage that was supported in many industrialized countries at the time. Second, legislation in the 1940s, including the 1942 Stabilization Act, limited the employer's freedom to raise wages but allowed employers to increase benefits, such as adding health care coverage. Third, in 1945 a law was enacted that prevented employers from changing benefit programs until the end of a labor contract. Fourth, in 1949 it was enacted that benefits should be considered part of the wage package so unions could negotiate health insurance under the labor contract. Fifth, in 1954 the Internal Revenue Service determined that employer contributions to purchase health insurance were not taxable as income.

At its peak, US employer-based health care coverage applied to nearly 70% of persons younger than 65 years. Over the years of growth of employer-based health care coverage, the amount of money that the employee paid for the health care premium decreased from about 50% of the total premium in 1960 to 15% in 2000. However, with the increasing cost of health care and a Financial Accounting Standards Board (FASB) ruling in 1990 that requires employers to have future liabilities of health care on their books, employer-sponsored health care coverage became more difficult for employers to maintain. Projections estimate that during the next 10 years, the number of companies providing health care coverage will decrease and the coverage provided will change. Benefits will be less generous, and the share that the employee contributes will increase. In addition, the employer-based benefits for retirees are rapidly decreasing as the cost of health care rises and the economy has weakened. As employer-based health insurance decreases, other funding mechanisms for health care will be needed. At this point, its funding is handled through other mechanisms.

Employee Retirement Income Security Act

The Employee Retirement Income Security Act (ERISA), enacted on Labor Day in 1974, is the federal statute that establishes **minimum standards for pension plans** in private industry and governs the federal income tax effects associated with employee benefit plans. Although initially intended to deal with pensions, its purveyance covers self-funded, employer-based health care benefit plans. ERISA was established to protect the interest of employee benefit plan participants and beneficiaries by requiring disclosure of information about the plan, establishing standards of conduct for plan beneficiaries, and providing appropriate remedies when needed. ERISA does not require employers to provide health care coverage to employees, dependents, or retirees, but when they do, the operation of the plan is regulated by ERISA.

Under the ERISA laws, employers are exempt from state regulation, an exemption that provides both advantages and disadvantages. Several amendments to ERISA have been made with respect to health benefits. For example, the **Consolidated Omnibus Budget Reconciliation Act of 1985** (COBRA) allows employees and beneficiaries the right to continue their coverage under the health benefit plans for a limited time after loss of employment or when a beneficiary is no longer eligible for coverage under the employee's health care plan. The length of time allowed for coverage is usually 12 to 18 months. The premium for this coverage can be quite high, however, because the employer usually sets the premium at the estimated cost of care for the individual or the individual's family.

The **Health Insurance Portability and Accountability Act** (HIPAA) enacted in 1996 prohibits health plans from refusing to cover an employee's preexisting medical condition in some circumstances. It also bars health plan benefits from certain types of discrimination and ultimately disallows the sharing of an individual's information with other business entities. Other amendments include the Newborns' and Mothers' Health Protection Act, the Mental Health Parity Act, and the Women's Health and Cancer Rights Act.

Self-Pay Health Insurance

"Self-pay" refers to the growing section of the US population who pay for their health care directly. They may be part of the 9% of the population who purchase insurance directly, either as their primary source of insurance (two-thirds of this percentage) or as a Medicare supplemental insurance (one-third). The other members of the self-pay group are part of the underinsured or uninsured population. A segment of this population, often its younger members, can afford health care insurance but make a choice not to purchase it and take the risk that they will stay healthy.

Insurance and the Underinsured and Uninsured

The most recent estimates report that more than 60 million people in the United States are either underinsured or uninsured. The underinsured group represents people who have some form of insurance but either their health care benefits are inadequate to cover the cost of care or the share of the cost that they have to pay is beyond their financial ability. The Census Bureau's 2005 Current Population Survey estimates that 45.8 million individuals in the United States are uninsured. The numbers of underinsured and uninsured persons are increasing and are affecting the health care payer and provider systems in the nation. The uninsured group is a dynamic population with, at any given time, 20% who have been without insurance for 3 months or less and 34% who have been uninsured for 6 months or less.

The uninsured have an increased likelihood of being poor and having low incomes, with estimates that more than 50% have incomes below 200% of the DHHS poverty guideline. It is not surprising that many of the uninsured population are not working or are working less than full time, work for employers who do not offer health care insurance as part of the wage package, and cannot afford to pay for coverage. Employers who do not offer coverage are more likely to have fewer than 100 employees. Despite their low income, however, many people do not meet the Medicaid eligibility criteria. Yet, not all uninsured individuals have low incomes. More than 10% of the uninsured have incomes greater then 500% of the DHHS poverty guideline. This statistic may seem surprising, considering that health insurance is so important, until some demographic characteristics of this population are considered.

About 80% of the uninsured are adults and about 65% are younger than 34 years. This may be because younger adults are more likely to have lower incomes than older adults and also are more likely to believe that they will not need health care. Also, older individuals are eligible for Medicare and children are more likely to be eligible for Medicaid and SCHIP. About two-thirds of uninsured adults do not have a college education and one-quarter have not graduated from high school. Half of the uninsured are white and half represent a mixture of race and ethnic minorities. Most of the uninsured persons in the United States are citizens; however, about 20% are not.

Key Trends

In large part because of the rise in costs, the number of employers offering health insurance as a benefit has declined. Although insurance is offered by 99% of firms with more than 200 employees, less than 50% of firms with 3 to 9 employees offer health benefits. Only 25% of all businesses offer such benefits to part-time workers. These changes in employer health care coverage have resulted in increased numbers of people spending time without health insurance. The number of uninsured (ie, individuals without health care coverage at some point during a given survey year) has increased by 5% to more than 45 million individuals, or 15% of the US population. This 5% increase from 2004 to 2007, the last year for which the data are available, is on top of a 15% increase in the prior 4 years.

While active employee coverage rates have declined, the number of employers who offer health coverage to retirees has decreased even more rapidly. Between 1988 and 2008, the percentage of large employers (with >200 workers) offering retiree benefits declined from 66% to 31%, although in recent years that figure has been fairly stable. Substantially, all these employers offered such benefits to retirees who were not yet 65 years old (ie, retirees who were not Medicare eligible), with 75% offering them to Medicare-eligible retirees. Medicare provides basic coverage to all persons over age 65 in the United States, yet most individuals still have supplemental insurance to manage the cost of self-pay components, either provided through their employer or purchased on their own.

The growth in the number of uninsured persons is a key concern for many people in the United States because of both the cost implications and the quality-of-life and health concerns. Studies have shown that uninsured persons have less access to providers and a correspondingly more difficult time receiving the care they may require. In a 2008 analysis of National Health Interview Survey data by the Kaiser Commission on Medicaid and the Uninsured, the commission noted that 27% of the uninsured postponed seeking care because of cost, compared with 6% to 10% for people covered by employer or government insurance programs. The uninsured also are more likely to access care through an emergency department at a hospital, one of the most costly ways to receive basic care and particularly so when low-cost preventive measures could have prevented many such encounters. The same study noted that 52% of the uninsured had no usual source of care, compared with just 10% of individuals who have coverage through a health plan.

- The cornerstone of the health care system in the United States, employer-based health care, provides coverage for more than 60% of persons younger than 65 years.
- The Employee Retirement Income Security Act (ERISA) was established to protect the interests of employee benefit plan participants and beneficiaries. It has undergone several amendments, such as the Consolidated Omnibus Budget Reconciliation Act of 1985 (COBRA), allowing plan coverage to continue after an employee's job is lost.

- Persons who self-pay for health insurance are among those who buy insurance to supplement Medicare coverage, those who are uninsured or underinsured, and those who personally purchase their primary insurance.
- In the United States, the uninsured and the underinsured together total about 60 million and are likely to not be working or to work for employers who do not provide health insurance.

Provider Reimbursement Mechanisms

Payers use various methods to reimburse providers for health care services. The primary concern for payers is the incentive environment that the reimbursement arrangement creates. Does the payment model promote high-quality care while minimizing unnecessary services? As part of their strategy, payers may choose to share or shift the risks of overutilization or high cost to the provider community. On the basis of how the payment models respond to changes in service utilization, they may be grouped as either variable or fixed reimbursement arrangements. New or updated models are continually being developed to create balanced risk-sharing and to promote best care.

Variable Reimbursement Arrangements

Two primary variable reimbursement models are available: discounted FFS and fee schedules. In these models, the provider is paid for each service performed. This reimbursement method helps ensure that payments are in relation to the resources used (ie, provision of more services results in higher payments), the economic reward it delivers for the provision of additional services may lead to unnecessary health care and cost.

Discounted FFS results when a payer contracts for a discount off the provider's standard fee schedule. The discounted FFS simplifies the administration and understanding of the plan but potentially promotes higher volumes of services, as previously described. The discount is ostensibly agreed to as a means to increase patient volumes: participation in a given network may allow access to a wider patient base (albeit for a lower price), as well as ensure ongoing access to the provider's own patients. It also allows the provider to maintain control over the charges for a given service, potentially offsetting the value of the discount.

Fee schedules are used as a means to control price risk by establishing a fixed price for each service performed (eg, a price for each current procedural terminology [CPT] code in a physician practice). Many fee schedules are built as a percentage of Medicare rates or are based on Medicare's resource-based relative value scale (RBRVS). The fee schedule strives to ensure that the payer pays the same fee for the same service, regardless of provider. These schedules differ by geographic area and may still be subject to negotiation. They give greater financial reward as more services are provided.

The 2 primary concerns with variable reimbursement models are the incentive for overutilization and the tendency to promote upcoding or unbundling. "**Upcoding**" refers to a slow upward creep in CPT coding (eg, from a routine office visit to an extended one). "**Unbundling**" refers to the practice of billing separately for services for which a bundled code exists (often found in a laboratory setting).

In situations where a health plan provides benefits for services performed by noncontracted providers, the plan may implement a usual, customary, or reasonable (UCR) fee schedule. This system compares the patient charge with the UCR charge for similar providers in the service area, creating an upper limit to the payment per service. A common example of a UCR fee schedule is limiting payment to the 90th percentile.

Fixed Reimbursement Arrangements

Fixed reimbursement models are most commonly used in a hospital environment or across physician and hospital services. They involve a predetermined payment for a given condition or treatment episode, regardless of the services used during the hospital stay or episode. Although payments are made for each case seen, the incentive is for the provider to reduce or minimize resource use per episode. The provider may record a profit or incur a loss (eg, when costs exceed the payment received) on any individual case, but overall, when the arrangement is well planned and care is delivered efficiently, the provider has an opportunity to increase profitability over time.

Diagnosis-Related Groups

The most common fixed-payment mechanism is the diagnosis-related group (DRG). The DRG has been part of the Medicare prospective payment system since its introduction in 1983 and provides a single payment for each hospital stay on the basis of diagnosis. Although outlier provisions may increase payment for costs beyond certain thresholds, the **DRG payment does not change on the basis of services used or length of stay**. This characteristic of DRGs creates an incentive for the hospital to minimize costly procedures and to discharge the patient as soon as possible. Many facilities engage in quality improvement efforts to optimize treatment and minimize resource use for high-volume or high-cost DRGs.

Medicare implemented a system of **Medical Severity Diagnosis- Related Groups** (MS-DRGs), effective in October 2007, to take into account the severity of a patient's condition in determining payment. This increased specificity results in increased reimbursement for facilities that treat patients who have a higher illness profile and in lowered reimbursement for those facilities whose patients have fewer complications or comorbidities (Figure 2).

Case Rate or Bundled Case Rate

A second common fixed-rate method is referred to as a case rate or bundled case rate. By nature, these rates are defined as a predetermined, fixed payment for all services related to a defined episode of care or procedure. They most commonly cover both inpatient and outpatient services, as in the case with a heart transplant. The charge does not change, regardless of length of stay or resource use. The case rate may cover services leading up to the primary procedure and tracking it sometimes for as long as a year. Because these episodes of care are most common on high-cost or high-risk procedures, outlier provisions are not uncommon for cases that become catastrophic or grossly exceed expected utilization.

A related method is the global fee, where a flat rate is negotiated for a set of multiple services. A common example in an obstetric practice is the fee for a vaginal delivery or for a cesarean section, both including all prenatal and postnatal care. Clearly, identifying the services included in the payment is critical to the successful use of these fees.

Per Diem Payment

A third fixed-rate method is the per diem payment, in which a fixed payment is made for each day's stay in a given facility, again regardless of resource use. Rates may be specific to the facility, such as a rehabilitation center or skilled nursing facility, or may be broken up within a hospital into rates for the intensive care unit (ICU), neurologic intensive care unit (NICU), general surgery, or general medicine. Although this payment method provides motivation to the hospital to manage its services, the hospital may be less likely to seek shortened stays. Accordingly, plans using this method implement strong length-of-stay guidelines as part of their utilization management programs.

HMOs were the primary initiators of the fixed payment method, known as "capitation." Although capitation is used most frequently with primary care providers, it is also common in specialty practices or for a global capitation encompassing both physician and hospital services in group practices or health systems. Capitation involves paying a set amount monthly for providing services to a defined set of patients, regardless of whether these patients were seen.

Because the provider is accepting the risk that his or her patients may have a higher-than-average illness burden (thus requiring more services), rates should be adjusted to patient demographic characteristics and (if possible) to the illness profile of the assigned population. Under this method, physician practices prosper when they are able to get or keep their patients healthy using low-cost preventive care programs.

The payment may allow the provider to educate patients on the importance of good health and establish nurse triage lines or find other creative ways to provide low-cost but appropriate care, thus minimizing unnecessary services. However, a concern with this method is that patients may

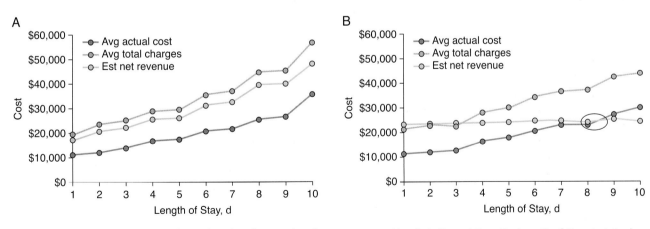

Figure 2 Inpatient Financials for Diagnosis-Related Group (DRG) 164 at a Large Hospital, Plotted Over the Length of Stay. A, Actual cost, total charges, and estimated revenue of a patient with a commercial fee-for-service (FFS) plan. Unlike a Medicare DRG, for a patient with a commercial FFS plan in DRG, the actual cost line does not cross the estimated net revenue line, regardless of length of stay. FFS revenue follows cost. B, Actual cost, total charges, and estimated revenue of a patient with Medicare coverage. The Medicare DRG payment remains flat, regardless of length of stay or underlying cost. For a Medicare patient in DRG 164, the per-case net operating income moves from positive to negative when length of stay exceeds 8 days, at which time the cost of care exceeds the allowable Medicare reimbursement (2008 Center for Medicare and Medicaid Services mean length of stay, 8.3 d; relative Medicare weight, 2.8081). DRG 164 indicates major chest procedure with complications and comorbidities.

not receive the care they need because the financial incentive is to minimize care. Providers and health plans alike should have an appropriate quality review program in place when capitation is used (Table 2).

Risk Pools, Bonus Payments, and Pay-for-Performance Plans

Each payment method creates a certain financial incentive for the provider of services. Risk pools or other incentive arrangements can be created to share the burden of utilization risk more equitably or to create an incentive for specific behaviors.

Risk Pools

Risk pools are a contractual pool of dollars available for reimbursement after certain targets (eg, a defined average length of stay, hospital days per 1,000 patients, overall per-member per-month [PMPM] costs) are met. The pool may be shared among all physicians in a specialty area or by only targeted groups participating in the arrangement. Similarly, bonus arrangements may be paid on the achievement of targets in other defined areas, such as immunization or mammography rates in quality or preventive care. Also related, withhold arrangements involve a payment holdback and are found in both FFS and fixed-payment (eg, capitated) environments. Under a withhold arrangement, a portion of the contractual amount is paid as usual, but a percentage is held back by the health plan, subject to meeting certain end-of-year targets or a like requirement.

Pay-for-Performance Plan

With an increasing focus on improving quality and safety as a means of reducing health care cost trends, pay-for-performance (P4P) plans are becoming increasingly common. These plans provide a financial reward for progressing toward goals in a defined set of quality metrics. This strategy is a marked departure from most payment methods, which essentially pay the same to all parties regardless of differences in quality.

Determining which measures to use, how to collect the data, and the role of risk adjustment add complexity to P4P plans. CMS has been a leader in establishing these programs, with bonus payments made to providers in the top percentile of their scoring method. Payment reductions will occur in the future for providers at the bottom of the scale. State Medicaid programs have also jumped on board with P4P plans; more than 50% of state programs had a P4P component in place in July 2006.

Notwithstanding agreement on the need to focus on quality, many experts see these programs as merely tinkering with a payment system that is fundamentally flawed. Primary concerns expressed include the array of metrics involved, a lack of consistency between plans, and the fact that payments are so modest as to be ineffective in changing behavior. An example of the differentiation comes from a PricewaterhouseCoopers study issued in 2007. Of 10 top commercial plans surveyed, more than 60 physician performance measures were found—but not a single physician performance measure was used in all 10 plans. Chapter 18 further describes P4Ps.

One other trend promoting high-quality care is the denial of payment for never events, a list of 28 serious adverse, reportable events identified by the National Quality Forum. As of October 1, 2008, CMS denies payment for select hospital-acquired conditions, which include never events such as a foreign object left in the patient during a surgical procedure and the administration of incompatible blood. Commercial payers have begun to follow suit.

- Variable reimbursement arrangements are either a discounted fee-for-service (FFS) schedule or a fee schedule, both of which pay the provider for only the service performed but also offer an economic reward for additional services performed—potentially leading to unnecessary care and costs.
- Fixed reimbursement arrangements provide a predetermined payment for a given condition or treatment episode, regardless of the services used during the hospital stay or episode, and encompass diagnosis-related groups (DRGs), a case rate or bundled case rate, and per diem payment or capitation.
- Risk pools involve a contractual pool of dollars available for reimbursement after certain targets are met and, similar to pay-for-performance (P4P) arrangements, reimburse providers for quality service and withhold reimbursement when quality is poor.

Health Care Cost Trends

One of the most important issues facing the health care industry is the rate of health care cost increases. Care costs are increasing substantially faster than the rate of general inflation and are consuming an ever-larger portion of the US economy (ie, gross domestic product [GDP]). These trends are leading to increased concern regarding insurance and affordability and, if cost goes unchecked, about whether it is unsustainable. Herein we look at key cost trends, reasons for cost increases, and the implications of this growth.

Rising Cost, a Key Health Care Trend

From 2000 to 2008, the average cost of health insurance for a family of four increased 119% (Figure 3). The pace of this increase far exceeded the pace of inflation and the

Table 2 Common Methods of Reimbursement for Health Care

Characteristic	Unit of Payment	Type of Health Plan	Reimbursement Considerations		
			Cost-Control Strategies by Plan	Financial Risk to Provider	Physician or Hospital Incentive
FFS and discounted FFS	Procedure	Indemnity, Medicare, Medicaid, PPOs, others	Utilization review	None	Deliver more services, increase charge master
Fee schedules	Procedure	Indemnity, Medicare, Medicaid, PPOs, others	Utilization review	Taking on price risk—fees may be below cost	Deliver more services
DRGs	Episode of illness	Indemnity insurers, Medicare, Medicaid, many managed care organizations	Prospective fees, utilization review	Delivering services beyond payment level	Admit more patients but provide fewer services, practice efficiently
Case rates and bundled case rates	Episode of illness or case	Indemnity insurers, Medicare, Medicaid, many managed care organizations	Prospective fees, utilization review	Delivering services beyond payment level	Admit more patients but provide fewer services; practice efficiently
Per diems	Days	Indemnity insurers, certain managed care organizations	Payment per day, LOS guidelines, utilization review	Delivering services beyond payment level	Retain patient longer; reduce resource use
Capitation and global capitation	Covered life	Many managed care organizations	Risk pools, withholdings, careful choice of network providers	Losing money, delivering services beyond payment level, seeing higher-risk patients	Deliver fewer services, practice most efficiently, promote healthy behaviors in patient base

Abbreviations: DRG, diagnosis-related group; FFS, fee for service; LOS, length of stay; PPO, preferred provider organization.
Data from Nash DB. The managed care manual. Boston (MA): Total Learning Concepts, Inc; c1997.

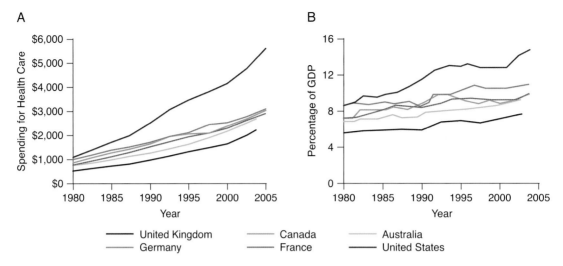

Figure 3 National Health Expenditures in the United States Compared With Other Countries, 1980-2003. A, Average spending on health care per capita ($US purchasing power parity). B, Total expenditures on health care as a percentage of gross domestic product (GDP). (Adapted from Zuckerman S, McFeeters J. Recent growth in health expenditures. March 2006. New York: The Commonwealth Fund; c2004-2009. [cited 22 Oct 2009]. Available at http://www.commonwealthfund.org/Content/Publications/Fund-Reports/2006/Mar/Recent-Growth-in-Health-Expenditures.aspx. Used with permission.)

growth in workers' earnings, which increased 29% and 34%, respectively, during the same time period. Figure 4 shows that, during the 20 years from 1988 to 2007, only a few years in the mid 1990s had health care inflation at a rate equal to or less than general inflation. Those years were influenced by unusual factors, such as industry reaction to a proposed national health insurance model while President Bill Clinton was in office and a simultaneous drive by employers to implement managed care plans. Health care spending passed $7,000 per person (per capita) in the United States in 2006.

Nationally, health care expenditures exceeded $2.1 trillion in 2006 and comprised 16% of the GDP. This percentage compares with 13.8% of the GDP in 2000 and just 5.2% of the GDP 40 years prior, in 1960. This rate of increase in health care expenditure far exceeds that of other countries. Health care spending per capita in the United States is more than double the spending of the country ranked next and, while all countries are experiencing growing health care costs, the US rate of growth is markedly higher.

Drivers of Cost Increases

Health care costs are affected by various complex and interrelated factors. In a PricewaterhouseCoopers study on the components of the change in medical costs between 2001 and 2002, researchers identified 5 diverse areas primarily responsible for cost increases, each comprising between 15% and 22% of the year-to-year change. New drugs, medical devices, and other advances were the largest single

component; however, even lesser factors in their study, such as litigation and defensive medicine (7%), were notable. Given the various issues involved, it is not difficult to see why the problem of rising costs has not yet been systematically addressed.

Costs are driven up by price increases or utilization increases, or a blend of the two. In the United States, it appears that utilization in general is the stronger of these 2 drivers. A report by the Congressional Budget Office (CBO) issued in June 2007 cited increased utilization as the reason for the 35% increase in Medicare physician expenditures between 1997 and 2005. The CBO found utilization increased 39% during that time, meaning that Medicare was actually paying *less* on a per-service basis than at the start of the period. Of note, when provider payment rates do not keep up with the cost of service (particularly with a large payer such as Medicare), it results in cost shifting, a phenomenon whereby the provider passes on higher charges to patients with other (eg, commercial) insurance.

Utilization increases are driven by a host of factors. The top factors are highlighted below.

Population

Lifestyle and aging are 2 primary components of utilization. Lifestyle factors include physical inactivity, obesity, smoking, and illicit drug use. Obesity is increasingly viewed as an epidemic, with physical inactivity more the norm than the exception in US society. To address the

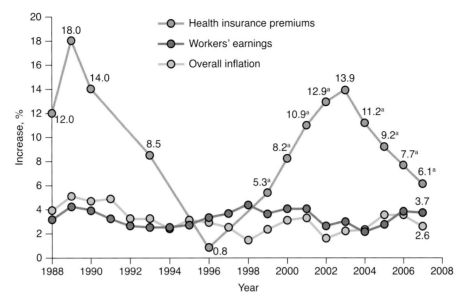

Figure 4 Increases in Health Insurance Premiums Compared With Other Indicators, 1988-2007. Figure charts the rise in health care insurance premiums in the past 20 years, comparing the premiums with earnings and inflation. Data on premium increases reflect the cost of health insurance premiums for a family of four. [a]Estimate is statistically different from the estimate for the previous year shown (*P*<.05). No statistical tests were conducted for the years before 1999. (Data from Employer health benefits: 2008 annual survey. Menlo Park [CA]: Henry J. Kaiser Family Foundation. c2008 [cited 5 Oct 2009]. Available from http://ehbs.kff.org/ pdf/7790.pdf. Used with permission.)

factors of lifestyle and aging, employers are increasingly implementing targeted educational and coaching programs to motivate and reward individuals for making better lifestyle decisions. The drive to implement consumerism and consumer-directed health plans also strives to create financial incentives for taking better care of oneself. In addition, the US population is aging, which leads to more health problems and a greater use of health services. As the baby boomers reach Medicare age, the impact on health care service use and cost will accelerate during the next 10 to 20 years.

Consumer Demand

Wealth and the spread of information and advertising are driving increased demand for services. Studies comparing the United States and other economies have found a strong correlation between wealth and health care spending. As a nation becomes wealthier, it chooses to spend more of its wealth on health care. In that environment, the health care industry continues to expand its knowledge and innovation to address conditions for which there is patient demand. Information and knowledge are being ever more rapidly disseminated, giving consumers a chance to identify and pursue new and expanded treatment options. Also, direct-to-consumer advertising by the pharmaceutical

industry grew more than 400% between 1996 and 2007, helping drive a 72% increase in prescriptions over that time.

The insulating impact of health insurance has increased dramatically over time also. Between 1970 and 2005, the share of personal health expenditures paid directly out of pocket by US consumers declined dramatically, from 40% to 15%. Moves to increase cost sharing in consumer-directed health insurance plans may reverse that trend. However, with expanded coverage—whether in public program coverage for more groups (eg, expanded eligibility for couples and those with incomes at a higher percentage of the federal poverty level) or in specific policy coverage to include alternative medicines and new treatments (eg, the implementation of Medicare Part D, which covers prescription drugs)—consumers generally have fewer financial barriers to the care they need or desire. To many consumers, the cost of care is just what they pay, without including the cost paid by a third party.

New Technology in Drugs, Devices, and Treatments

Advances in technology, drugs, and treatments could prove to be either cost additive or cost reducing in the long term. Conversely, to date they have both driven increased demand and utilization by expanding treatment possibilities to

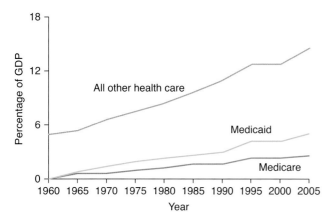

Figure 5 Trends in Health Care Costs as a Percentage of Gross Domestic Product (GDP), 1960-2005. Costs are projected for the different major payers in the 21st century. (Data from Congressional Budget Office [Internet]. The long-term outlook for health care spending. 2007 Nov. [cited 22 Oct 2009]. Available from http://www.cbo.gov/ftpdocs/87xx/doc8758/11-13-LT-Health.pdf)

conditions previously untreated and added higher-cost treatments that at times provided only marginal health improvement. (Marginal health improvement in the face of higher-cost treatments is particularly true in the pharmaceutical industry, where financial incentives as drugs approached patent expiration led to strong efforts to expand the life of a drug through minor improvements that have little impact on the end treatment outcome.) New imaging technologies, such as positron emission tomographic scans, come at a high price. New biologics and other specialty medications can require more than $100,000 per month for an effective treatment.

Other factors driving increased utilization include waste and fraud, litigation and defensive medicine, and the growth in chronic disease (in part due to the lifestyle factors noted earlier). Government health care mandates, of which there were more than 1,500 identified already by 2002, also drive increased coverage and use of health care services. Other regulatory impacts include laws and policies, such as HIPAA, that add a substantial administrative record-keeping requirement to the provider (and payer) system.

- Health care costs exceeded $2.1 trillion in 2006 and comprised 16% of the gross domestic product (GDP). The cost increases faster than inflation nationally and the costs of other countries' health care globally.
- The drivers behind the increased costs of health care include changes in age and lifestyle of the US population and the resulting increased health costs per capita; increased demand, in part because of the rise in information distribution and pharmaceutical advertising; and technological advances in drugs, treatments, and devices.

Implications of Current Rate of Growth

In 2006, health care expenditures in the United States were more than triple the percentage of the GDP than they were in 1960 (Figure 5). Over that 46-year period, health care expenditures increased more than 2.2% per year, more rapidly than inflation. In a study by the CBO in November 2007, these costs were projected forward 75 years. Using their best estimates, the CBO researchers projected that national spending on health care would be 49% of GDP by 2082 and, if historical trends were unchanged, would theoretically reach 99% of the GDP in 2082. Clearly, this trend is unsustainable; reaching even the lower figure would place great pressure on other portions of the economy and on the health care industry itself.

- Cost projections cite an increase in national health care spending of at least 49% by 2082.

SUGGESTED READING

Blumenthal D. Employer-sponsored health insurance in the United States: origins and implications. N Engl J Med. 2006 Jul 6;355(1):82-8.

Congressional Budget Office [Internet]. The long-term outlook for health care spending. 2007 Nov. [cited 22 Oct 2009]. Available from http://www.cbo.gov/ftpdocs/87xx/doc8758/11-13-LT-Health.pdf.

Employer health benefits: 2008 annual survey. Menlo Park (CA): Henry J. Kaiser Family Foundation. c2008 [cited 5 Oct 2009]. Available from http://ehbs.kff.org/pdf/7790.pdf.

Fronstin P. Sources of health insurance and characteristics of the uninsured: analysis of the March 2006 current population survey. Washington (DC): Employee Benefits Research Institute. October 2006. [cited 5 Oct 2009]. Available from http://www.ebri.org/pdf/briefspdf/EBRI_IB_10a-20061.pdf

Gorman RS. Managed care primer. Phoenix (AZ): Print Solutions, Inc. 1998.

Kaiser Commission on Medicaid and the Uninsured [Internet]. Washington (DC): Kaiser Family Foundation. The uninsured and the difference health insurance makes. 2008 Sep. [cited 5 Oct 2009]. Available from http://www.kff.org/uninsured/upload/1420-10.pdf.

Kongstvedt PR. The managed health care handbook. 2nd ed. Gaithersburg (MD): Aspen Publishers. c1993.

Nash DB. The managed care manual. Boston (MA): Total Learning Concepts; c1997.

Nash DB. The physician's guide to managed care. Gaithersburg (MD): Aspen Publishers; c1994.

Prescription drug trends. [Internet]. 2008 Sep. [cited 5 Oct 2009]. Washington (DC): Kaiser Family Foundation. Available from http://www.kff.org/rxdrugs/upload/3057_07.pdf.

PricewaterhouseCoopers. The factors fueling rising health-care costs. Sep 2002. [cited 5 Oct 2009]. Available from:

http://www.sickoflawsuits.org/content/pdfs/PwCFinalReport.pdf.

PricewaterhouseCoopers. The factors fueling rising healthcare costs. Sep 2006. [cited 5 Oct 2009]. Available from: http://www.savoyassociates.com/Docs/The%20Factors%20Fueling%20Rising%20Healthcare%20Costs%202006%20(PriceWaterhouseCoopers%20Report).pdf.

Questions and Answers

Questions

1. Which of the following agencies administers the largest programs for heath care in the United States?
   a. Centers for Disease Control and Prevention
   b. Centers for Medicare and Medicaid Services
   c. Food and Drug Administration
   d. Kaiser Permanente
   e. Blue Cross Blue Shield national network

2. What percentage of health care in the United States is financed through employer-based health insurance?
   a. 50%
   b. 15%
   c. 62%
   d. 42%
   e. 80%

3. In which of the following payment mechanisms might a person anticipate that the result would be a decrease in the average length of hospital stay?
   a. Fee for service
   b. Per diem
   c. Discounted fee schedule
   d. Diagnosis-related group (capitated)
   e. Contracted fee for service

4. Which of the following agencies is not administered by the US Department of Health and Human Services?
   a. Centers for Disease Control and Prevention
   b. World Health Organization
   c. Indian Health Service
   d. Administration for Children and Families
   e. National Institutes of Health

5. Which of the following care delivery structures consists of health care providers and health care sites contracting to payer systems to provide services at specified rates?
   a. Preferred provider organization
   b. Centers for Medicare and Medicaid Services
   c. Independent practice association
   d. Health maintenance organization
   e. Point-of-service plan

6. Individual states are responsible for funding which of the following agencies?
   a. Medicare
   b. Medicaid
   c. Food and Drug Administration
   d. Administration for Children and Families
   e. Agency for Health Care Research and Quality

7. Which of the following statements is true about the Employment Retirement Income Security Act (ERISA)?
   a. ERISA governs all health care benefit plans
   b. ERISA requires that all employers provide health care benefits
   c. ERISA exempts employers from state health plan regulation
   d. ERISA, will be replaced by the Health Insurance Portability and Accountability Act in 2010
   e. ERISA exempts employees from federal health plan regulations

Answers

1. Answer b.

The Centers for Medicare and Medicaid Services administers the largest programs for health care. Medicare is federally funded and federally administered. The 4 major divisions of Medicare cover hospital, physician, and medication expenses. Medicaid is a state-funded program that receives some federal funds.

2. Answer c.

The number of people relying on employers for health care coverage is large—about 160 million in the United States—but the number is expected to decline in the future. More than 60 million people in the United States are either underinsured or uninsured, and that number is expected to increase, in part because of fewer employers offering health care coverage or offering the level of benefits they provided in the past.

3. Answer d.

The diagnosis-related group used by Medicare pays a specific amount of money for hospitalized patients depending on the diagnosis. Therefore, the less money required in caring for the patient, the larger the profit margin. The other forms of payment do not support managing utilization, and there is no measure of quality or value.

4. Answer b.

The World Health Organization, an agency of the United Nations, has its headquarters in Geneva, Switzerland, and has regional offices around the world. WHO is charged with coordinating international health care initiatives and has been instrumental in addressing the effects of infectious diseases in developing countries.

5. Answer a.

PPOs were developed to organize physicians, other health care providers, hospitals, and other health care delivery sites into a bargaining unit and a health care delivery unit to manage the health care cost and to encourage payers to use their services.

6. Answer b.

Although Medicaid programs receive some federal funding, they are the primary responsibility of the individual state.

7. Answer c.

ERISA was set up in 1974 to establish minimal standards for pension plans in private industry. It regulates health care benefit plans. The regulation exempts the employer from following state-specific regulations.

18

MEDICAL QUALITY MANAGEMENT

Andrew Majka, MD, and Prathibha Varkey, MBBS, MPH, MHPE

Introduction

The past 2 decades have seen unprecented advances in medicine and technology. However, the health care system continues to perform far below acceptable levels for ensuring safety and addressing patient needs. The publication *To Err Is Human*: *Building a Safer Health System* from the Institute of Medicine (IOM) galvanized health care system response and the public demand for change when the United States learned that medical errors cause 44,000 to 98,000 deaths every year. The abyss between what providers know should be done for patients and what is actually done amounts to more than $9 billion per year in lost productivity and nearly $2 billion per year in hospital costs.

Despite a complex medical environment, providers rely largely on paper tools, memory, and hard work to improve the care given to patients. However, it is difficult to create reliable and sustained improvement in health care with use of traditional methods. Improvement often requires deliberate redesign of processes through human factors knowledge (ie, how people interact with products and processes), as well as tools known to assist improvement. The clear ethical imperative to enhance the quality and safety of health care and meet external accreditation requirements and patient expectations calls providers to address quality of care issues systematically.

What Is Quality of Care?

The US Agency for Healthcare Research and Quality defines quality health care as "doing the right thing, at the right time, in the right way, for the right person—and having the best possible results." Quality was first studied as an industrial process in 1931 by Walter A. Shewhart. His concepts include the identification of customer needs, reduction of variation in processes, and minimization of inspection cost. W. Edwards Deming, influenced by Shewhart's work, recognized quality as a primary driver for industrial success and subsequently transferred these methods to post–World War II Japanese engineers and executives. These methods, applied strategically, propelled Japanese manufacturing into marked automobile industry growth and subsequent worldwide recognition for quality.

- Quality of care is defined broadly as delivering the best care to every patient, every time, and accomplishing the best possible outcome.

How Is Quality Measured?

The measurement of defects is integral to quality improvement (QI). A systematic measurement of quality shows that improvement efforts lead to change in the primary end point in the desired direction, contribute to unintended results in different parts of the system, and determine whether new efforts are needed to bring a process back into an acceptable range.

With the use of samples of success as the numerator and total opportunities as the denominator, events can be graphed along a control chart to evaluate performance over time (Figure 1). An average line can be used in the run chart to clarify movement of the data away from the average.

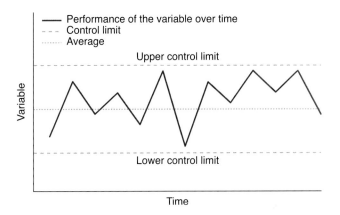

Figure 1 A Run Chart for Graphing Events Along a Control Chart to Evaluate Performance Over Time. Adapted from Varkey P, Reller MK, Resar RK. Basics of quality improvement in health care. Mayo Clin Proc. 2007 Jun;82(6):735-9. Used with permission.

Two other horizontal lines—the upper control limit and the lower control limit—also can be used in a control chart. As long as data points plot within the control limits, the process is assumed to be in control and no further action is necessary.

Avedis Donabedian, often considered the father of quality measurement, described quality design in relation to structure, process, and outcomes. **Structural measures** assess the availability and quality of resources, management systems, and policy guidelines and are often critical for sustaining processes over time. This type of assessment is used primarily for licensing and hospital accreditation. An example of a health care structural component is the decision to use intensivists in the intensive care unit to decrease the death rate.

Process measures use the actual process of health care delivery as the indicator of quality through analysis of the activities of physicians or other heath care providers, to determine whether medicine is practiced in accordance with clinical practice guidelines. For example, a **process measure** may be the proportion of diabetic patients who receive an annual retinal examination. **Outcome indicators** measure the end result of health care and are often dependent not only on medical care but also on genetic, environmental, and behavioral factors. They are usually based on group results and not individual cases, and thus they do not indicate the quality of care delivered to an individual patient. Examples of outcome measures are mortality data and patient satisfaction data.

Improvement Tools

Historically, health care has been focused on quality assurance (ie, a system for evaluating service delivery or product quality) and quality control (ie, a system for verifying and maintaining the desired quality level). However, any of these methods used alone is not adequate to enhance outcomes. Checking for defects and recommending changes without recognizing the effects of these changes on other parts of the organization may improve 1 process but harm others. Consequently, the best organizations are now combining quality assurance with proactive QI.

Continuous QI (CQI) is built on the principle that opportunity for improvement exists in every process every time. Within an organization, CQI requires a commitment to constantly improve operations, processes, and activities in order to meet patient needs in an efficient, consistent, and cost-effective manner. The CQI model emphasizes the view of health care as a process and focuses on the system, rather than on the individual, when improvement opportunities are considered.

Regardless of whether CQI is part of the organizational improvement philosophy or not, QI methods can be used to accomplish improvement goals. The most common QI methods used in health care are Plan-Do-Study-Act (PDSA), Six Sigma, and Lean. The choice of method depends on the nature of the improvement project. For most methods, users will find similar techniques. Most methods typically include an iterative testing of ideas and redesign of process or technology based on lessons learned. More recently, experts have been using principles from the different methods (eg, use of "Lean-Sigma" methods) for the same project, thus making the distinctions between the methods less relevant.

The PDSA Cycle

The PDSA cycle is the most commonly used approach for rapid-cycle improvement in health care. This method involves a trial-and-learning approach where a hypothesis or a suggested solution for improvement is made and testing is carried out on a small scale before any changes are made to the whole system.

A logical sequence of the 4 repetitive phases (Figure 2) is carried out over a course of small cycles, which eventually leads to exponential improvements. In the **Plan** phase, ideas for improvement are detailed, tasks assigned, and expectations confirmed with the testing team. Measures of improvement are then selected. In the **Do** phase, the plan is implemented and any deviation from the plan is documented. These deviations are often called "defects." The defects are then analyzed in the **Study** phase. In this phase, the results from the test cycle are studied and questions are asked regarding what went right, what went wrong, and what will be changed in the next test cycle. In the **Act** phase, lessons learned from the Study phase are incorporated into the test of change, and a decision is made on the continuation of the test cycles. For the next cycle, the phases are followed again in the same steps. Sidebar 1 outlines a case study of PDSA methods.

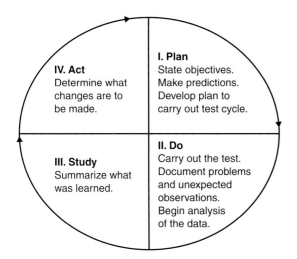

Figure 2 The Plan-Do-Study-Act Cycle. Adapted from Langley GJ, Nolan KM, Nolan TW, Norman CL, Provost LP. The improvement guide: a practical approach to enhancing organizational performance. San Francisco: Jossey-Bass Publishers, c1996. Used with permission.

Langley et al developed "**The Model for Improvement**" to assist persons contemplating a QI. In this model, the researchers asked 3 important questions to focus a person's efforts before the start of a project. The model recommends setting a focused aim, articulating time frames clearly, and

identifying measurable goals at the start of a project, all 3 of which can then be incorporated into the PDSA process.

Six Sigma

Originated by Motorola in the mid 1980s, Six Sigma is a rigorous statistical measurement method designed to reduce cost, decrease process variation, and eliminate defects. Sigma is a statistical unit reflecting the number of standard deviations between a given process and perfection. For example, at the level of 6 sigma, a process has about 3.4 defects per million opportunities (DPMO) and is virtually error free (99.9996%).

When the DPMO has been calculated, sigma values can be looked up in tables found in common statistical books or software packages. Teams can then identify the level of intended magnitude of improvement. Six Sigma is achieved through a series of steps: define, measure, analyze, improve, and control (**DMAIC**). The **Define** step, the first action, entails the creation of a project charter. The charter defines the customer's needs; the project scope, goals, success criteria, and team members; and the project deadlines. In the **Measure** step, a data collection plan for the process is developed, and data are collected from several sources to determine the depth of defects or errors (the DPMOs) in the system. Control charts are created to study the process further. In the **Analyze** step, the third action, data analysis occurs; deviation from standards is identified, and sources of process variation are used to test a hypothesis. In the **Improve** step, creative solutions and implementation plans are developed. In the final action, the **Control** step, the process is controlled by the implementation of policies, guidelines, and error-proofing strategies to make it impossible to revert to the former process. Quality controls are developed for ongoing monitoring of the new process.

Organizations that use a combination of Lean and Six Sigma methods, or Lean-Sigma, incorporate a testing phase during the Improve step. In this step, teams create solutions, develop and conduct tests of change, learn from the tests, improve the change, and then test it again, eventually finding the solution that fits best. By the time a solution is ready to be rolled out, it has gone through many tests of change and has a greater chance of acceptance. Sidebar 2 contains a case study of the Six Sigma method.

The Lean Method

Taiichi Ohno, a Toyota engineer, revolutionized thinking about process inefficiency, or waste, in the early 1950s, leading to the creation of the Toyota Production System. Application of this system led to use of the term "Lean" in many industries, including health care. Lean is driven by the identified needs of the customer and aims to improve processes by removing non–value-added activities. These activities, also referred to as waste, do not add to the business

Sidebar 2 Case Study of the Six Sigma Methodology

The Charleston Area Medical Center (CAMC), Charleston, West Virginia, used Six Sigma to evaluate and improve its rate of surgical site infections for colon and vascular surgical procedures. At the start of the project, the surgical infection rate was 0 sigma (660,828 defects per million opportunities). A multidisciplinary team of surgeons, an anesthesiologist, safety personnel, an epidemiologist, the chief of nursing, and 2 Six Sigma specialists was assembled to assist with the project. A business case was developed, and data were collected through a detailed abstraction tool. After careful analysis, a preoperative order set was developed, with a checklist that included recommended antibiotics and weight-based dosages. Education of team members, use of physician report cards, and prompting of surgeons by anesthetists and nurses (if a patient arrived in the preoperative holding area without an antibiotic order) were some of the other interventions implemented during the project. At the report's publication, the surgical site infection rate at CAMC had decreased by 91% (2.86 sigma), with a potential annual savings in excess of $1 million.

profit margin or the customer experience, and the customer is often not willing to pay for them. Seven different types of waste were identified by Ohno: 1) overproduction or underproduction, 2) waste inventory, 3) rework or rejects (eg, assembly mistakes), 4) waste of motion (eg, poor work area ergonomics), 5) waste of waiting time (eg, a patient's wait for an appointment), 6) waste of processing (eg, outdated policies and procedures), and 7) waste due to transport or handling (eg, transporting a patient unnecessarily). Lean tools maximize value-added steps in the best possible sequence to deliver continuous flow. Delivery of services or products occurs both when the customer needs them and how the customer requested the delivery.

One of the more commonly used tools in Lean is **value stream mapping** (VSM). This tool graphically displays the process of services or product delivery, using inputs, throughputs, and outputs. A current VSM (cVSM) is typically done at the beginning of a project, and opportunities for improvement are highlighted. Thereafter, front-line staff generate ideas for improvement. There is an expectation that the improvement team will test their ideas using Kaizens—highly choreographed, rapid-change events in which improvement ideas are expeditiously tested and implemented. Future-state VSMs (fVSMs) are often designed during the Kaizen workshops to depict new ideas.

To create an organized, cost-efficient workplace that has clear work processes and standards, Lean experts often recommend **the 5S strategy**, which involves 1) sorting out items in the immediate work area and keeping only those items that are needed frequently, 2) shine, which includes cleaning the workplace and inspecting equipment to look for abnormal wear, 3) set work items accomplished in order, after the efficiency of the work flow is optimized through VSM, 4) standardization of work-flow processes, and 5) sustainment of the gains accomplished from the

previous 4 steps. Sidebar 3 provides a case study of the Lean method.

- Continuous quality improvement (QI) builds on the belief that improvement can occur in every process, every time, within the health care system and requires the commitment to improve and thus to meet the patient's needs efficiently, consistently, and in a cost-effective manner.
- Plan-Do-Study-Act (PDSA) incorporates a trial-and-learning approach where a hypothesis or suggested solution for improvement is made, a plan developed, and testing carried out on a small scale and in orderly repetition before a change is made throughout the system.
- Six Sigma is a measurement method designed to decrease cost and process variation and to eliminate defects in health care delivery through a process of 5 steps—define, measure, analyze, improve, and control (DMAIC)—to close the gap between a given process and perfection.
- The Lean method is driven by identified needs of the customer and various aims to improve processes through removing non–value-added activities and to manage value-added activities in the best possible sequence for continuous flow.

Commonly Used QI Strategies

Most of the published literature about QI suggests the use of multipronged approaches for success, as opposed to single interventions. Several commonly used QI strategies are listed below:

1. **Academic detailing** uses trained care providers (eg, pharmacists, physicians) to conduct face-to-face visits

Sidebar 3 Case Study of Lean Methodology

Using Toyota Production System techniques, Park Nicollet Medical Center, Minnesota, in 2004 decreased patient waiting times, allowing the center's new ambulatory clinic to eliminate waiting rooms. Before the implementation of Lean, patients were scheduled to see their physician in batches, which led to the need for waiting rooms. After Lean methods were in place, patients were checked in with use of a concept of continuous flow. Appointments were scheduled in 10-minute intervals with the appointments for the nurse, the physician, and the diagnostic testing services scheduled in sequence. Park Nicollet Medical Center also addressed surgical case cart content standardization using Lean concepts. By agreeing on a set of standard instruments for surgical procedures, the medical center reduced its instrument counts by 60%. As a result, the staff sterilize 40,000 fewer instruments each month, saving thousands of dollars for the center's hospital. Its clinic also saved about $7.5 million in 2004 using Lean.

to encourage adoption of a desired behavior pattern. It has been shown to be effective in enhancing provider knowledge and changing prescribing behaviors, although it has generally proved ineffective in enhancing patient outcomes in a sustained fashion.

2. **Opinion leaders** are members of the local system who are usually able to influence others either on a broad range of issues or in a single area of acknowledged expertise. These leaders may have no leadership title. Peer feedback from local opinion leaders has been shown to have a modest effect on enhancing quality of care and has been used as part of multifaceted QI strategies in several institutions.

3. **Audit and feedback** entail a summary of the clinical performance of an individual provider, practice, or clinic that is transmitted to the respective entity. Audit and feedback are often done in conjunction with reports that contain anonymous performance rates of comparable clinics or providers. Based on the timeliness and type of feedback, this strategy has showed small-to-modest benefits in the improvement of targeted processes or outcomes, especially when combined with achievable benchmark feedback.

4. **Reminder systems** prompt providers to remember information relevant to a particular encounter, patient, or service. They are often effective when integrated into the work flow and are available at the point of care delivery.

5. **Re-engineering and process redesign** consist of improving an existing process or system in such a way that the improvements allow expanded opportunities to be met or existing problems to be solved. This approach broadens the reach of the project by allowing additional uses, generating lower costs, or delivering improvements in usability. Because of the nature of the process, this strategy has often yielded novel product or service innovations that go beyond the realm of improvement and result in the redesign of existing structures or processes.

Financial Incentives

The use of financial incentives for achieving increased or desired level of compliance with deliberate processes of care has shown some evidence of achieving target goals. There is less evidence that negative incentives, such as the withholding of salary or year-end bonus for not achieving the target performance level, are an effective means of enhancing quality of care.

Pay for Performance

Pay for performance (P4P) is an emerging movement in health insurance where providers are rewarded for meeting preestablished targets for the delivery of health care services. Although focus on P4P began with examining single performance indicators (eg, the checking of hemoglobin A_{1c} every 3 months for patients with diabetes mellitus) or single aspects of care (eg, preventive services), health plans currently monitor performance on numerous conditions and types of care, such as lipid control, ophthalmologic annual evaluations, microalbumin urinary assessments and foot care for patients with diabetes mellitus, or the use of aspirin, angiotensin-converting enzyme inhibitors, and β-blockers and adequate lipid control in patients with acute myocardial infarction.

In recent studies, hospitals that engaged in public reporting and P4P achieved modestly greater improvements in quality than hospitals engaged in public reporting only. However, results of other research suggest that practicing physicians continue to be skeptical about P4P incentives and the public reporting of performance. Many of them worry that, because of these initiatives, some physicians will avoid patients who have clinically complex conditions or are not compliant.

- Financial enticements are becoming more prevalent in a reward system of positive incentives, versus ineffective negative incentives, for health care providers who meet care industry goals.
- Pay for performance (P4P) is a current concept in health insurance that rewards care providers as they meet projected targets of care and its delivery.

Outcomes Research

Outcomes research aims to measure and enhance the quality of care and focuses on the end results of health care and its delivery for patients. Methods to quantify end results of care include those related to morbidity, death, physiologic measures, symptoms, patient satisfaction measures, and quality of life. Development of outcome instruments for specific diseases has been a key research area in the past few decades. When outcome measurements are used appropriately, they provide evidence on benefits, risks, and results of treatments from the angle of the physician and the patient together so that both physician and patient can make more informed decisions about treatment choices, especially for conditions that are chronic or do not substantially enhance cure rates (eg, cancer).

Patient Satisfaction and Functional Status Measures

The key argument for patient satisfaction measures is that the patient is the final pathway of what the experience of care has been. Thus, patient satisfaction measures should help physicians understand the quality of care delivered.

Lack of comparability of patient satisfaction data across different institutions still is an obstacle because patient surveys in different institutions are typically measured by different entities for different purposes using different instruments. Patient satisfaction measures are used by health plans, hospitals, and medical practice groups throughout the country. Picker Institute, Press Gainey, and Professional Research Consultants are a few examples of commonly used consultant groups that assist with patient satisfaction surveys.

There also exist several measurement systems that integrate a patient's opinion of health with the outcome. One such measurement is the **quality-adjusted life-years (QALYs)**. It is the arithmetic product of life expectancy and a measure of the remaining quality life-years. The equation for calculating this measurement is $QALY = X \times Q$, where X is the number of years lived and Q is the health-related quality of life attributed to the relevant year of life. Perfect health has a Q value of 1 and death has a Q value of 0.

The QALY method can be used to determine the number of months of reasonable-quality life that a patient would gain with a certain treatment. Factors that influence QALYs include the patient's pain level, mobility, and general mood. Thus, a QALY calculation takes into account both the quantity and the quality of life generated through health care interventions. Although QALYs are far from perfect as measures of outcome, they help with resource allocation decisions and the need for investment in new technologies and therapies.

The health survey **SF-36** is a short-form questionnaire that contains 36 questions. It provides an 8-scale profile of functional health and well-being scores. In addition, it gives psychometrically based physical and mental health summary measures and a preference-based health utility index. The 8 areas measured for functional health in the SF-36 are vitality, physical functioning, bodily pain, general health perceptions, physical role functioning, emotional role functioning, social role functioning, and mental health.

QI Versus Research

Often, confusion exists about whether a project is QI or research. Most QI projects have data collection in small samples, frequent changes in protocols and interventions, the discarding of poor ideas, and the pursuance of ideas that work. This constantly changing baseline makes it problematic to think of QI as traditional research. The concepts of QI projects and QI research are not mutually exclusive. Clearly, the object of most QI projects is to efficiently address the need of a local situation. By comparison, research projects seek to address problems in a manner that will provide results that have more generalizability and, hopefully, are publishable.

A QI project also can be considered research when 1) the tested intervention involves a deviation from established practices, 2) individual patients are the participants, 3) randomization or blinding is conducted, and 4) participants are subject to additional risks or burdens beyond usual clinical practice to give results generalizability. Further, the activity should collect baseline data with large data sets to permit appropriately powered statistical testing. Methods such as randomized controlled trials, controlled studies, preintervention and postintervention studies, and time series are commonly used in QI research.

- Patient satisfaction, or the end result of health care and its delivery, is frequently measured by health plans, hospitals, and medical practice groups nationwide as an estimate of quality care.
- Several measurement systems integrate a patient's opinion of care received with its outcome, including measurement of quality-adjusted life-years (QALY), or the balance of quality time after receiving care.

Evidence-Based Medical Practice

The practice of evidence-based medicine uses the best available evidence from clinical care research for making decisions about care delivery. Therefore, evidence-based medical care is integral to the definition of quality and often has a key role in utilization management, benchmarking, and variation of care. The Box notes the hierarchy of evidence for prevention and treatment decisions.

In the IOM's report *Crossing the Quality Chasm: A New Health System for the 21st Century*, effectiveness is listed

Box The Hierarchy of Strength in the Evidence for Prevention and Treatment Decisions

1. N-of-1 randomized trial. The patient and clinician are blinded to whether the patient is receiving active or placebo medication. The patient makes quantitative ratings of troublesome symptoms during each period, and the N-of-1 randomized control trial continues until both the patient and the clinician conclude that the patient is or is not obtaining benefit from the target intervention

2. Systematic review of randomized trials

3. Single randomized trial

4. Systematic review of observational studies addressing patient-important outcomes

5. Single observational study addressing patient-important outcomes

6. Physiologic study (eg, studies of blood pressure, cardiac output, exercise capacity, or bone density)

7. Unsystematic clinical observation

Adapted from Guyatt G, Rennie D, Meade MO, Cook DJ. Users' guides to the medical literature: a manual for evidence-based clinical practice. 2nd ed. New York: McGraw-Hill Medical; JAMA & Archives Journals; c2008. Used with permission.

as one of 6 specific aims for improving health care. Effective care is based on systematically obtained evidence to determine whether an intervention produces better results (ie, outcomes) than the alternatives, including doing nothing. This effective care requires an avoidance of underuse, overuse, and misuse, all of which could lead to patient harm. Unfortunately, many aspects of patient care involve scant or no evidence of effectiveness or ineffectiveness. Physicians must also rely on clinical expertise and on patient values and preferences in making decisions about care. Access and information available at the point of care become especially important in these situations.

Clinical Practice Guidelines

Clinical practice guidelines (CPGs) are systematically defined statements to assist practitioner and patient decisions about appropriate health care for clinical circumstances. They provide clinical advice and can take the form of an algorithm, a computer-based protocol, and policy documents. The importance of CPGs is that no strong evidence is available on many health care decisions, and with the use of CPGs, several unnecessary variations in practice can be discouraged. CPGs are tools for decision making and need to be adapted to local processes and culture. Their flexibility allows legitimate differences in interpretation and helps generate ownership and accountability for the guidelines.

Although not welcomed by all physicians, CPGs are gaining legitimacy. Recognition of the value of evidence-based guidelines is increasing. The recent phenomenon of Minute Clinics in retail stores, for example, is a direct result of agreed-on treatment practice guidelines for such common conditions as urinary tract infection, acute pharyngitis, and acute upper respiratory tract infections.

Management of Demand and Disease

Demand management consists of activities and interventions designed to improve the appropriateness of the use of health care resources. It typically is conducted by health plans or by employers to assist patients with chronic disease and can be coordinated with case management, disease management, and other utilization management processes. However, caution needs to be taken not to confuse the patient by duplicating processes and interventions. The following activities are often included in the implementation of disease management programs:

1. Providing health information to the patient
2. Offering preventive services that follow evidence-based guidelines
3. Providing case management, disease management, and other supportive services to the patient
4. Evaluating the health risks of the patient

5. Partnering with community resources to promote the use of local and national programs that can improve health and wellness
6. Monitoring the utilization of patient services to identify the need for intervention, such as care coordination

Case management programs target individuals with chronic or catastrophic disease. They are typically designed for individual patients who receive an individualized care plan. The case management program helps the patient proceed through the complex health care systems and avoid the fragmentation or poor utilization of services. With case management, communication with the care providers and the patient is frequent, such as the appropriate referral to specialists, hospitals, and ancillary services.

Disease management is a system of coordinated health care interventions and communications for populations with conditions for which patient self-care efforts can considerably improve health care outcomes. A typical disease management program has the following 6 components: 1) population identification processes, 2) evidence-based practice guidelines, 3) collaborative practice models that include the physician and the support service providers, 4) patient self-management education, 5) process and outcomes measurement evaluation and management, and 6) routine reporting and feedback loops with the patient, the physician, and the other stake holders while being cognizant of the Health Insurance Portability and Accountability Act (HIPAA).

The patient-centered **medical home** is an outgrowth of these principles and was developed as a concerted effort of the American College of Physicians, the American Academy of Family Physicians, the American Academy of Pediatrics, and the American Osteopathic Association (AOA). The mainstays of the patient-centered medical home model include a personal physician, a physician-directed medical practice that coordinates the patient's care, whole-person orientation to expand patient centeredness in social and cultural needs, coordinated or integrated care for not only medical needs but also the patient's social, cultural, spiritual, and emotional needs, and a focus on quality and safety.

It is hoped that this kind of model facilitates partnerships between the individual patient, the patient's personal physicians, and, when needed, the patient's family. Care is facilitated by registries, information technology, and a health information exchange about the patient's condition that includes medications, medical history, and ongoing medical problems, with the assistance of electronic medical records that are easily retrieved across medical systems. These components help ensure that patients receive the indicated care when and where they need and want it in a culturally and linguistically appropriate manner. The Centers for Medicare and Medicaid Services

(CMS) has legislation requiring implementation of this concept.

- Sound medical practice incorporates prevention and treatment decisions that are based on evidence showing their effectiveness, which is an attribute of quality care.
- Clinical practice guidelines (CPGs) are tools for provider decision making, particularly regarding the delivery of medical care for which no clear evidence of outcome exists. They may be adapted to local processes and culture.
- Management of health care demand, cases, and disease covers activities and interventions designed to improve the appropriateness of the use of health care resources and extends to the concept of a patient-centered medical home that supplies personal physicians and a physician-directed medical practice that coordinates and provides whole-patient care.

Accreditation Organizations and Systems

Joint Commission

Many agencies accredit health care organizations. The Joint Commission is a private-sector, US-based, nonprofit organization and is the **national accrediting body for most hospitals** (ie, general, psychiatric, children's, and rehabilitation hospitals). Nursing homes, long-term-care facilities, addiction services, and independent and freestanding medical laboratories, as well as rehabilitation centers, can also be accredited by the Joint Commission.

The commission is the most well-known accrediting body because a hospital that meets its accreditation is deemed to meet the Medicare conditions of participation needed for Medicare and Medicaid reimbursement. The Joint Commission charges hospitals fees for doing their evaluation. The commission provides the concerned organization its accreditation decision, the date the decision was awarded, and any standards that need improvement. The accreditation is not automatically renewed, so a full survey is required at least every 3 years.

Utilization Review Accreditation Commission

The Utilization Review Accreditation Commission (URAC) was developed to improve the quality and accountability of health care organizations. URAC **accredits medical management organizations** (eg, those focused on disease management or case management, call centers), health plans (eg, health maintenance organizations [HMOs], preferred provider organizations), and the health Web sites of hospitals. The commission also reviews HIPAA privacy and HIPAA security for accreditation. Organizations seeking URAC accreditation must maintain at least 2 QI projects. An accreditation period is for 2 to 3 years, after which the organization must go through the review process again to maintain its accredited status. As with other accrediting agencies, an on-site visit reviews the policies and procedures of the applicant organization to determine whether it is operating to its stated policies.

Commission on Accreditation of Rehabilitation Facilities

The Commission on Accreditation of Rehabilitation Facilities (CARF) is an international nonprofit organization that provides accreditation standards and surveys for organizations working in the human services field. **Durable medical equipment, prosthetics, orthotics, and supplies** must be accredited by CARF to have Medicare and Medicaid billing privileges. Comprehensive, integrated inpatient rehabilitation programs are also reviewed. These programs provide medical rehabilitation for persons who have had a stroke, a brain or spinal cord injury, a traumatic injury, or pain that cannot be controlled by medication alone. Nursing homes, continuing-care retirement communities, assisted-living facilities, service networks for the aged, and adult day services can be accredited also.

Community Health Accreditation Program

Community Health Accreditation Program (CHAP) is an independent, nonprofit accrediting body that is an alternative to the Joint Commission. CHAP is used for **assessing community-based health care organizations**. The CMS granted deeming authority to CHAP for home care.

Health Care Facilities Accreditation Program

This accreditation organization was founded by the AOA. It is a voluntary agency recognized by federal and state governments, as well as insurance carriers and managed care organizations. The program **accredits acute care hospitals**, as well as hospital laboratories.

National Committee for Quality Assurance

The National Committee for Quality Assurance (NCQA) is an independent nonprofit organization whose mission is to improve health care quality. The NCQA develops the **Healthcare Effectiveness Data and Information Set (HEDIS)**, a tool to measure performance on dimensions of care and service and to allow consumers, purchasers, and CMS to compare health plan and medical group performance with other plans and provider groups, as well as with regional and national benchmarks. The dimensions of care and service include the following:

1. Guidelines for effectiveness of care measures
2. Adult body mass index measurement
3. Weight assessment and counseling for nutrition and physical activity of children and adolescents
4. Childhood immunization status
5. Lead screening in children
6. Breast cancer screening
7. Cervical cancer screening
8. Colorectal cancer screening
9. Chlamydia screening in women
10. Glaucoma screening in older adults

CMS requires HMOs to have these data for the Medicare Advantage program applicable to its Medicare HMO enrollees. HEDIS measures are in a standard format so it is easy to compare data for benchmarking, purposes and to identify trends in improvement.

Baldridge National Quality Program

The Baldridge National Quality Program criteria provide a systems perspective for understanding performance management. It offers a validated practice instrument that an organization can use to evaluate itself. The program was created in 1987 by public law for the promotion of quality improvement through organizational and personal learning, improvement in **overall organizational effectiveness and capabilities**, and delivery of value to customers, thereby contributing to market success. The National Institute of Standards and Technology, an agency of the US Department of Commerce, manages the Baldridge National Quality Program. Organizations are measured against 7 categories: leadership; strategic planning; customer and market focus; measurement, analysis, and knowledge management; workforce focus; process management; and results.

- The Joint Commission is a well-known, nonprofit, and important national accrediting agency for most hospitals, and its accreditation award deems the hospital as meeting the Medicare conditions of participation required for Medicare and Medicaid reimbursement.
- The Utilization Review Accreditation Commission (URAC) accredits medical management organizations, health plans (eg, preferred provider organizations), and the health Web sites of hospitals; reviews compliance with the Health Insurance Portability and Accountability Act (HIPAA); and requires that an accredited hospital be operating at least 2 quality improvement (QI) plans.
- An international nonprofit organization, the Commission on Accreditation of Rehabilitation

Facilities (CARF) provides accreditation standards and surveys for organizations working in human services and extends its accreditation potential to comprehensive, integrated rehabilitation programs and such facilities as nursing homes and assisted-living establishments.

- The Community Health Accreditation Program (CHAP) is an independent, nonprofit accrediting body that is an alternative to the Joint Commission, having received authority from the Centers for Medicare and Medicaid Services (CMS) to deem home care compliance and assess community-based health care organizations.
- The Health Care Facilities Accreditation Program, a voluntary agency recognized by federal and state governments plus insurance carriers and managed care organizations, accredits acute care hospitals and hospital laboratories.
- The National Committee for Quality Assurance (NCQA) develops the Healthcare Effectiveness Data and Information Set (HEDIS), a means to measure performance of care and service and to allow consumers, purchasers, and CMS to compare health plan and medical group performance data with other plans, provider groups, and regional and national benchmarks.
- The criteria of the Baldridge National Quality Program, managed by the National Institute of Standards and Technology, provide a systems perspective for understanding performance management and promotion of QI of organizations.

Acknowledgment

A substantial portion of this chapter is adapted and reproduced from Varkey P, Reller MK, Resar RK. Basics of quality improvement in health care. Mayo Clin Proc. 2007 Jun; 82(6):735-9. Used with permission.

SUGGESTED READING

Audet AM, Doty MM, Shamasdin J, Schoenbaum SC. Measure, learn, and improve: physicians' involvement in quality improvement. Health Aff (Millwood). 2005 May-Jun;24(3):843-53.

Berwick DM. Developing and testing changes in delivery of care. Ann Intern Med. 1998 Apr 15;128(8):651-6.

Committee on Quality Health Care in America, Institute of Medicine. Crossing the quality chasm: a new health system for the 21st century. Washington (DC): National Academy Press; c2001.

The Joint Commission: Helping health care organizations help patients [Internet]. [cited 12 Oct 2009]. Available from http://www.jointcommission.org.

Langley GJ, Nolan KM, Nolan TW, Norman CL, Provost LP. The improvement guide: a practical approach to enhancing organizational performance. San Francisco: Jossey-Bass Publishers, c1996.

Lindenauer PK, Remus D, Roman S, Rothberg MB, Benjamin EM, Ma A, et al. Public reporting and pay for performance in hospital quality improvement. N Engl J Med. 2007 Feb 1;356(5):486-96. Epub 2007 Jan 26.

Rolnick SJ, Margolis KL, Fortman KK, Maciosek MV, Grimm RH Jr. How acceptable are financial incentives and written feedback for improving hypertension control? Perspectives from physicians, clinic administrators, and patients. Am J Manag Care. 2002 May;8(5):441-7.

Varkey P, Reller MK, Resar RK. Basics of quality improvement in health care. Mayo Clin Proc. 2007 Jun;82(6): 735-9.

Questions and Answers

Questions

1. Which of the following measures is the most valid outcome measure for the effectiveness of hypertension treatment?
   a. Number of antihypertensive prescriptions
   b. Prevalence of heart disease in the population
   c. Incidence of stroke in the population
   d. Cost of hypertension-related hospitalizations for the population
   e. Number of clinic visits related to hypertension per year

2. From the following list of activities, which is the best example of a quality improvement project?
   a. Randomized trial on the effect of an upgraded colonoscope
   b. Patient survey to assess the prevalence of depression in the population
   c. Use of a new heart-lung machine for surgery when it has been shown to be efficacious in animals
   d. Reduction in patient no-show rates at an ambulatory clinic
   e. Prospective trial of a modified pneumonia vaccine to reduce rates of pneumonia among elderly persons

3. At the 6 sigma level, a process has which of the following rates?
   a. 3.4 defects per million opportunities (DPMO)
   b. 1.2 DPMO
   c. 6.8 DPMO
   d. 0 DPMO
   e. 6.0 DPMO

4. Which of the following tools is commonly used in the Lean method to display process inputs, throughputs, and outputs?
   a. Flow stream mapping
   b. Lean value streams
   c. Flow streams
   d. Value stream mapping
   e. Swim lane mapping

5. You are the medical director of a 150-bed community hospital. The board of the hospital's quality committee asks you to identify an organization that the hospital should request for accreditation review. Which of the following organizations would be most suitable for accreditation of your hospital?
   a. Utilization Review Accreditation Commission (URAC)
   b. National Committee for Quality Assurance (NCQA)
   c. Joint Commission
   d. Baldridge National Quality Program
   e. Healthcare facilities accreditation program

6. Your medical group is trying to develop guidelines for effective and quality health care. The group has organized several work segments to look at developing or adopting outside treatment guidelines. It has decided to adopt 1 accepted, evidence-based performance standard. Which of the following measures would you accept as the initial performance measure?
   a. Pay for performance
   b. Establishment of a Minute Clinic in a local retail shop
   c. Healthcare Effectiveness Data and Information Set (HEDIS) guidelines
   d. A Baldridge National Quality Program review
   e. SF-36

Answers

1. **Answer c.**

   Outcome indicators measure the end result of health care and are often dependent not only on medical care but also on genetic, environmental, and behavioral factors. Effective hypertension control should ideally prevent new cardiovascular events in a population, including stroke and myocardial infarction. Since the incidence of stroke in the population measures new cases of stroke, this is the best outcome measure in this instance. The other choices do not measure outcomes related to the effectiveness of hypertension treatment.

2. **Answer d.**

   If the tested intervention involves a deviation from established practices, individual patients are the participants, randomization or blinding is conducted, and participants are subject to additional risks or burdens beyond the usual clinical practice, then the project is considered a research project and not a quality improvement project. Reducing the number of no-shows at an ambulatory clinic addresses the need of the local situation and aims at redesigning or enhancing processes, constituting the principles of quality improvement. Hence, it is the correct answer.

3. **Answer a.**

   Sigma is a statistical unit reflecting how far a given process deviates from perfection. At the level of 6 sigma, a process has about 3.4 DPMO and is virtually error free (99.9996%). After the DPMO has been calculated, sigma values can be looked up in tables that can be found in common statistical books or software packages. Teams can then identify the level of intended magnitude of improvement.

4. **Answer d.**

   One of the more commonly used tools in the Lean method is called value stream mapping (VSM). This tool helps to display the process of services or the product delivery that is using inputs, throughputs, and outputs. A current VSM (cVSM) is typically done at the beginning of a project, opportunities for improvement are highlighted, and front-line staff generate ideas for improvement. Expectation is placed with the improvement team to test their ideas using Kaizens, or highly choreographed rapid-change events in which improvement ideas are quickly tested and implemented within the workshop. Future-state VSMs (fVSMs) are often designed during the Kaizen workshops to depict new ideas.

5. **Answer c.**

   One factor that needs consideration when choosing an accreditation organization is what characteristics private and public or government health plans require for the community hospital to bill their patients for services provided. The Joint Commission is the important national accrediting agency for most hospitals, and its accreditation award deems the hospital as meeting the Medicare conditions of participation required for Medicare and Medicaid reimbursement. It would be the best accrediting agency for this hospital. The NCQA is an independent nonprofit organization whose mission is to improve health care quality; it does not do accreditation. It publishes the Healthcare Effectiveness Data and Information Set, which allows consumers, purchasers, and the Centers for Medicare and Medicaid Services to compare health plan performance. The Utilization Review Accreditation Commission (URAC) accredits medical management organizations, health plans (eg, preferred provider organizations), and the health Web sites of hospitals but does not accredit hospitals. The Health Care Facilities Accreditation Program, a voluntary agency recognized by federal and state governments plus insurance carriers and managed care organizations, accredits only acute care hospitals and hospital laboratories. The criteria of the Baldridge National Quality Program, managed by the National Institute of Standards and Technology, provide a systems perspective for understanding performance management and promotion of quality improvement of organizations but are not used for accreditation.

6. **Answer c.**

   The HEDIS guidelines are a tool of evidence-based dimensions of care that have demonstrable favorable outcomes for quality patient care. Pay for performance is endorsed by health plans and insurance companies to reward compliance of treatment guidelines with agreed-on incentives to encourage use of those guidelines. Minute Clinics are operational units typically operated by nurse practitioners for "simple" illnesses, such as urinary infections, that have agreed-on treatment protocols.

INDEX

Note: Page numbers followed by *f, t,* and *b* indicate *figures, tables,* and *boxes,* respectively.